Cancer Clinical Pharmacology

Cancer Clinical Pharmacology

EDITED BY

Jan H. M. Schellens
The Netherlands Cancer Institute, Amsterdam, The Netherlands

Howard L. McLeod
Department of Medicine, Washington University Medicine School, St Louis, Missouri, USA

David R. Newell
Northern Institute for Cancer Research, University of Newcastle, Newcastle upon Tyne, UK

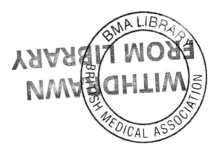

OXFORD
UNIVERSITY PRESS

*This book has been printed digitally and produced in a standard specification
in order to ensure its continuing availability*

OXFORD
UNIVERSITY PRESS

Great Clarendon Street, Oxford OX2 6DP

Oxford University Press is a department of the University of Oxford.
It furthers the University's objective of excellence in research, scholarship,
and education by publishing worldwide in

Oxford New York

Auckland Cape Town Dar es Salaam Hong Kong Karachi
Kuala Lumpur Madrid Melbourne Mexico City Nairobi
New Delhi Shanghai Taipei Toronto
With offices in
Argentina Austria Brazil Chile Czech Republic France Greece
Guatemala Hungary Italy Japan South Korea Poland Portugal
Singapore Switzerland Thailand Turkey Ukraine Vietnam

Oxford is a registered trade mark of Oxford University Press
in the UK and in certain other countries

Published in the United States
by Oxford University Press Inc., New York

ISBN 978-0-19-262966-1

Printed and bound by CPI Antony Rowe, Eastbourne

Contributing Authors

Sharyn D. Baker
Institute for Drug Development, Cancer Therapy and Research Center, San Antonio, Texas, USA

Jos H. Beijnen
Department of Pharmacy and Pharmacology, The Netherlands Cancer Institute/Slotervaart Hospital, Amsterdam, The Netherlands

Alan V. Boddy
Northern Institute for Cancer Research, University of Newcastle, Newcastle upon Tyne, UK

Jim Cassidy
Cancer Research UK Dept. of Oncology, Glasgow University, UK

Etienne Chatelut
Institut Claudius Regaud, Université Paul-Sabatier, Toulouse, France

Luca Gianni
Division of Medical Oncology A, Istituto Nazionale Tumori, Milan, Italy

D. Paul Harkin
Department of Oncology, The Queen's University of Belfast, Belfast City Hospital, Belfast, UK

Steven W. Johnson
University of Pennsylvania Cancer Center, Philadelphia, Pennsylvania, USA

Patrick G. Johnston
Department of Oncology, The Queen's University of Belfast, Belfast City Hospital, Belfast, UK

Wandena S. Lakhai
Department of Pharmacy and Pharmacology, The Netherlands Cancer Institute/Slotervaart Hospital, Amsterdam, The Netherlands

Jan Liliemark
Department of Experimental Haematology, Karolinska Institute, Stockholm, Sweden

Alberta Locatelli
Division of Medical Oncology A, Istituto Nazionale Tumori, Milan, Italy

Per E. Lønning
Department of Oncology, University of Bergen, Haukeland University Hospital, Bergen, Norway

Howard L. McLeod
Department of Medicine, Washington University Medicine School, St Louis, Missouri, USA

Gérard Milano
Oncopharmacology Unit, Centre Antoine, Nice, France

Peter J. O'Dwyer
University of Pennsylvania Cancer Center, Philadelphia, Pennsylvania, USA

Curt Peterson
Department of Clinical Pharmacology, University Hospital of Linköping, Linköping, Sweden

Jacques Robert
Institut Bergonie, Comprehensive Cancer Center, Bordeaux, France

Hilde Rosing
Department of Pharmacy and Pharmacology, The Netherlands Cancer Institute/Slotervaart Hospital, Amsterdam, The Netherlands

Eric K. Rowinsky
Institute for Drug Development, Cancer Therapy and Research Center, San Antonio, Texas, USA

Jan H.M. Schellens
The Netherlands Cancer Institute, Amsterdam, The Netherlands

James P. Stevenson
University of Pennsylvania Cancer Center, Philadelphia, Pennsylvania, USA

Timothy W. Synold
Department of Medical Oncology, City of Hope National Medical Center, Duarte, California, USA

Lucia Viganò
Division of Medical Oncology A, Istituto Nazionale Tumori, Milan, Italy

Preface

This book provides an overview of current insights into clinical pharmacology in the field of medical and haematological oncology. It is intended to serve students of medicine and pharmacy, and fellows in oncology, haematology and internal medicine. Furthermore, since cancer clinical pharmacology is a vast and rapidly expanding subject, the book is also likely to be useful for oncology health care professionals. We aim to provide a scientific basis for anticancer therapy in patients with solid tumour and haematological malignancies. Coverage includes basic principles of pharmacology and tumour biology, bioanalytical aspects, pharmacokinetics and pharmacodynamics of anticancer agents, and clinical pharmacology of individual anticancer agents, including the most important recently registered novel anticancer drugs. We hope that the text will be sufficiently concise that the reader will need only a limited amount of time to understand the clinical pharmacology and application of the main current anticancer agents. We encourage readers to give us their comments and thoughtful criticism that will help us improve any future editions.

January 2005

Jan H.M. Schellens
Howard L. McLeod
David R. Newell

Acknowledgements

We are grateful to all the professionals who knowingly or unknowingly have provided us with valuable insights into the practice of clinical pharmacology and medical oncology. We owe a debt of gratitude to our teachers and our medical educators who devote their energies to improving patient care in oncology. We thank all authors and co-authors who have conscientiously integrated their skills to prepare the individual chapters of this book. The editors take full responsibility for the content of the book.

Contents

1 | Bioanalytical methods for anticancer drugs

Jos H. Beijnen and Hilde Rosing

Introduction

Most anticancer agents exhibit a narrow therapeutic window with small margins between toxic and subtherapeutic exposure. Inter-individual pharmacokinetic and pharmacodynamic variabilities are usually substantial and may explain why some patients experience chemotherapy as a relatively mild treatment while others suffer from severe side effects. Antitumour activity also varies greatly in cohorts of patients even though they are treated with the same dose of anticancer agent. Clinical pharmacological research aims to obtain more insight into these variabilities by analysing concentration–time profiles, usually in plasma (pharmacokinetics), after drug administration. The ultimate goal is to define and adjust dosages for the individual patient which yield the optimal effect (minimal toxicity with maximal antitumour activity). Thus drug analysis in a biological matrix is pivotal and indispensable for pharmacokinetic research. In the technical jargon of the pharmacologist, *bioanalysis is defined* as the quantitative measurement of a drug (and its metabolites) in biological samples (plasma, urine, tissue, etc.) after administration. Bioanalysis can be considered as a mature scientific field. It encompasses the development, validation and implementation of generally sophisticated analytical methodologies. An understanding of the chemistry and physicochemical properties of the analyte, as well as the basics of analytical chemistry and equipment, are prerequisites. Analytical chemists and pharmacists are pre-eminently prepared for this task during their academic education.

In oncology, bioanalysis plays a pivotal role during both the preclinical and clinical stages of *development* of an anticancer drug. An initial insight into the pharmacokinetic properties (absorption-distribution-elimination-metabolism) of a potential new anticancer drug can be obtained during animal toxicology studies. The information collected is very helpful in the further design and dose escalation strategies in early clinical phase I trials.[1,2] The study of the pharmacokinetics of the drug is the primary objective of phase I clinical trials. The outcome of these investigations is used in the further development of a drug. For instance, when a compound appears to have a long terminal half-life a prolonged infusion schedule may not be necessary. The occurrence of non-linear kinetics cautions the clinical investigator in the dose escalation steps.

Pharmacokinetic research is also receiving increasing attention in phase II and III trials. Pharmacokinetic–pharmacodynamic (toxicity–antitumour activity) relationships, including relationships with patient demographics (*population kinetics*), can be investigated using data collected from large numbers of patients. For example, Bruno and coworkers have performed a very elegant investigation of *docetaxel* in a large phase II evaluation programme. Their reports[3,4] are considered as landmark conceptual publications of population kinetics in oncology. Population kinetics form the fundamentals for the ultimate goal of *individualized* 'tailor-made' chemotherapy.[5] However, in view of the narrow therapeutic index of most anticancer drugs and the many proven pharmacokinetic–pharmacodynamic relationships, it is surprising that *therapeutic drug monitoring (TDM)* is still uncommon for most anticancer drugs in daily use. An exception is high-dose *methotrexate* treatment where measurement of drug levels is vital to enable leucovorin rescue to be started in time; absence of monitoring of methotrexate plasma levels in these cases can be considered to be medical mal-practice. The reason why there are still so few examples of 'TDM-anticancer drugs' may be due to the fact that is very difficult to establish the right pharmacokinetic target parameter, particularly in combination therapies. Furthermore, the real supplementary value of TDM in therapeutic outcome has not yet been demonstrated per-suasively by, for instance, performing comparative ran-domized trials of classic dosing (in mg/m²) versus adaptive dosing. However, two recent trials have demonstrated the advantages of adaptive dosing and therefore are extremely important and supportive for the TDM con-cept. Evans and coworkers[6] performed a prospective com-parison of conventional fixed-dose (mg/m²) chemotherapy with AUC (area under the plasma concentration–time curve) targeted individualized chemotherapy, including methotrexate, in childhood acute lymphoblastic leu-kaemia. The relapse-free survival in the *individualized* cohort was significantly better than that in the con-ventional therapy group. In a recent French study by Milano's group it was demonstrated that an individual *5-fluorouracil* adaptive dosing strategy improved the therapeutic index compared with standard dosing (g/m²).[7] Objective response rates were comparable in both treat-ment groups; however, toxicity was significantly reduced in the adaptive dosing group. These comparative trials are obviously of great importance for the further devel-opment and justification of the concept of pharmaco-kinetically guided dose adaptation.

The basis of the concepts discussed above is that drug levels are measured and that the outcomes of the analysis are reliable, and thus are precise and accurate.

In this chapter we aim to provide an overview of aspects that are relevant for anticancer drug analysis in biological matrices. High-pressure liquid chromatogra-phy (HPLC) is by far the most frequently used tech-nique, and thus will be discussed in more detail, including assay validation. More detailed information can be found elsewhere.[8–11]

Analytical methods

A variety of methods can be used for the analysis of anticancer drugs in biological matrices. Preferably, it should be feasible to perform the analysis in a hospital laboratory environment, particularly when the analyti-cal method is used for routine TDM purposes. There-fore the method should be robust but also kept as simple as possible. However, in those cases when phar-macokinetic monitoring is used in a particular clinical

investigation, for example to investigate a putative drug–drug interaction, the collected samples could be transported to and analysed in a central laboratory which has experience with more complicated methods and equipment. Thus the final choice of method can be very arbitrary and based on the available equipment and experience within the laboratory. However, in most cases the research question, the expected performance of the analytical methodology and the compound under investigation determine the choice of the method. In par-ticular, sensitivity, measurement of metabolites, analy-sis time, physicochemical and spectroscopic properties of the drug, etc. dictate the strategy to be followed during development of the method.

Microbiological assays are the oldest techniques. Quantification of *mitomycin C* in plasma and urine was initially (in the early 1960s) performed by measuring the antimicrobial activity of samples against *Bacillus sub-tilis*. The advantage of this method is that no sample pre-treatment is required. The first biodeterminations of *paclitaxel* were accomplished using a biochemical assay based on the ability of the drug to induce the formation of tubulin polymers that hydrolyse guanosine 5′-triphos-phate (GTP) at 0°C. The lower limit of quantification of this method was approximately 100 ng/ml.[12] Biochemical assays may give information about the pharmacological activity of a drug, but they are often too labour intensive to support pharmacokinetic studies in which it is neces-sary to analyse a large number of samples. With the advent of novel compounds in oncology, exploiting novel targets including angiogenesis inhibitors, telom-erase inhibitors and compounds which interfere with growth signal transduction pathways, interest in these methods has revived as they can be used as surrogate pharmacodynamic endpoint parameters in dose-finding studies. Classical dose escalation to achieve maximal tolerated dosages are probably inappropriate for these compounds. For instance, dose selection for a drug that acts as a farnesyltransferase inhibitor should be based on the extent of inhibition of the target enzyme rather than on the highest dose that can be tolerated by the patient.

Immunoassays are very useful for routine analysis of TDM drugs like anti-epileptics, aminoglycosides, cardiac agents, etc. A *fluorescence polarization immuno-assay (FPIA)* for methotrexate, which is easy to imple-ment in a hospital laboratory, is commercially available (FPLx from Abbott). The advantages of this method-ology are that it only requires a small sample volume (e.g. 75 μl), a short analysis time and a high sensitivity and that there is no need for a sample pretreatment procedure. Another advantage of FPIA over radioimmunoassays (RIAs) is that an FPIA operates without radiolabelled reagents. Continuous attention must be paid to cross-reactivity with these types of analytical techniques. However, the cross-reactivity of 7-hydroxy-methotrexate, the major metabolite of methotrexate in plasma, is less than 1%.

The bioanalytical technique of first choice for platinum-based anticancer drugs is still flameless atomic absorption spectrometry *(AAS)*.[13] A more sensitive, but more expensive, method is inductively coupled plasma–mass spectrometry *(ICP–MS)*.[14] However, AAS and ICP–MS are non-specific methods because they only determine elemental platinum. The intact drug can be quantified by liquid chromatographic methods. The analysis of platinum–DNA adducts in white blood cells has been investigated with the aim of obtaining better insight into drug exposure and activity at DNA level. After isolation of the cells the platinum content can be measured by AAS. A ^{32}P-post-labelling assay has also been developed which measures guanine–guanine (G–G) and adenine–guanine (A–G) intrastrand platinum adducts separately.[15] The method is very sensitive (100 attomole platinum per microgram DNA for G–G adducts; 50 attomole platinum per microgram DNA for A–G adducts). The question remains as to how platinum adduct levels in white blood cells correlate with anti-tumour activity.[16,17]

Capillary electrophoresis is a relatively new technique in the field of bioanalysis. The principle of the method is that charged molecules migrate between the cathode and the anode in a liquid-filled fused silica capillary tube. Separations between analytes are based on differences in electrophoretic mobility by charge, size and mass. Major advantages in this technology are the high resolution power and its potential for direct analysis of biological samples without pretreatment. However, a drawback is that quantitative determinations are cumbersome and only relatively small samples (nanolitre range) can be loaded into this microanalytical system. When a limited amount of sample is available, capillary electrophoresis may be an option. High-sensitivity detectors must be used to compensate for the loss of sensitivity due to the low loading capacity. A module equipped with a laser-induced fluorescence detector has been used for the analysis of methotrexate and anthracyclines.[18,19] However, capillary electrophoresis is still in its infancy for widespread bioanalytical purposes.

Chromatographic methods, particularly HPLC, are by far the most commonly employed technologies in the field of bioanalysis, including the analysis of anticancer agents. Gas–liquid chromatography (GC) is used for volatile thermal stable compounds. Detector technologies are based on flame ionization (including nitrogen/phosphorus selective), electron capture and mass spectrometry. Most anticancer agents do not meet the requirements needed for successful GC analysis. However, this is not the case for the oxazaphosphorines, cyclophosphamide, ifosfamide and trofosfamide for which GC methods have been designed.[20] The enantiomers of ifosfamide and two metabolites 2- and 3-dechloroethyli-fosfamide can be resolved on a Chirasil-L-val gas chromatographic column. Indications for a stereospecific metabolism of ifosfamide have been found.[21]

Nuclear magnetic resonance (NMR) and positron emission tomography (PET) are novel sophisticated techniques with several potential applications for monitoring anticancer drugs and metabolites. The major advantages of these techniques are that they are non-invasive and can provide a vast pool of pharmacokinetic data, in principle from every tissue or fluid in the human body. So far they are only available and operational for specific research problems in specialized centres.[22,23]

High-performance liquid chromatography

High-performance liquid chromatography (HPLC) is undoubtedly the most commonly used technique for the quantitative determination of anticancer agents in biological matrices. It is a powerful and versatile tool and is applicable to almost every case. The system is simple, comprising a pump which pumps a fluid (mobile phase), at a carefully controlled flow rate, through a column filled with solid material (stationary phase) which interacts with the analytes. After separation and elution the analytes pass through a detector coupled to a data processing system. HPLC usually operates under high-pressure conditions so that an ingenious device (the injector) is required to bring the sample into the eluent flow. There are many types of chromatography [e.g. adsorption (normal phase, reversed phase), size exclusion, ion-pair and ion-exchange] allowing most analytes, even enantiomeric mixtures, to be separated. Reversed phase chromatography is most frequently employed.

Sample pretreatment

Plasma is most frequently used as the matrix for pharmacological research. Other matrices are urine, bile, tissues, cerebrospinal fluid, saliva etc. Frequently, plasma cannot be injected directly into the liquid chromatography system. In particular, proteins in plasma tend to accumulate within the column and denature the stationary phase at the expense of system performance. The first signs are increased column pressure, peak broadening and diminished separation efficiency. As well as proteins, biological matrices contain many other endogenous compounds, such as carbohydrates, lipids, salts, etc., that may all interfere with the analysis. Thus sample pretreatment is necessary to eliminate proteins, in particular, from the matrix. The following sample pretreatment procedures, focused on the removal of proteins, are used most frequently in bioanalysis: (i) protein precipitation, (ii) liquid–liquid extraction and (iii) solid-phase extraction, and combinations of these methods. Drugs are present in plasma as either free or protein bound, and an equilibrium exists between them. The sample pretreatment procedures described above release the bound drug and the sum of bound and free drug is determined.

Protein precipitation (denaturation) can be effectively performed with organic solvents, such as acetonitrile or methanol, or a strong acid like perchloric acid.[24] After centrifugation a protein pellet and a supernatant remain for further analysis. Because of interference this relatively rough technique is usually inadequate for the analysis of very low drug concentrations, but it can be useful for measurements of higher drug levels, and is rapid and easy to use. However, recovery problems can arise when the analytes adsorb to the protein pellet and/or are lost by inclusion. Therapeutic plasma levels of *suramin* are considered to be

between 200 and 300 µg/ml. The drug is highly bound (>95%) to proteins. After protein precipitation with acetonitrile (100 µl plasma + 200 µl acetonitrile), the drug is released from this binding (extraction recovery 82%) and can be quantified in the extract by HPLC. The assay is not very sensitive, with a lower limit of quantification of 5 µg/ml, but it is sufficient for its intended use in TDM.[25]

Sample pretreatment by methanol extraction with protein precipitation is a crucial part of the bioanalysis of topotecan. The topotecan molecule possesses an unstable lactone moiety which hydrolyzes at physiological pH with the formation of a hydroxy acid (Fig. 1.1).[26] This is a reversible reaction; ring closure can be achieved by lowering the pH. Both the conversion rate and the equilibrium constant are dependent on pH.[26] The hydroxy acid analogue of topotecan is considered inactive. The equilibrium is fixed by immediate treatment of plasma samples with cold methanol (below −30°C). After rapid cooled centrifugation (4°C) a clear methanolic extract remains. The lactone form of topotecan is stable in a methanolic extract at −70°C for at least 15 months; if it is stored at −30°C for the same period, about half the drug is converted into its hydroxy acid congener. The extracts are injected into the HPLC system for analysis. On acidification of the samples topotecan is quantitatively converted into its lactone form, after which total levels can be analysed. The difference between the total topotecan (lactone + hydroxy acid forms) and the lactone level gives the hydroxy acid concentrations. The native fluorescence of the compound (excitation wavelength, 361 nm; emission wavelength, 527 nm) is very intense, allow-

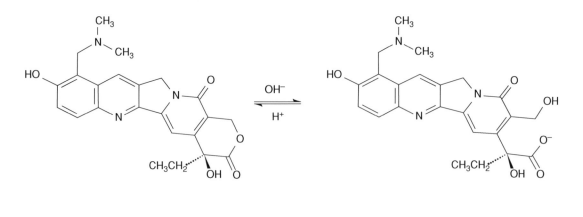

(a)   (b)

Figure 1.1.   Chemical structures of topotecan in (a) its lactone form and (b) its open-ring form (hydroxy acid).

ing analyte concentrations to be measured down to 50 pg/ml.[27]. The methanol precipitation step to fix the lactone–hydroxy acid equilibrium also appears to be an effective sample pretreatment procedure for other camptothecin derivatives, such as 9-aminocamptothecin[28] and irinotecan,[29] and for camptothecin itself [30]

Liquid–liquid extractions are classic but efficient separation techniques and are still preferable to other methods in some cases. The polarity of the organic phase and the pH are the main determinants for recovery. A concentration step can be incorporated by evaporating the organic solvent and dissolving the analyte residue in a small volume. However, the procedure is labour intensive, sometimes involving many sample-handling steps; furthermore, the environmental effect of large volumes of organic solvents is a disadvantage. Liquid–liquid extraction can be used for drug analysis in tissues. We have used this for *doxorubicin* and doxorubicinol and their aglycone metabolites. After homogenization, addition of blank plasma to supplement the sample and a borate buffer (pH 9.5), liquid–liquid extraction with chloroform-1-propanol (4:1) was performed. With this procedure 20 different tissues could be extracted for doxorubicin and its metabolites.[31] The cardioprotective agent *dexrazoxane* (ICRF-187) was isolated from plasma by a combination of protein precipitation (with acetonitrile) followed by a liquid–liquid extraction with 10% 2-methyl-2-propanol in chloroform.[32]

Solid phase extraction (SPE) has become very popular as sample pretreatment procedures. This approach utilizes small disposable extraction columns filled with a sorbent. A variety of sorbents are available, exploiting adsorption (normal phase, reversed phase, wide-pore reversed phase), ion exchange and size exclusion chromatography, allowing almost every analyte to be separated from endogenous matrix components. Solid phase extractions usually comprise four steps.

1. The column is conditioned/activated.

2. The sample is loaded onto the column and aspirated through the column, extracting the analytes.

3. The column is washed to remove any interference.

4. The analytes are selectively eluted.

Method development and optimization usually include changing the sorbent, the composition of washing solutions and eluents, the pH of solvents, etc. It is important to check for variability between batches and between columns from different suppliers as this may have a major influence on the performance of the SPE.[33,34] A recent development is the use of mixed stationary phases which offers more chromatographic interactions to obtain the desired selectivity.

Sample pretreatment is often the most tedious part of the analytical procedure. However, automation and computerization using robots to perform SPEs are becoming more common. We have used an automated SPE system in the analysis of the experimental anticancer drugs *carzelesin and docetaxel* and their metabolites.[35,36] Dilute plasma samples are automatically loaded on SPE columns using a robot [automated sample preparation with extraction columns (ASPEC)]. Preconditioning, sample loading, washing and elution are all automatically executed. The SPE eluate can be injected on-line directly into the HPLC system or, when a concentrated sample is required for increased sensitivity, it can be processed further (e.g. evaporation of the organic solvent and reconstitution of the residue in a small volume of eluent). There are examples of direct injection of serum or plasma into liquid chromatographic systems using analytical columns which do not adsorb proteins. The stationary phase material has pores which are too small for proteins to enter but are still accessible by smaller analyte molecules which can interact within the pores in a reversed phase manner [internal-surface reversed phase (ISRP)]. Other developments in automated isolation procedures of drugs from biological matrices are on-line microdialysis sampling and on-line column-switching techniques.

Derivatization of the analyte can be part of the sample pretreatment. Pre-column derivatization is usually employed to improve the detection of the analyte. We used this technique for the purpose of improving detectability in the bioanalysis of aplidine, a novel experimental marine-derived antitumour agent. *Aplidine* was derivatized with 4′-hydrazino-2-stilbazole, yielding a highly fluorescent derivative which could be analysed down to the nanogram per millilitre level.[37] Other reasons for derivatization are to improve chromatographic properties, to introduce a chiral group and to convert enantiomers into diastereomers facilitating chromatographic separation, and to improve stability of the analyte. For example, 4-hydroxyifosfamide is a metabolic product of the prodrug ifosfamide and is a precursor of the cytotoxic alkylating ifosforamide mustard. The most difficult problem in the analysis of 4-hydroxyifosfamide is its instability in biological fluids. However, the compound can be stabilized by reacting it with semicarbazide at 4°C, yielding a stable semicarbazone derivative which prevents further de-composition. Apart from an improving stability, the derivatization leads to a product with sufficient UV absorptivity at 230 nm for HPLC detection.[38]

In the case of covalently protein bound platinum, plasma samples are ultrafiltrated to separate the free levels from the bound fraction.[39] An alternative is to precipitate proteins with ethanol and to use the super-natant for free drug analysis. The method is rapid and cheaper than making plasma ultrafiltrates. Ma *et al.*[40] have compared the two procedures and found that ethanol extraction is as effective as ultrafiltration.

Chromatography

Apart from the sample pretreatment procedure, the most important way of achieving the desired separation between the analyte and potential interferences is by the correct choice of stationary column material and mobile phase used in an isocratic or gradient mode. Reversed phase chromatography is most commonly employed and utilizes a stationary phase (e.g. octade-cyl-, phenyl-, octyl-, butyl-, or ethyl-bonded phases) which is less polar than the mobile phase. The quality of commercial columns (e.g. consistency of the silica support) has improved substantially over the past decade. During assay development the following parameters need optimization: selection of stationary phase, column dimensions, composition of mobile phase including pH, buffers, ion pair reagent, percentage organic modifier, etc. Reversed phase chromatography was used for the analysis of *paclitaxel* and its metabo-lites in plasma.[41] The optimized system provided sepa-ration of the parent compound and three hydroxylated metabolites. Figure 1.2 shows typical chromatograms of plasma samples from a patient without [Fig. 1.2(a)]

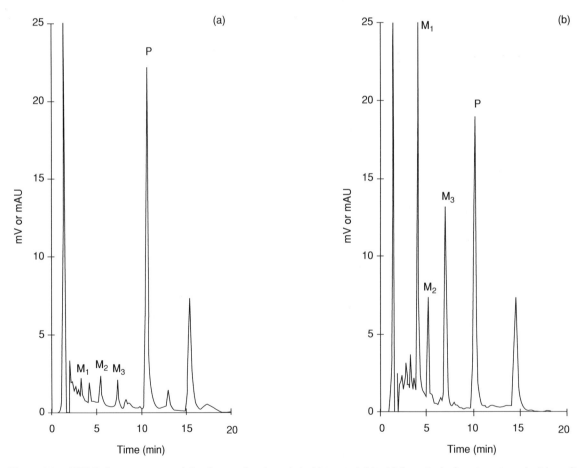

Figure 1.2. HPLC chromatograms of the plasma of patients (a) without and (b) with hepatic dysfunction, treated with pacli-taxel 175 mg/m^2 as a 3 h i.v. infusion. Samples were taken 1 h after the start of the infusion. P = paclitaxel; M$_{1-3}$ = metabolites

and a patient with [Fig. 1.2(b)] liver dysfunction, demonstrating a clear differences in metabolite levels.

Regulatory bodies have put much effort into the perception that racemic drugs are mixtures of compounds and that each drug enantiomer must be treated as a different compound. *Enantiomers* often differ in pharmacological and toxicological properties. Chiral bioanalysis has also been used in oncology. Chromato-

Table 1.1 HPLC detection modes and typical detection limits

UV–visible	10 ng/ml
Fluorescence	1 ng/ml
Electrochemistry	0.5 ng/ml
Mass spectrometry	0.01 ng/ml

Table 1.2 Selected overview of bioanalytical methods for registered anticancer drugs in plasma

Drug	Sample pretreatment	Method	Limit of quantitation	Metabolites	Reference
Amsacine	LL	HPLC–UV	20 ng/ml	No	65
Azathioprine	SPE	HPLC–UV	5 ng/ml	Yes	66
Bleomycin	PP	HPLC–FL	70 ng/ml	Yes	67
Busulfan	LL (+derivatization)	GC–MS	10 ng/ml	No	68
Capecitabine	PP	HPLC–MS	50 ng/ml	Yes	104
Carboplatin	UF	AAS	0.024 µM	No	39
Carmustine	II	HPLC–UV	50 ng/ml	No	69
Chlorambucil	SPE	HPLC–UV	30 ng/ml	Yes	70
Cisplatin	UF	HPLC–ECD	3 ng/ml	No	71
Cyclophosphamide	II	GC–N/PD	50 ng/ml	Yes	72
Cytarabine	SPE	CE–UV	120 ng/ml	No	73
Dacarbazine	UF	HPLC–UV	5 µg/ml	Yes	74
Daunorubicin	SPE	HPLC–FL	0.1 ng/ml	Yes	75
Docetaxel	SPE	HPLC–UV	10 ng/ml	Yes	35
Doxorubicin	LL	HPLC–FL	0.5 ng/ml	Yes	76
Etoposide	LL	HPLC–ECD	2 ng/ml	Yes	77
Epirubicin	SPE	HPLC–FL	1 ng/ml	Yes	78
5-Fluorouracil	PP	HPLC–UV	120 ng/ml	Yes	79
Fotemustine	SPE	HPLC–UV	20 ng/ml	No	80
Hydroxycarbamide	PP	HPLC–ECD	1.5 µg/ml	No	81
Gemcitabine	PP	HPLC–UV	50 ng/ml	Yes	82
Idarubicin	LL	HPLC–FL	1 ng/ml	Yes	83
Imatinib	PP	HPLC–MS	30 ng/ml	Yes	103
Ifosfamide	LL	GC–N/PD	2 ng/ml	Yes	84
Irinotecan	PP	HPLC–FL	1 ng/ml (0.5 ng/ml SN-38)	Yes	29
Lomustine	LL	GC–MS	1 ng/ml	No	85
Melphalan	PP	HPLC–UV	50 ng/ml	No	86
Mercaptopurine	SPE	HPLC–UV	2 ng/ml	No	66
Methotrexate	PP	HPLC–UV	20 ng/ml	Yes	87
Mitomycin C	LL	HPLC–UV	1 ng/ml	No	88
Mitoxantrone	PP/SPE	HPLC–VIS	1 ng/100 µl	No	80
Nimustine	SPE	HPLC–UV	50 ng/ml	No	90
Paclitaxel	SPE	HPLC–UV	10 ng/ml	Yes	41
Procarbazine	LL	GC–MS	10 ng/ml	Yes	91
Suramin	PP	HPLC–UV	5 µg/ml	No	25
Teniposide	LL	HPLC–UV	50 ng/ml	No	92
Thiotepa	LL	GC–N/PD	5 µg/ml	Yes	72
Tioguanine	UF	HPLC–UV	200 ng/ml	No	93
Topotecan	PP	HPLC–FL	0.05 ng/ml	No	27
Vincristine	SPE	HPLC–ECD	0.3 ng/ml	No	94
Vinblastine	LL	HPLC–FL	1 ng/ml	Yes	95
Vindesine	SPE	HPLC–FL	2.5 ng/ml	No	96
Vinorelbine	LL	HPLC–FL	2.0 ng/ml	No	105

Abbreviations: LL, liquid–liquid extraction; PP, protein precipitation; SPE, solid phase extraction; UF, ultrafiltration; UV, UV detection; VIS, visible light detection; FL, fluorescence detection; ECD, electrochemical detection; AAS, atomic absorption spectrometry; GC, gas–liquid chromatography; MS, mass spectrometry detection; N/PD, nitrogen/phosphorus selective detection; CE, capillary electrophoresis.

graphic resolution of cyclophosphamide enantiomers, existing by virtue of an asymmetrically substituted phosphorus atom, has been achieved by precolumn chiral derivatization.[42] In some cases achiral–chiral chromatography combinations with column switching are employed as for the stereoisomers of leucovorin and its metabolite 5-methyltetrahydrofolate. After protein precipitation with perchloric acid, the supernatant is injected onto an achiral system where the total amount of (6R,6S)-*leucovorin*, eluting as a single peak, is determined. The column effluent containing this folinate peak was on-line directed onto a chiral column for the determination of the ratio of the diastereomers by a column-switching technique. Separation of (6R)-leucovorin and 6(S)-leucovorin is achieved using a column with bovine serum albumin (Resolvil BSA-7).[43] Coupling achiral and chiral systems has also been used for the HPLC separation of the (+)(R) and (–)(S) enantiomers of ifosfamide.[44,45]

Detection

The major detection modes in HPLC are given in Table 1.1 with typical detection limits. UV–visible detectors were the first to be used in HPLC systems and are still very useful for many applications in pharmacological studies in oncology (Table 1.2). Diode array detectors allow complete UV spectra to be recorded during chromatographic analysis and can be very helpful to confirm peak purity and for the structural identification and confirmation of metabolic products.

High sensitivity and selectivity can be obtained by fluorescence detection. When the analyte exhibits native fluorescence properties these can be exploited, e.g. with the camptothecins.[27–29] A fluorophore can be introduced into the analyte by chemical derivatization when the drug shows no native fluorescence. This has been done for the

marine derived, cyclic depsipeptide aplidine using derivatization with trans-4'-hydrazine-2-stilbazole.[101]

Liquid chromatography coupled with mass spectrometry (LC–MS) offers many advantages in the bioanalytical field.[46–48] Its unique capability lies in its increased sensitivity, selectivity, and specificity, and the possibilities for on-line structural confirmation of analytes and metabolite identification as has been demonstrated for paclitaxel.[49] The high costs and complexity of the methodology of the early machines, such that they could only be operated by 'super-specialists', prevented their widespread implementation in the field for many years. However, new developments in *LC–MS* technology, particularly the introduction of novel interface technologies, have made this technique (rugged, reliable, easy to use) accessible to a larger number investigators. The main functions of these devices, which is placed between the chromatograph and the mass analyser, are ionization of the analytes, removal of solvent, and transfer of sample. Several interfaces, of which the *thermospray* and electrospray types are the most popular, are commercially available. In the thermospray interface the eluent flows from a resistively heated capillary into a heated ion chamber. At the capillary temperature the solvent partially vaporizes, leading to a stream of electrically charged droplets which continuously vaporize and shrink during passage through the chamber which is evacuated and heated. This process is enhanced when the analyte emerges in an ionic form and when volatile electrolytes (e.g. ammonium acetate) are used in the eluent. In those cases where no ions are generated (because of the use of non-polar solvents or the absence of electrolytes in the eluent) ionization can be effected by a (plasma) discharge electrode in the interface chamber ('discharged-assisted thermospray'). Analyte ions are subsequently led through a small orifice into the high-vacuum mass analyser. The Heated Nebulizer

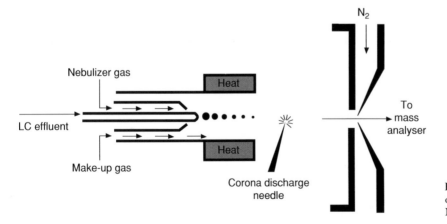

Figure 1.3. Schematic diagram of an LC–MS interface (Heated Nebulizer).

interface is an example of a thermospray interface. The nebulizer and make-up gases support vaporization and aerosol formation. Ionization of the analyte molecules in the gas phase occurs by a corona discharge (Fig. 1.3).

Ionization of electrospray interfaces, like those in thermospray devices, occurs at atmospheric pressure. The eluent is expelled from a stainless-steel capillary used as a sheath electrode, which is held at a high voltage (up to 6 kV), yielding a spray of highly charged droplets which are directed towards an electrode. We have used an LC–MS system of this type. It is composed of a liquid chromatograph coupled through an *atmospheric pressure ionization (API) interface* to a triple quadrupole tandem mass spectrometer (Sciex, API 365). The API interface is equipped with novel and simple, although very subtle, 'curtain gas' technology (see Fig. 1.3, where the Heated Nebulizer interface also has the curtain gas device). The curtain gas (nitrogen) crosses the ion current, desolvates the ions and thereby protects analyser components from contamination. The ions are then drawn through a lens towards the mass analyser. A very small orfice separates the atmospheric pressure for the vacuum of the mass analyser. High-capacity turbopumps maintain the high vacuum of the mass spectrometer.

In a tandem mass spectrometer (MS²), which comprises two mass spectrometers separated by a collision cell, it is possible to analyse a mass-selected ion in the first analyser and then, after a reaction in the collision

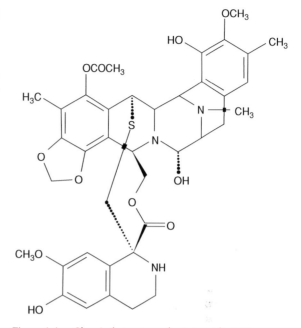

Figure 1.4. Chemical structure of *ecteinascidin 743*.

cell, in the second analyser. In the collision cell the ions selected by the first analyser react with a gas (helium, argon or nitrogen) and are detected by the second analyser.

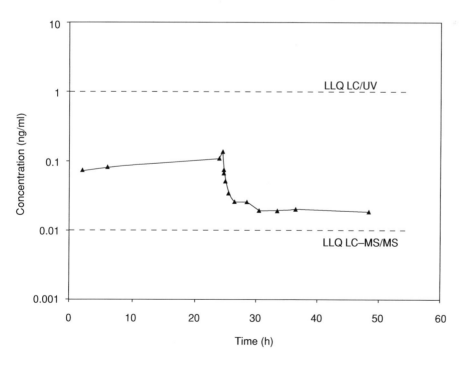

Figure 1.5. Plasma concentration–time curves of *ET-743* administered by a 24 h i.v infusion at a dosage of 100 µg/m². Limits of quantitation (LLQ) of the LC/UV and LC–MS/MS methods are shown by the dotted lines.

LC–MS/MS was used for the bioanalysis of *ecteinascidin 743 (ET-743)*. The complex structure of this compound is shown in Figure 1.4. This new marine-derived anticancer drug is currently under investigation in phase I and II clinical trials. The dosages are of the order of micrograms per square metre. With a conventional HPLC–UV method the limit of quantitation was 1 ng/ml.[50] With this method it was possible to detect maximal blood levels of the drug when administered in short 1-h infusions. However, this method is not suitable for drug analysis during 24-h infusion schedules (phase I dosages ranging from 50 to 1800 µg/m²). With miniaturized HPLC coupled to electrospray ionization tandem mass spectrometry the lower limit of quantitation is 100-fold lower (10 pg/ml), allowing us to record full pharmacokinetic curves at all tested dosages.[51] Figure 1.5 shows the lower limits of quantitation of both methods in relation to the kinetic curves of ET-743. Sample pretreatment procedures (SPE) are identical for both methods, but the LC part of the LC–MS/MS system had to be made MS compatible. Therefore we used a mobile phase composed of water–methanol and volatile buffers (ammonium acetate and formic acid).[51]

Spisulosine (ES-285; (2S, 3R)-2-amino-3-hydroxy-octadecane) is another marine derived, investigational anticancer agent. It is currently studied in phase I clinical trials. The molecule has no UV-VIS absorbance, fluorescence, nor electrochemical activity. The drug, however, can be quantitatively measured in plasma by coupled liquid chromatography and tandem mass spectrometry. Sample pretreatment is simple and carried out by protein precipitation with acetonitrile, containing isotopically labeled (d_3) ES-285 as internal standard. After centrifugation, aliquots of 10 µL of the supernatant are injected directly onto an Inertsil ODS-3 column. Multiple reaction monitoring chromatograms obtained on an API 365 triple-quadrupole mass spectrometer were used for quantification. In this setting the lower limit of quantification was 10 ng/mL in human, mouse, rat and dog plasma.[99]

A recent study by De Jonge et al[102] showed that HPLC coupled with electrospray ionization tandem mass spectrometry is also very suitable to quantitate simultaneously cyclophosphamide, 4-hydroxycyclophosphamide, thiotepa and tepa in human plasma.

Validation

Bioanalytical results can have far-reaching consequences. On the basis of the analytical outcomes decisions are made for an individual patient to continue or to stop therapy or the dose may be reduced or increased, etc.

During clinical drug development the analytical results may even determine whether the new chemical entity 'survives'. Thus it is clear that the analytical results must be precise and accurate. Assay validation aims to characterize analytical methods and guarantees that only reliable methods are used in clinical studies. It is a golden rule that clinical samples are subjected to analysis only after proper validation and approval of the assay. The importance of this is demonstrated in the following case study.[52]

Twenty-three different laboratories participated in a placebo-controlled trial of zidovudine in HIV-infected patients. Quality control specimens were sent to each participating laboratory with the request to quantitate *zidovudine* levels. Results obtained by HPLC ranged from 0 to 350 ng/ml. Later it was found that blank plasma samples containing no zidovudine had been distributed. We have experience with the assay and it is clear that most laboratories had looked at the wrong peak in the chromatograms; zidovudine elutes near an endogenous compound.[53] Laboratories measuring the drug by RIA and FPIA provided the correct values. The impact of these findings was great because a high percentage of subjects from the placebo group (15%) were initially reported to have positive zidovudine assays and were wrongly suspected of using zidovudine. It is not clear whether the assays were validated according to current guidelines, and it is not clear whether if this was the case it would have prevented this ignominious failure. Nevertheless this example justifies the need for a thorough validation of the assay procedure before clinical samples are analysed. For 10 years, assay validation consisted only of obtaining a calibration curve and recovery determination. In recent years a more rigorous approach has been introduced, and guidelines on how to validate a bioanalytical assay are now available. The Washington Conference Report has given this a great impulse.[54] Although meaningful pragmatic guidance is provided, a detailed 'recipe' for performing the validation and for interpreting the results and defining criteria is not given. Thus in every analytical situation the researcher must have the experience to be able to interpret his or her own results. An overview of definitions of validation parameters is given in Table 1.3.

Selectivity and specificity are determined by assaying blank samples from different individuals and samples spiked with drugs (concomitant medications) at relevant therapeutic concentrations that could be present in patient samples. Drug metabolites, degradation products and pharmaceutical vehicles should all be tested.[33]

Table 1.3 Definition of method validation parameters (97)

Validation parameter	Definition
Selectivity	A method is selective when it distinguishes the analyte from degradation products, related compounds and/or matrix components
Specificity	A method is specific when it only determines the analyte of interest
Accuracy	The closeness of test results to the nominal value (also indicated as 'bias')
Repeatability	The closeness of test results obtained from a series of measurements of the same homogenous sample under the assay conditions (also indicated as: 'within-day' or 'intra-assay' precision)
Reproducibility	The closeness of test results obtained from a series of measurements under a maximum variety of conditions over a long time interval (also indicated as: 'between-day' or 'inter-assay' precision)
Limit of detection	The lowest concentration of the analyte in the sample that can be detected but not quantified under the experimental conditions
Limit of quantification	The lowest concentration of the analyte in the sample that can be measured with acceptable accuracy and precision under the experimental conditions
Linearity	A method is linear when it provides test results which are proportional to the concentration of the analyte in the sample in a given range, directly or after mathematical transformation
Range	The range of an analytical method is the interval between the upper and lower limits of quantitation for which it has demonstrated that the analytical procedure has a suitable level of precision, accuracy and linearity

Accuracy and precision are determined by analysing independently prepared samples with known nominal concentrations and quantifying them using calibration standards. This test must be performed with various analyte concentrations equally divided over the concentration range of interest and on different days. The ratio of the measured to nominal concentrations times multiplied by 100 provides the accuracy, and the between-run precisions are obtained by one-way analysis of variance (ANOVA) for each test concentration, with the run day as the classification variable.

Linearity of an assay must be demonstrated by analysis of calibration standards in three separate analytical runs. The variance over the calibration range is usually not constant, but the accuracy of the low concentrations can be increased by weighted regression (e.g. by plotting the reciprocal of the squared concentration versus the ratio of the peak areas of analyte and internal standard). The *F* test for lack of fit gives the linearity of the calibration curves and provides more information than the correlation coefficient, which only indicates whether a relationship between parameters exist (e.g. concentration and detector response) and does not give linearity.[55] Recoveries of sample pretreatment procedures can be concentration dependent. In order to obtain insight into the recovery yield over the whole concentration range of interest, the slope of the processed calibration curve is divided by the slope of a calibration curve from non-processed standards. This ratio multiplied by 100 gives the percentage recovery over the tested concentration range.

It is of utmost importance to know the stability characteristics of the analytes (parent drug, metabolites, internal standard) both in the solid state as in stock solutions and in dilutions. For bioanalytical purposes the following *sample stabilities* are generally relevant: (i) during *sample handling* on the ward (blood withdrawal, centrifugation, short-term storage); (ii) during prolonged storage (usually at −20 or −70°C); (iii) after freeze–thawing; (iv) during sample pretreatment; (v) during storage in an autosampler prior to analysis, stock solution dilutions, etc. It is important to remember that compounds can be less stable in biological matrices than in aqueous solutions.[56–58]

The robustness of an analytical method is an important issue. It is evident that methods must be easy to *repeat by* other laboratories. For HPLC methods robustness can be tested by, for example, changing analytical and SPE columns (another lot number, another supplier) and also by changing the technician who performs the analysis. However, there is no general rule for testing robustness. When the most critical parts of an analytical assay have been identified, it is clear that these should be part of the evaluation of robustness.

Validation is necessary for each biological matrix. Changing from plasma to urine analysis requires that a complete validation programme must be executed because of the different nature of these matrices.

This also holds for tissues. Results from validation experiments of doxorubicin and metabolites in several murine tissues demonstrated the importance of validation in all relevant specimens since accuracy and precision were highly matrix dependent. The largest deviations from *doxorubicin* nominal values were found for liver and small intestine.[31]

An HPLC method developed for *topotecan* determination in human plasma appeared to be unsuitable for dog and rat plasma because of endogenous interference. After recognition that the column temperature had a very selective effect on the chromatography of topotecan and interferences, an adapted method was developed and validated for dog and rat plasma.[59] This emphasizes the importance of checking the performance of the method carefully when another matrix is subjected for analysis. The effects of additives in the pharmaceutical formulation should also be investigated. We noted that Cremophor EL, part of the Taxol® formulation (paclitaxel in Cremophor EL + ethanol, 1:1), has a major impact on the performance of SPE columns and the recovery of *paclitaxel*.[33]

Detailed information and strategies for method validation are difficult to present, because each compound has different requrements.[60]. Practical elaboration of the validation parameters discussed above for paclitaxel[41], docetaxel,[35] ET-743,[50 51] dexrazoxane,[32] irinotecan,[29] topotecan,[27] 9-aminocamptothecin,[28] carzelesin,[36] and ABT-518,[100] which have served as examples here, can be found in the literature.

Samples and sampling

Plasma is the most commonly used biological matrix. It allows the determination of the most relevant pharmacokinetic parameters (AUC, half-life, clearance, and distribution volume) and is easy accessible. It is assumed that *plasma concentration* gives an adequate representation of drug concentration and exposure at the target (e.g. a tumour). However, this assumption is questionable, particularly for compounds with a very large distribution volume. *Tumour tissue* is difficult to access. In those cases where tissue is available, the analytical data must be handled with caution. Van Tellingen *et al.*[61] used HPLC to measure teniposide concentrations in resected brain tumour specimens (malignant gliomas and brain metastases). From albumin measurements it became clear that a substantial fraction of the resected brain tissues contained whole blood. Shortly after drug infusion, when the plasma concentrations are high, most of the drug measured in the tumour specimens originated from blood. It was only possible to discern a real tissue uptake of teniposide in samples taken 24 h after drug administration when plasma concentrations declined to 0.2 µg/ml. The study revealed that an accurate determination of drug tissue concentration is hindered by concurrent plasma levels. Therefore it is essential to include a suitable procedure to establish the contribution of drug in blood.[61] Tissue concentrations (in µg/g) that are less than the plasma concentration (in µg/ml) from a concomitantly taken blood sample must be interpreted with great caution. Validation work done in different tissue samples has also demonstrated that there is a large difference between matrices.[31] Separate validation data must be available for each matrix.

Leucocytes, which form platinum adducts after treatment with a platinum-containing drug, are used as a DNA source. Theoretically, this matrix is attractive because it seems a step closer to the place where the drug works, at the DNA level; however, it remains to be seen whether it really has a better predictive value than platinum levels in plasma ultrafiltrates.[16,17] A disadvantage is that a relatively large blood volume (15 ml) is necessary for the analysis. On the other hand, it is not necessary to take as many serial samples to construct a classic plasma kinetic curve because of the kinetics of adduct formation.

For obvious reasons *saliva* has attracted interest as a biological matrix for drug monitoring. Sampling is non-invasive and patient-friendly. As saliva is rapidly formed by ultrafiltration of plasma, only the non-protein bound fraction of a drug can be expected in saliva. Thus, theoretically, carboplatin saliva concentrations could be a perfect reflection and replace platinum analysis in plasma ultrafiltrate. Platinum concentrations in saliva were found to be about 50-fold lower than in plasma ultrafiltrate, however, the profile was very erratic with a large variation and therefore appeared not to be a reliable replacement for plasma ultrafiltrate analysis.[62] The saliva concentrations for topotecan were of the same order of magnitude as the plasma concentrations. However, the large variability in plasma-to-saliva ratios also precludes the use of this matrix.[63]

Blood sampling is a major issue in the cascade of events finally leading to an analytical outcome. When things go wrong during sampling on the ward none of the subsequent precautions are relevant. A classic error is to take samples from the same infusion line that was used to administer the drug. When sampling from double lumen catheters, it is important to use the right lumen for drug administration and blood sampling.[64]

Conclusions

Bioanalysis, the quantitative determination of a drug (and its metabolites) in biological matrices, plays a pivotal role in almost every phase of the development of a pharmaceutical product. Important decisions are made on the basis of the outcomes of these investigations. Thus it is clear that bioanalytical assays must be extensively validated before clinical samples can be measured. The characteristics and performance of an assay are revealed by validation, and after successful validation the assay can be expected to provide reliable data. HPLC continues to be popular for the bioanalysis of anticancer drugs. This is because it is a versatile analytical tool applicable for almost every drug. It is expected that the combination of liquid chromatography and mass spectrometry will undergo rapid expansion in the near future.

References

1. Collins JM, Zaharko DS, Dedrick RL, Chabner BA (1986) Potential roles for preclinical pharmacology in phase I clinical trials. *Cancer Treat Rep*, **70**, 73–80.
2. Collins JM, Grieshaber CK, Chabner BA (1990) Pharmacologically guided phase I clinical trials based upon preclinical drug development. *J Natl Cancer Inst*, **82**, 1321–6.
3. Bruno R, Vivier N, Vergniol JC, *et al.* (1996) Population pharmacokinetic model for docetaxel: model building and validation. *J Pharmacokinet Biopharm*, **2**, 153–73.
4. Bruno R, Hille D, Riva A, *et al.* (1998) Drug metabolism and pharmacokinetics/pharmacodynamics of docetaxel in phase II studies in patients with cancer. *J Clin Oncol*, **16**, 187–96.
5. van Warmerdam LJC, van den Bemt BJF, ten Bokkel Huinink WW, Maes RAA, Beijnen JH (1995) Dose individualisation in cancer chemotherapy: pharmacokinetic and pharmacodynamic relationships. *Cancer Res Ther Control*, **4**, 277–91.
6. Evans WE, Relling MV, Rodman JH, Crom WR, Boyett JM, Pui CH (1998) Conventional compared with individualized chemotherapy for childhood acute lymphoblastic leukemia. *N Eng J Med*, **338**, 499–505.
7. Fety R, Rolland F, Barberi-Heyob M, *et al* (1998) Clinical impact of pharmacokinetically-guided dose adaptation of 5-fluoro-uracil: results from a multicentre randomized trial in patients with locally advanced head and neck carcinomas. *Clin Cancer Res*, **4**, 2039–45.
8. Niessen WMA, van der Greef J (1992) *Liquid Chromatography–Mass Spectrometry*. New York: Marcel Dekker.
9. Riley CM, Lough WJ, Wainer IW. (1994) *Pharmaceutical and Biomedical Applications of Liquid Chromatography*. Oxford: Elsevier.
10. Richens A, Marks V (1981) *Therapeutic drug monitoring*. New York: Churchill Livingstone.
11. Reid JM, Ames MM (1998) Assay methodology. In Grochow LB, Ames, MM (eds) *A Clinician's Guide to Chemotherapy Pharmacokinetics and Pharmacodynamics*. Baltimore, MD: Williams & Wilkins, 497–513.
12. Hamel E, Linn CM, Johns DG (1982) Tubulin-dependent biochemical assay for the antineoplastic agent taxol and application to measurement of the drug in serum. *Cancer Treat Rep*, **66**, 1381–6.
13. Hodes TJM, Underberg WJM, Los G, Beijnen JH (1992) Platinum antitumor agents: a review of bioanalysis. *Pharm Weekbl Sci*, **14**, 61–77.
14. McKay K (1993) New techniques in the pharmacokinetic analysis of cancer drugs II. The ultratrace determination of platinum in biological samples by inductively coupled plasma-mass spectrometry. *Cancer Surv*, **17**, 407–14.
15. Welters MJ, Maliepaard M, Jacobs-Bergmans AJ, *et al.* (1997) Improved ^{32}P-postlabelling assay for the quantification of the major platinum-DNA adducts. *Carcinogenesis*, **18**, 1767–74.
16. Schellens JHM, Ma J, Planting AST, *et al.* (1996) Relationship between exposure to cisplatin, DNA adduct formation in leucocytes and tumour response in patients with solid tumours. *Br J Cancer*, **73**, 1569–75.
17. Fisch MJ, Howard KI, Einhorn LH (1996) Relationship between platinum-DNA adducts in leukocytes of patients with advanced germ cell cancer and survival. *Clin Cancer Res*, **2**, 1063–7.
18. Reinhoud NJ, Tjaden UR, Irth H, van der Greef J (1992) Bioanalysis of some anthracyclines in human plasma by capillary electrophoresis with laser-induced fluorescence detection. *J Chromatogr B Biomed Appl*, **574**, 327–34.
19. Roach MC, Gozel P, Zare RN (1988) Determination of methotrexate and its major metabolite, 7-hydroxy-methotrexate using capillary zone electrophoresis and laser-induced fluorescence detection. *J Chromatogr*, **426**, 129–40.
20. Kaijser GP, Beijnen JH (1998) Oxazaphosphorines: cyclophosphamide and ifosfamide. In Grochow LB, Ames, MM (eds) *A Clinician's Guide to Chemotherapy Pharmacokinetics and Pharmacodynamics*. Baltimore, MD: Williams & Wilkins, 229–58.
21. Kaijser GP, Beijnen JH, Bult A, Keizer HJ, Underberg WJM (1997) Chromatographic analysis of the enantiomers of ifosfamide and some of its metabolites in plasma and urine. *J Chromatogr B Biomed Appl*, **690**, 131–8.
22. Maxwell RJ (1993) New techniques in the pharmacokinetic analysis of cancer drugs III. Nuclear magnetic resonance. *Cancer Surv*, **17**, 415–23.
23. Tilsley DWO, Harte RJA, *et al.* (1993) New techniques in the pharmacokinetic analysis of cancer drugs IV. Positron emission tomography. *Cancer Surv*, **17**, 425–42.

24. Blanchard J (1981) Evaluation of the relative efficacy of various techniques for deproteinizing plasma samples prior to high-performance liquid chromatographic analysis. *J Chromatogr*, **226**, 455–60.

25. Beijnen JH, van Gijn R, de Clippeleir JJM, Vlasveld LTh, Horenblas S, Underberg WJM (1990) Rapid determination of suramin in micro-volumes of plasma by using ion-pair high performance liquid chromatography. *J Drug Dev*, **3**, 21–6.

26. Underberg WJM, Goossen RMJ, Smith BR, Beijnen JH (1990) Equilibrium kinetics of the new experimental antitumour compound SK&F 104864-A in aqueous solution. *J Pharm Biomed Anal*, **8**, 681–3.

27. Rosing H, Doyle E, Davies BE, Beijnen JH (1995) High-performance liquid chromatographic determination of the novel antitumor drug topotecan and topotecan as the total of the lactone plus carboxylate forms, in human plasma. *J Chromatogr B Biomed Appl*, **668**, 107–15.

28. van Gijn R, Herben VMM, Hillebrand MJX, ten Bokkel Huinink WW, Bult A, Beijnen JH (1998) High-performance liquid chromatographic analysis of the investigational anticancer drug 9-aminocamptothecin, as the lactone form and as the total of the lactone and the carboxylate forms, in micro-volumes of human plasma. *J Pharm Biomed Anal*, **17**, 1257–65.

29. Herben VMM, Mazee D, van Zomeren DM, *et al.* (1998) Sensitive determination of the carboxylate and lactone forms of the novel antitumour drug irinotecan and its active metabolite SN-38 in plasma by high-performance liquid chromatography. *J Liquid Chromatogr Relat Technol*, **21**, 1541–58.

30. Beijnen JH, Rosing H, Ten Bokkel Huinink WW, Pinedo HM (1993) High-performance liquid chromatographic analysis of the antitumour drug camptothecin and its lactone ring-opened form in rat plasma. *J Chromatogr B Biomed Appl*, **617**, 111–17.

31. van Asperen J, van Tellingen O, Beijnen JH (1998) Determination of doxorubicin and metabolites in murine specimens by high-performance liquid chromatography. *J Chromatogr B Biomed Appl*, **712**, 129–43.

32. Rosing H, van Gijn R, ten Bokkel Huinink WW, Beijnen JH (1997) High-performance liquid chromatographic analysis of the cardioprotective agent dexrazoxane in human plasma and urine. *J Liquid Chromatogr Relat Technol*, **20**, 583–601.

33. Huizing MT, Rosing H, Koopmans FP, Beijnen JH (1998) Influence of Cremophor EL on the quantification of paclitaxel in plasma using high-performance liquid chromatography with solid-phase extraction as sample pretreatment. *J Chromatogr B Biomed Appl*, **709**, 161–5.

34. Vendrig DEMM, Holthuis JJM, Erdelyi-Toth V, Hulshoff A (1987) Solid-phase extraction of vinblastine and vincristine from plasma and urine: variable drug recoveries due to non-reproducible column packings. *J Chromatogr*, **414**, 91–100.

35. Rosing H, Lustig V, Koopman FP, ten Bokkel Huinink WW, Beijnen JH (1997) Bioanalysis of docetaxel and hydroxylated metabolites in human plasma by high-performance liquid chromatography and automated solid-phase extraction. *J Chromatogr B Biomed Appl*, **696**, 89–98.

36. van Tellingen O, Pels EM, Henrar REC, *et al.*(1994) Fully automated high-performance liquid chromatographic method for the determination of carzelesin (U-80,244) and metabolites (U-76,073 and U-76,074) in human plasma. *J Chromatogr*, **652**, 51–8.

37. Sparidans RW, Henrar REC, Jimeno J, Faircloth G, Floriano P, Beijnen JH (1998) Bioanalysis of aplidine, a new marine antitumor depsipeptide, in plasma by high-performance liquid chromatography after derivatization with 4′-hydrazino-2-stilbazole. *Ann Oncol*, **9** (Suppl 2), 50.

38. Kerbusch T, Huitema ADR, Kettenes-van den Bosch JJ, *et al.* (1998) High-performance liquid chromatographic determination of stabilized 4-hydroxyifosfamide in human plasma and erythrocytes. *J Chromatogr B Biomed Appl*, **716**, 275–84.

39. van Warmerdam LJC, van Tellingen O, Maes RAA, Beijnen JH (1995) Validated method for the determination of carboplatin in biological fluids by Zeeman atomic absorption spectrometry. *Fresenius J Anal Chem*, **351**, 1820–4.

40. Ma J, Stoter G, Verweij J, Schellens JHM (1996) Comparison of ethanol plasma-protein precipitation with plasma ultrafiltration and trichloroacetic acid protein precipitation for the measurement of unbound platinum concentrations. *Cancer Chemother Pharmacol*, **38**, 391–4.

41. Huizing MT, Sparreboom A, Rosing H, van Tellingen O, Pinedo HM, Beijnen JH (1995) Quantification of paclitaxel metabolites in human plasma by high-performance liquid chromatography. *J Chromatogr B Biomed Appl*, **674**, 261–8.

42. Reid JM, Stobaugh JF, Sternson LA (1989) Liquid chromatographic determination of cyclophosphamide enantiomers in plasma by precolumn chiral derivatization. *Anal Chem*, **61**, 441–6.

43. Sips JHM, van Tellingen O, Nooijen WJ, Rodenhuis S, Ten Bokkel Huinink WW, Beijnen JH (1994) The pharmacokinetics of reduced folates after intraperitoneal and intravenous administration of folinic acid. *Cancer Chemother Pharmacol*, **35**, 144–8.

44. Kaijser GP, Korst A, Beijnen JH, Bult A, Underberg WJM (1993) The analysis of ifosfamide and its metabolites [review] *Anticancer Res*, **13**, 1311–24.

45. Masurel D, Wainer IW (1989) Analytical and preparative high performance liquid chromatographic separation of the enantiomers of ifosfamide, cyclophosphamide and trofosfamide and their determination in plasma. *J Chromatogr*, **490**, 133–43.

46. Gelpi E (1995) Biomedical and biochemical applications of liquid chromatography–mass spectrometry. *J Chromatogr A*, **703**, 59–80.

47. Loo JA (1995) Bioanalytical mass spectrometry: many flavours to choose. *Bioconjug Chem*, **6**, 644–65.

48. Burlingame AL, Boyd RK, Gaskell SJ (1996) Mass spectrometry. *Anal Chem*, **68**, 599R–651R.

49. Royer I, Alvinerie P, Armand JP, Ho LK, Wright M, Monsarrat B (1995) Paclitaxel metabolites in human plasma and urine: identification of 6-alpha-hydroxy-taxol, 7-epitaxol and taxol hydrolysis products using liquid chromatography/atmospheric pressure chemical ionization mass spectrometry. *Rapid Commun Mass Spectrom*, **9**, 495–502.

50. Rosing H, Hillebrand MJX, Jimeno JM, *et al.* (1998) Analysis of Ecteinascidin 743, a new potent marine-derived anticancer drug, in human plasma by high-performance liquid chromatography in combination with solid-phase extraction. *J Chromatogr B Biom*ed Appl, **710**, 183–9.

51. Rosing H, Hillebrand MJX, Jimeno JM, *et al.* (1998) Quantitative determination of ecteinascidin 743 in human plasma by miniaturized high-performance liquid chromatography coupled with electrospray ionization tandem mass spectrometry. *J Mass Spectrom*, **33**, 1134–40.

52. Krøgstad DJ, Eveland MR, Lim LL-Y, Volberding PA, Sadler BM (1991) Drug level monitoring in a double-blind multicenter trial: false-positive zidovudine measurements in AIDS clinical trials group protocol 019. *Antimicrob Agents Chemother*, **35**, 1160–4.

53. Underberg WJM, Underberg-Chitoe UK, Bekers O, Meenhorst PL, Beijnen JH(1989) A rapid, simple and accurate method for the bioanalysis of zidovudine. *Int J Pharm*, **50**, 175–9.

54. Shah VP, Midha KK, Dighe S, *et al.* (1992) Analytical methods validation: bioavailability, bioequivalence and pharmacokinetic studies. *J Pharm Sci*, **81**, 309–12.

55. Thompson M (1990) Abuse of statistics software packages. *Anal Proc*, **27**, 142–6.

56. Beijnen JH, van der Nat JM, Labadie RP, Underberg WJM (1986) Decomposition of mitomycin and anthracycline cytostatics in cell culture media. *Anticancer Res*, **6**, 39–44.

57. Bouma J, Beijnen JH, Bult A, Underberg WJM (1986) Anthracycline antitumor agents. A review of physicochemical, analytical and stability properties. *Pharm Weekbl Sci*, **8**, 109–33.

58. Beijnen JH, Lingeman H, van Munster HA, Underberg WJM (1986) Mitomycin antitumour agents: a review of their physicochemical and analytical properties and stability. *J Pharm Biomed Anal*, **4**, 275–95.

59. Rosing H, Doyle E, Beijnen JH (1996) The impact of temperature in the high-performance liquid chromatographic analysis of topotecan in rat and dog plasma. *J Pharm Biomed Anal*, **15**, 279–86.

60. Lang JR, Botlon SM (1994) A comprehensive method validation strategy for bioanalytical applications in the pharmaceutical industry. In Riley, CM, Lough, WJ, Wainer IW (eds) *Pharmaceutical and Biomedical Applications of Liquid Chromatography.* Oxford: Elsevier, 345–67.

61. van Tellingen O, Boogerd W, Nooijen WJ, Beijnen JH (1997) The vascular compartment hampers accurate determination of teniposide penetration into brain tumor tissue. *Cancer Chemother Pharmacol*, **40**, 330–4.

62. van Warmerdam LJC, van Tellingen O, Ten Bokkel Huinink WW, Rodenhuis S, Maes RAA, Beijnen JH (1995) Monitoring carboplatin concentrations in saliva: a replacement for plasma ultrafiltrate measurements? *Ther Drug Monit*, **17**, 465–70.

63. van Warmerdam LJC, Rosing H, ten Bokkel Huinink WW, Maes RAA, Beijnen JH (1995) Do topotecan concentrations in saliva reflect plasma concentrations? *J Oncol Pharm Pract*, **1**, 41–5.

64. Huitema ADR, Holtkamp M, Tibben MM, Rodenhuis S, Beijnen JH (1999) Sampling technique from central

venous catheters proves to be critical for pharmacokinetic studies. *Ther Drug Monit*, **21**, 102–4.

65. Jurlina JL, Paxton JW (1983). High performance liquid chromatographic method for the determination of 4′-(9-acridinylamino)methanesulfon-manisidide in plasma. *J Chromatogr* **276**, 367–74.

66. Van Os EC, McKinney JA, Zins BJ, Mays DC, Shriver ZV, Sandborn WJ, Lipsky JJ (1996) Simultaneous determination of azathioprine and 6-mercaptopurine by high performance liquid chromatography. *J Chromatogr B Biomed Appl* **679**, 147–54.

67. Mahdadi R, Kenani A, Pommery N, Pommery J, Hénichart, JP, Lhermitte M (1991). High-performance liquid chromatography assay of bleomycin in human plasma and rat hepatocytes. *Cancer Chemother Pharmacol* **28**, 22–6.

68. Ehrsson H, Hassan M (1983). Determination of busulfan by GC-MS with selected ion-monitoring. *J Pharm Sci* **72**, 1203–5.

69. Jones RB, Matthes SM, Dufton C, Shpall EJ, Bearman SI, Ross M, Cagnoni P (1998). Nitrosoureas, In Grochow, L.B. and Ames, M.M. (eds). *A Clinician's Guide to Chemotherapy Pharmacokinetics and Pharmacodynamics, Williams & Wilkins, Baltimore,* 331–344.

70. Oppitz MM, Musch E, Malek M, Rub HP, von Unruh GE, Loos U, Muhlenbruch B (1989). Studies on the pharmacokinetics of chlorambucil and prednimustine in patients using a new high-performance liquid chromatographic assay. *Cancer Chemother Pharmacol* **23**, 208–12.

71. Treskes M, De Jong J, Leeuwenkamp OR, Van der Vijgh WJF (1990). Sensitive determination of cisplatin in body fluids with HPLC and on-line reductive electrochemical detection. *J Liquid Chromatogr* **13**, 1321–38.

72. Huitema ADR, Tibben MM, Kerbusch T, Zwikker JW, Rodenhuis S, Beijnen JH (1998). Simultaneous determination of N,N′,N″-triethylenethiophosphoramide, cyclophosphamide and some of their metabolites in plasma using capillary gas chromatography. *J Chromatogr B Biomed Appl* **716**, 177–86.

73. Lloyd DK, Cypess AM, Wainer IW (1991). Determination of cytosine-beta-D-arabinoside in plasma using capillary electrophoresis. *J Chromatogr* **568**, 117–24.

74. Fiore D, Jackson AJ, Didolkar MS, Dandu VR (1985). Simultaneous determination of dacarbazine, its photolytic degradation product, 2-azahypoxanthine and the metabolite 5-aminoimidazole-4-carboxamide in plasma and urine by high-pressure liquid chromatography. *Antimicrob Agents Chemother* **27**, 977–9.

75. De Jong J, Maessen PA, Akkerdaas A, Cheung SF, Pinedo HM, Van der Vijgh WJF (1990). Sensitive method for the determination of daunorubicin and all its known metabolites in plasma and heart by high-performance liquid chromatography with fluorescence detection. *J Chromatogr B Biomed Appl* **529**, 359–68.

76. Beijnen JH, Meenhorst PL, Van Gijn R, Fromme M, Rosing H, Underberg WJM (1991). HPLC determination of doxorubicin, doxorubicinol and four aglycone metabolites in plasma of AIDS patients. *J Pharm Biomed Anal* **9**, 995–1002.

77. Holthuis JJM, Römkens FMGM, Pinedo HM, van Oort WJ (1983). Plasma assay for the antineoplastic agent VP 16–213 (Etoposide) using high-performance liquid chromatography with electrochemical detection. *J Pharm Biomed Anal* **1**, 89–97.

78. Dobbs NA, Twelves CJ (1991). Measurement of epidoxorubicin and its metabolites by high performance liquid chromatography using an advanced automated sample processor. *J Chromatogr B Biomed Appl* **572**, 211–7.

79. Jung M, Berger G, Pohlen U, Pauser S, Reszka R, Buhr HJ (1997). Simultaneous determination of 5-fluorouracil and its active metabolites in serum and tissue by high-performance liquid chromatography. *J Chromatogr B Biomed Appl* **702**, 193–202.

80. Gordon BH, Richards RP, Kiley MP, Gray AJ, Ings RM, Campbell DB (1989). A new method for the measurement of nitrosoureas in plasma: an h.p.l.c. procedure for the measurement of fotemustine kinetics. *Xenobiotica* **19**, 329–39.

81. Havard J, Grygiel J, Sampson D (1992). Determination by high performance liquid chromatography of hydroxyurea in human plasma. *J Chromatogr* **584**, 270–4.

82. Freeman KB, Anliker S, Hamilton M, Osborne D, Dhahir PH, Nelson R, Allerheiligen SRB (1995). Validated assays for the determination of gemcitabine in human plasma and urine using high performance liquid chromatography with ultraviolet detection. *J Chromatogr* **665**, 171–81.

83. Beijnen JH, Neef C, Bouma J, Paalman ACA, Underberg WJM (1988). Analysis of 4-demethoxydaunorubicin and metabolites in plasma and urine. *Chem Pharm Bull* **36**, 3503–11.

84. Kaijser GP, Beijnen JH, Bult A, Wiese G, de Kraker J, Keizer HJ, Underberg WJM (1992). Gas chromatographic determination of 2- and 3-dechloroethylifosfamide in plasma and urine. *J Chromatogr B Biomed Appl* **583**, 175–82.

85. Smith RG, Blackstock SC, Cheung LK, Loo TL (1981). Analysis of nitrosourea antitumor agents by gas chromatography-mass spectrometry. *Anal Chem* **53**, 1205–8.

86. Chang SY, Alberts DS, Melnick LR, *et al.* (1978). High pressure liquid chromatographic analysis of melphalan in plasma. *J Pharm Sci* **67**, 679–83.

87. Van Tellingen O, Van der Woude HR, Beijnen JH, Van Beers CJT, Nooyen WJ (1989). Stable and sensitive method for the simulateneous determination of N^5-methyltetrahydrofolate, leucovorin, methotrexate and 7-hydroxymethotrexate in biological fluids. *J Chromatogr B Biomed Appl* **488**, 379–88.

88. Den Hartigh J, Van Oort WJ, Bocken MCYM, Pinedo HM (1981). HPLC determination of the antitumor agent mitomycin C in human blood plasma. *Analytica Chimica Acta* **127**, 47–56.

89. Varossieau FJ, Beijnen JH, Los G, Nagel JD, McVie JG (1992). Micro-determination of the antitumor drug mitoxantrone using HPLC and on-line sample pre-concentration. *J Drug Dev* **5**, 107–12.

90. Tatsuhara T, Tabuchi F, Yamane M, Hori T (1990). Rapid and simple method for the determination of nimustine hydrochloride in human blood and brain by high-performance liquid chromatography. *J Chromatogr B Biomed Appl* **526**, 507–14.

91. Gorsen RM, Weiss AJ, Manthei RW (1980). Analysis of procarbazine and metabolites by gas chromatography-mass spectrometry. *J Chromatogr* **221**, 309–18.

92. Holthuis JJM, Van Oort WJ, Pinedo HM (1981). A sensitive HPLC method for the determination of the antineoplastic drugs VP 16–213 and VM 26 in biological fluids. *Analytica Chimica Acta* **130**, 23–30.

93. Breithaupt H, Goebel G (1981). Quantitative high-pressure liquid chromatography of 6-thioguanine in biological fluids. *J Chromatogr Sci* **19**, 496–9.

94. Bloemhof H, van Dijk KN, de Graaf SSN, Vendrig DEMM, Uges DRA (1991). Sensitive method for the determination of vincristine in human serum by high-performance liquid chromatography after on-line column extraction. *J Chromatogr* **572**, 171–9.

95. Van Tellingen O, Beijnen JH, Baurain R, ten Bokkel Huinink WW, Van der Woude HR, Nooyen WJ (1991). High-performance liquid chromatographic determination of vinblastine, 4-O-deacetylvinblastine and the potential metabolite 4-O-deacetylvinblastine-3-oic acid in biological fluids. *J Chromatogr* **353**, 47–53.

96. Vendrig DEMM, Teeuwsen J, Holthuis JJM (1988). Determination of vinca alkaloids in plasma and urine using ion-exchange chromatography on silica gel and fluorescence detection. *J Chromatogr* **434**, 145–55.

97. Rosing H, Man WY, Doyle E, Bult A, Beijnen JH (2000). Bioanalytical liquid chromatographic method validation. A review of current practices and procedures. *J Liq Chromatogr Rel Technol*, **23**, 329–54.

98. Van Kesteren Ch, De Vooght MMM, López-Lázaro L, Mathôt RAA, Schellens JHM, Jimeno JM, Beijnen JH (2003). Yondelis (trabectedin, ET-743): the development of an anticancer agent of marine origin. *Anticancer Drugs* **14**, 487–502.

99. Stokvis E, Nan-Offeringa L, Rosing H, López-Lázaro L, Acena JL, Miranda E, Lyubimov A, Levine BS, D≤Aleo C, Schellens JHM, Beijnen JH (2003). Quantitative analysis of ES-285, an investigational marine anticancer drug, in human, mouse, rat, and dog plasma using coupled liquid chromatography and tandem mass spectrometry. *J Mass Spectrom* **38**, 548–54.

100. Stokvis E, Rosing H, Crul M, Rieser MJ, Heck AJR, Schellens JHM, Beijnen JH (2004). Quantitative analysis of the novel anticancer drug ABT-518, a matrix metalloproteinase inhibitor, plus the screening of six metabolites in human plasma using high-performance liquid chromatography coupled with electrospray tandem mass spectrometry. *J Mass Spectrom* **39**, 277–88.

101. Sparidans RW, Schellens JHM, López-Lázaro L, Jimeno JM, Beijnen JH (2004). Liquid chromatographic assay for the cyclic depsipeptide aplidine, a new marine antitumor drug, in whole blood using derivatization with trans-4′-hydrazino-2-stilbazole. *Biomed Chromatogr* **18**, 16–20.

102. De Jonge ME, van Dam SM, Hillebrand MJX, Rosing H, Huitema ADR, Rodenhuis S, Beijnen JH (2004). Simultaneous quantification of cyclophosphamide, 4-hydroxy-cyclophosphamide, N′,N″,N‴-triethylenethiophosphoramide (thiotepa) and N′,N″,N‴-triethylenephosphoramide

(tepa) in human plasma by high-performance liquid chromatography coupled with electrospray ionization tandem mass spectrometry. *J Mass Spectrom* **39**, 262–71.

103. Parise RA, Ramanathan RK, Hayes MJ, Egorin MJ (2003). Liquid chromatographic-mass spectrometric assay for quantitation of imatinib and its main metabolite (CGP 74588) in plasma. *J Chromatogr B* **791**, 39–44.

104. Xu Y, Grem JL (2003). Liquid chromatography-mass spectrometry method for the analysis of the anticancer agent capecitabine and its nucleoside metabolites in human plasma. *J Chromatogr B* **783**, 273–85.

105. Robieux I, Vitali V, Aita P, Freschi A, Lazzarini R, Sorio R. Sensitive high-performance liquid chromatographic method with fluorescence detection for measurement of vinorelbine plasma concentrations. *J Chromatogr B* **675**, 183–7.

2 | Principles of pharmacokinetics

Etienne Chatelut

Introduction

Pharmacokinetics is the study of the fate of a drug between the time of its administration to an organism and the time it is eliminated from the body. Pharmacokinetic studies require an understanding of both the mechanisms and the kinetics of three main processes, absorption, distribution, and elimination, and it is mainly the last of these that will be addressed in this chapter. Pharmacokinetic information is accumulated during the development of a drug, and at each stage of drug development the collected pharmacokinetic data should be used to guide the design to the following phase. After a drug is approved, the therapeutic management of patients may also benefit from the use of pharmacokinetic data. Specifically, clinical pharmacokinetics are of special interest in oncology because of the narrow therapeutic index of cytotoxic drugs and the large inter-individual differences in pharmacokinetic parameters that are observed.

Pharmacokinetic parameters

In humans, the blood is usually the most accessible fluid and is widely used for deriving pharmacokinetic parameters. In most cases, the drug concentrations are determined in *plasma* and, unless stated otherwise, the discussion in this chapter relates to data so derived.

Pharmacokinetic parameters can be divided into two groups. The first group is composed of those which describe in some form the plasma concentration–time profile and have units of time, concentration, or time multiplied by concentration. The second group is composed of parameters which define the rate or extent of pharmacokinetic processes (e.g. absorption, distribution, and elimination). The secondary parameters are obtained from the plasma concentration–time profile by taking into account also the dosage and the schedule of administration. Given these individual parameters and the target plasma concentrations required, optimal doses and schedules of administration can be identified.

Parameters relative to the plasma concentration–time profile after a single administration

Figure 2.1 shows the concentration–time curve following intravenous bolus administration of a drug. The maximum concentration is observed immediately after completion of the administration. Indeed, dilution of the dose within (at least) the plasma compartment is essentially instantaneous. A semilogarithmic plot of these data indicates an initial rapid decline of the plasma concentration which precedes a terminal linear phase. The first phase corresponds to the sum of the distribution and elimination processes. Immediately after a bolus administration, the drug is 'diluted' in an initial (or central) compartment from which it distributes into other tissues which constitute the peripheral compartment (see later in the chapter). Once an equilibrium is achieved between drug in tissue and in the central compartment, the decline of the plasma concentration C is due only to the elimination process and is described by a mono-exponential function:

$$C = B\exp(-\beta t) \tag{2.1}$$

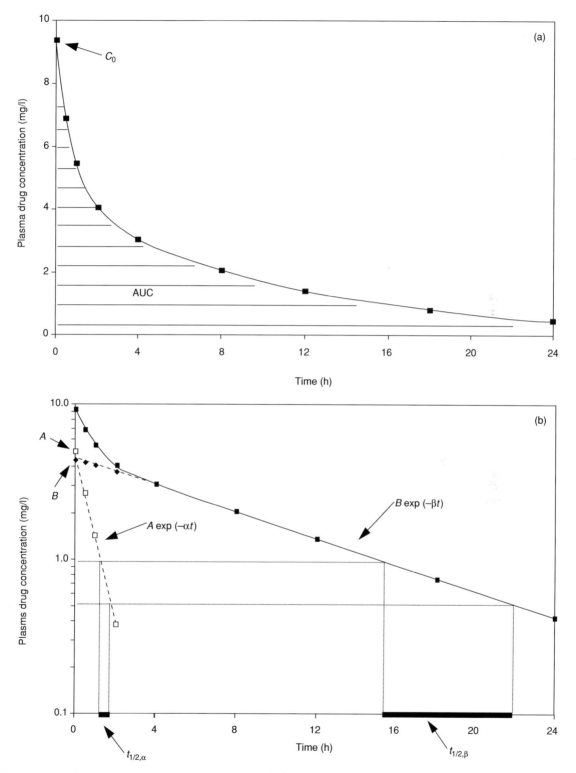

Figure 2.1. (a) Plasma concentration after an intravenous bolus injection: AUC, area under curve; C_0, concentration at time zero. (b) The data in (a) replotted with a logarithmic y-axis. The data (solid squares) are described by a bi-exponential equation: $C = A\exp(-\alpha t) + B\exp(-\beta t)$; $t_{1/2,\alpha}$ is the distribution half-life and $t_{1/2,\alpha}$ is the elimination half-life.

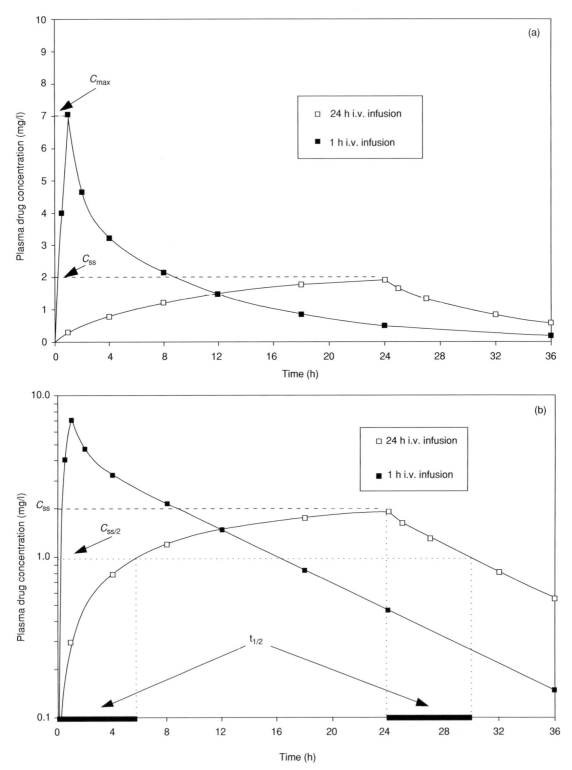

Figure 2.2. (a) Plasma concentration after intravenous infusion: C_{max}, maximum concentration; C_{ss}, concentration at steady state. (b) The data in (a) replotted with a logarithmic *y*-axis: After one half-life ($t_{1/2}$), the concentration has reached 50% of the plateau value corresponding to the 24 h infusion C_{ss}.

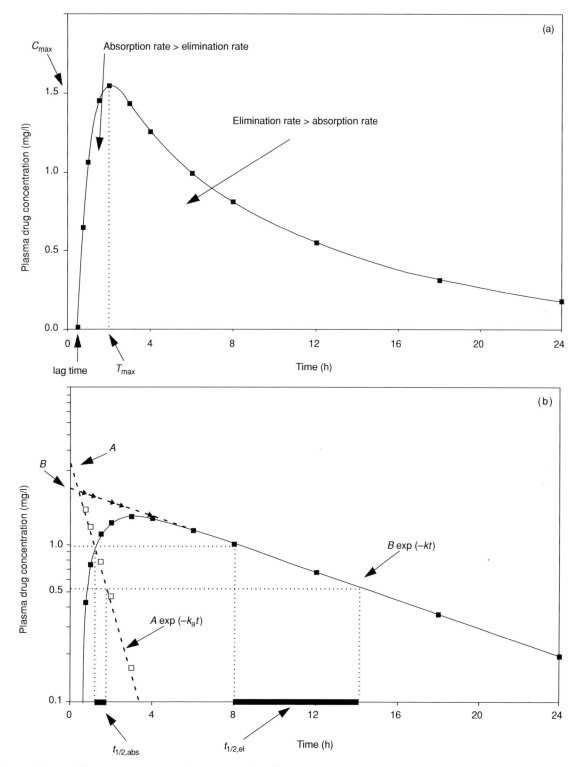

Figure 2.3. (a) Plasma concentration after extravascular administration: C_{max}, maximum concentration; T_{max}, time to peak concentration; lag time, time between extravascular administration and the apparent onset of absorption. (b) data shown in (a) replotted with a logarithmic y-axis. The data (solid squares) are described by the equation $C = B\exp(-kt) - A\exp(-k_a t)$; $t_{1/2,abs}$ and k_a, half-life and rate constant of absorption; $t_{1/2,el}$ and k, half-life and rate constant of elimination.

where β is the terminal disposition rate constant of the drug, corresponding graphically to the slope of the linear decay in Figure 2.1(b). The terminal half-life $(t_{1/2,\beta} = \ln2/\beta)$ is the time taken for the plasma concentration, as well as the amount of the drug in the body, to fall by one-half. A half-life corresponding to the distribution process $(t_{1/2,\alpha})$ can be determined as the time taken for the 'residual' concentration to fall by one-half, where the residual concentration at time t is the difference between the observed concentration and the theorical concentration corresponding to $B\exp(-\beta t)$. For some drugs, no initial phase of distribution is observed in the plasma concentration–time profile, i.e. the drug is immediately distributed in a single compartment, and the plasma concentration–time profile is said to be described by a '*single-compartment model*'. Description of the pharmacokinetics of a drug by a single-compartment model does not imply that the drug is homogeneously distributed in the body (which is very rare), but only that the equilibrium between the plasma compartment and the other tissues is 'instantaneous'. Alternatively, the concentration–time profile of a drug may follow a tri-exponential function, indicating that it distributes from the central compartment to two peripheral compartments. The latter compartments differ from one another in the rate at which equilibrium is reached.

The *area under the concentration–time curve (AUC)* represents the total systemic exposure to the drug, as illustrated in Figure 2.1(a). The AUC is an important parameter as it represents, in a single value, drug exposure. However, it should be noted that toxicity and/or activity may be a function of concentration, time or concentration and time (i.e. the AUC).

Figure 2.2 shows the concentration–time curve of a drug administered at the same dose to the same patient by *intravenous infusions* of duration 1 h or 24 h. The *maximum plasma concentrations C_{max}* are lower than those observed after intravenous bolus dosing because both elimination and distribution processes occur during infusion. Consequently, at the end of the infusion, the distribution phase is shortened after the 1 h infusion and is not seen after the 24 h infusion. For this duration of infusion, C_{max} corresponds to the steady-state concentration C_{ss}, the level of which is determined by the ratio of the rates of infusion and elimination. The plasma concentration of drugs that follow mono-exponential kinetics (and those that distribute rapidly relative to elimination) increases during the infusion according to the equation

$$C = C_{ss}[(1 - \exp(-kt)] \qquad (2.2)$$

where k is the elimation rate constant which describes the decline in drug plasma concentration following cessation of the intravenous infusion [(Fig. 2.2(b)]. One half-life $(t_{1/2} = \ln2/k)$ after the beginning of the infusion, the plasma concentration is $C_{ss}/2$, and after 3.3 half-lives the plasma concentration reaches 90% of C_{ss}, when it is usual to consider that steady state has been attained.

After extravascular administration of a drug (Figure 2.3), the concentration–time curve is divided into two phases. Initially, the plasma drug concentration increases because the rate of absorption of the drug from the site of administration (enteric, intramuscular, or subcutaneous depending on the route) is greater than that of elimination. The time of the peak concentration corresponds to the time at which the two rates are equal, after which the rate of elimination exceeds the rate of absorption and the plasma concentration decreases. After *oral administration* of a drug, an additional pharmacokinetic parameter relative to the concentration–time curve may be defined: the lag time. The *lag time* is the delay between the time of ingestion and the appearance of the drug in the plasma; it corresponds to the time taken for the drug to adopt a diffusable form and reach the intestinal site of absorption. Usually, there is no lag time after *intramuscular* or *subcutaneous administration*. As with intravenous infusions, most drugs distribute during the absorption phase so that when C_{max} is reached it is much lower than that after intravenous bolus of the same dose, and the decline in plasma concentration usually follows a mono-exponential function (see later).

Pharmacokinetic parameters

Bioavailability

Bioavailability F is a parameter specific to extravascular administration and is defined as the fraction of the drug dose that reaches the general circulation unchanged. Bioavailability is determined by administering the drug to a patient (or a healthy volunteer) by the intravenous and extravascular routes, and then comparing the AUC obtained after extravascular administration (AUC_{ev}) with that obtained after intravenous administration (AUC_{iv}), taking into account the extravascular and intravenous dosages (D_{ev} and D_{iv}, respectively), according to the equation

$$F = (AUC_{ev}/AUC_{iv})\ (D_{ev}/D_{iv}). \qquad (2.3)$$

Usually, F is close to 100% when a drug is given by *intramuscular or subcutaneous injection* because the metabolism at these sites of injection is limited. However, after *oral ingestion*, F may vary from zero to 100% for different drugs. Factors that can limit the oral bioavailability of a drug include poor solubility of the drug in the gastrointestinal tract contents, poor absorption through the gastrointestinal tract epithelium, and extensive metabolic conversion of the drug within the gut and/or liver. The last of these is known as the *first-pass effect*.

Clearance

Clearance (CL) is defined as the rate of elimination of the drug relative to its plasma concentration C:

$$CL = (\text{rate of elimination})/C. \qquad (2.4)$$

CL is expressed as volume per unit of time. CL does not indicate how much of the drug is being removed but, rather, the (virtual) volume of plasma that would have to be completely free of drug to account for the overall loss of compound.

Calculation of the time-averaged or total plasma CL after a single intravenous administration of a drug is based on the following equation, obtained by integrating eqn (2.4) from time zero to infinity):

$$CL = \text{dose}/AUC \qquad (2.5)$$

After extravascular administration, the dose should be replaced by the bioavailable dose to give the apparent clearance:

$$CL = (F \times \text{dose})/AUC. \qquad (2.6)$$

During continuous intravenous infusion, the steady state is reached when the rate of elimination equals the rate of infusion. By substituting the rate of infusion and C_{ss} for the rate of elimination and C, respectively, in eqn (2.4), CL can be calculated as follows:

$$CL = (\text{rate of infusion})/C_{ss} \qquad (2.7)$$

It should be noted that eqns (2.5)–(2.7) indicate that the plasma exposure of a patient to a drug depends only on the dose (or the bioavailable dose in the case of extravascular administration) and CL.

In order to appreciate how physiopathological factors can influence CL, total CL should be considered as a result of all processes of elimination that may occur in the kidney, liver (by metabolism and/or biliary excretion) and other organs. Total CL is the result of the addition of these separate clearances:

$$CL = CL_{renal} + CL_{hepatic} + CL_{other}. \qquad (2.8)$$

Renal clearance may be the result of three processes: first, glomerular filtration which is dependent on both the glomerular filtration rate (characteristic of the patient, and depending on the blood flow and the number of functional nephrons) and the unbound fraction f_u of the drug in plasma (see below), since protein-bound drug is not filtered; secondly, drugs may be actively secreted across the tubular membranes through carrier-mediated mechanisms; finally, drugs may be passively reabsorbed depending mainly on their hydrophobicity. After a single dose of a drug, calculation of the *renal clearance* requires complete urinary recovery (i.e. collection of urine for at least five plasma elimination half-lives) and measurement of the fraction f_e of the dose collected unchanged in urine:

$$CL_{renal} = f_e CL. \qquad (2.9)$$

Hepatic clearance includes both metabolic and biliary excretory clearance. Since complete recovery of both drug metabolites and drug excreted in bile is not achievable in most clinical situations, $CL_{hepatic}$ cannot be directly measured. However, hepatic clearance cannot exceed $(1 - f_e)CL$, but approaches it when other routes of elimination are not important. Three main factors determine hepatic clearance: hepatic blood flow, the unbound fraction f_u of the drug in plasma and the intrinsic clearance CL_{int}. The term CL_{int} represents the ability of the enzymatic and biliary transport systems of the hepatocytes to clear the drug since the drug is present within the hepatocytes, and the amount of drug available to enter the hepatocytes depends on the first two factors (i.e. hepatic blood flow and f_u).

Volume of distribution

The volume of distribution V of a drug is the volume that would be required to contain all the drug present in the body at the same concentration as in the plasma:

$$V = (\text{amount of drug in body})/C \qquad (2.10)$$

where C is the plasma concentration. V rarely corresponds to a physiological compartment, but nevertheless reflects the extent of distribution. Indeed, the concept of volume of distribution considers the body as a single homogeneous compartment that is rarely respected. V (only) indicates the fraction of drug in the body in plasma:

fraction of drug in the body in plasma $= V_{plasma}/V$ (2.11)

where V_{plasma} is the plasma volume. The plasma volume is about 5 litres in adults and the volume of total body water is approximately 40 litres. Many drugs exhibit volumes of distribution far in excess of this latter value, which does not mean that the drug distributes within the *total body water*, but that it is present in (at least) one particular tissue at a much higher concentration than in plasma. Some drugs distribute homogeneously within a physiological volume, and in such cases V approaches the value of this physiological volume. For example, V for aminoglycosides that do not distribute within the intracellular compartment has a value not far in excess of 12 litres which correspond to the extra-cellular fluid volume. The volume of distribution of a drug is largely dependent on its partition coefficient (oil/water) and the unbound fraction f_u in plasma. However, complexity arises from the fact that f_u and the partition coefficient are not independent parameters. For example, a drug may have a small volume of distribution because it is hydrophilic and hence unable to diffuse into tissues, or because it is very hydrophobic and tightly bound to plasma proteins.

After bolus intravenous administration, the initial volume of distribution is given by

$$V_{\text{initial}} = \text{dose}/C_0 \tag{2.12}$$

where C_0 corresponds to the initial concentration which is usually derived by back-extrapolation. Most of the drug subsequently distributes into a larger volume that increases with time until the end of the distribution phase(s) [Figure 2.1(b)]. The volume of distribution during the elimination (or final) phase when the distribution is completed (V_{area}) is given by

$$V_{\text{area}} = \text{dose}/(\beta \times \text{AUC}) \tag{2.13}$$

where β is the terminal disposition rate constant of the drug. Equation (2.13) can also be used to calculate the volume of distribution after extravascular administration, but the dose must be corrected for bioavailability.

By substituting CL for dose/AUC in eqn (2.13), the *terminal half-life* can be expressed as a function of both CL and V_{area}:

$$t_{1/2,\beta} = \ln2/\beta = (\ln2)V_{\text{area}}/\text{CL}. \tag{2.14}$$

The relationship in eqn (2.14) is useful because it shows that β, the terminal rate of decline of the plasma concentration (and of the amount of drug in the body), depends not only on the body's ability to eliminate the drug but also on the extent of the drug's distribution. The greater the volume of distribution, the slower is the decline of plasma concentration. Indeed, organs of elimination can only clear drugs from the plasma with which they are in direct contact.

It should be noted that V_{area} and V_{initial} have the same value for drugs whose distribution is described by a single-compartment model. The terminal rate of decline of the plasma concentration (β) and the corresponding half-life ($t_{1/2,\beta}$) now become the unique rate of decline (k), also called the *elimination rate constant*, and the unique half-life ($t_{1/2}$), respectively.

Pharmacokinetic parameters and multi-dose regimens

Repeated administrations of a dose at time intervals τ (dosage interval) can be considered as equivalent to a continuous intravenous infusion at a rate $F(\text{dose})/\tau$, on average. Then the average plasma concentration C_{av} increases up to a steady-state concentration $C_{\text{av,ss}}$ that is reached when the mean rate of elimination within the dosing interval approximates the rate of administration ($F \times \text{dose})/\tau$. As for continuous intravenous infusion, $C_{\text{ss,av}}$ depends on CL (and F in the case of extravascular administration) but not on the volume of distribution:

$$C_{\text{av,ss}} = (F \times \text{dose})/(\text{CL} \times \tau) \tag{2.15}$$

However, the time necessary to reach the steady-state depends on $t_{1/2}$ of the drug, and hence on both clearance and volume of distribution [see eqn (2.14)], and the dosage interval:

$$n = 3.3(t_{1/2}/\tau) \tag{2.16}$$

where n is the number of doses (rounded to the superior whole number) necessary to obtain a C_{av} that is >90% of $C_{\text{av,ss}}$.

Unlike continuous intravenous infusion, intermittent drug administration produces fluctuations of plasma concentration around the C_{av} (Figure 2.4). The fluctuation between C_{max} and C_{min} depends on both the dosing interval τ and the half-life $t_{1/2} = \ln2/k$ of the drug. If the drug is given by intravenous bolus (or if the absorption process is extremely rapid relative to elimination), the fluctuation can defined as follows

$$C_{\text{max}}/C_{\text{min}} = 1/\exp(-kt). \tag{2.17}$$

If the drug distributes slowly from an initial volume of distribution to a larger volume, the fluctuation of plasma concentrations will be higher (and will exceed the fluctuation of tissue concentrations). However, after extravascular administration, slow absorption of the drug often blunts the fluctuations.

In all cases, the ratio of plasma concentration (or amount of drug in the body) when steady state is

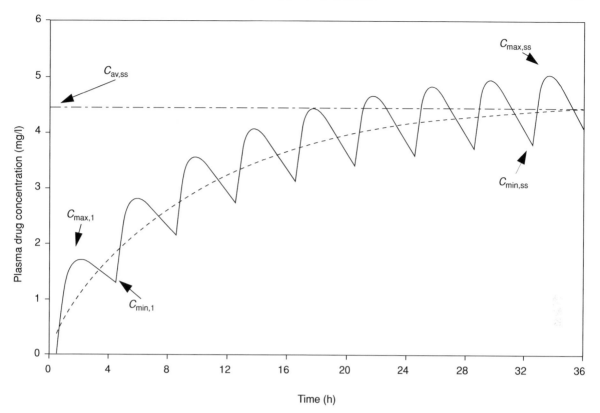

Figure 2.4. Plasma concentration after repeated administration (every 4 h): $C_{max,1}$ and $C_{max,ss}$, maximum concentration after the first administration and at steady state; $C_{min,1}$ and $C_{min,ss}$, minimum concentration after the first administration and at steady state; $C_{av,ss}$, average concentration over the dosing interval at plateau.

reached to that after the first dosage is given by the accumulation index R_{ac}:

$$R_{ac} = C_{av,1}/C_{av,ss} = C_{max,1}/C_{max,ss} = C_{min,1}/C_{min,ss}$$
$$= 1/[1 - \exp(-k\tau)]. \qquad (2.18)$$

Alternative data for pharmacokinetic analysis

In some circumstances total plasma parent drug concentrations do not allow calculation of the pertinent pharmacokinetic parameters. Three main alternatives will be briefly discussed below.

Blood concentration

If a drug is concentrated in erythrocytes and has an extremely low concentration in plasma, the pharmacokinetic parameters obtained from plasma concentration–time data (as described above) will be limited

significance. The recommendation for these drugs is to measure the drug in blood in order to determine blood pharmacokinetic parameters (e.g. blood clearance and blood volume of distribution).

Unbound plasma drug concentration

Many drugs are bound reversibly to plasma proteins, mostly to plasma albumin for acidic drugs and to α_1-acid glycoprotein for basic drugs. Since only the unbound drug is in equilibrium with peripheral tissues, binding of a drug to plasma proteins can limit concentrations in tissues such that the unbound drug plasma concentration is often more closely related to the pharmacological activity. For drugs with low unbound fraction f_u (e.g. <0.1) and for which plasma protein binding exhibits a large variability within and among patients, it may be useful to measure the unbound plasma concentration and then calculate the corresponding clearance CL_u and volume of distribution V_u. However, drugs which bind to plasma proteins usually also bind to tissue macromolecules, and there is often rapid re-equilibration between free and bound plasma and tissue levels. In such cases, total plasma drug concentrations are a suitable measure of drug exposure.

Metabolite plasma concentration

Some metabolites have pharmacological properties and in these cases determination of metabolite pharmacokinetic parameters based on plasma metabolite concentration may be as important as determining the parameters of the parent drug. Specific example will be given in the relevant chapters.

Pharmacokinetic analysis of plasma concentration–time data

Importance of the sampling scheme

In general terms a pharmacokinetic analysis consists of 'drawing' the most probable continuous curve (as shown in Figs 2.1–2.3) from discontinuous data (e.g. plasma concentration at time points corresponding to each blood samples). However, some pharmacokinetic processes may be overlooked when sampling is too sparse. An obvious example is illustrated in Figure 2.1 where, if the first blood sample had not been taken until 4 h post bolus injection, the distribution phase would not have been detected and the plasma AUC would have been underestimated. After extravascular injection, the maximum observed plasma concentration and the corresponding peak time are strongly dependent on the sampling protocol: the more sparse it is, the larger the difference between the observed and actual maximum concentrations is likely to be.

Non-compartmental analysis

This method does not require the fitting of an equation to the observed plasma concentration–time data. Assessment of the AUC is performed by the trapezoidal rule, assuming a linear relationship between observations. The log-trapezoidal rule, in which decline in concentration between each pair of observation is assumed to be exponential, may be a more accurate alternative. Whichever method is used (trapezoidal or log-trapezoidal), estimation of AUC requires an intensive sampling protocol (usually 12–20 samples are obtained within the administration period and for 24–48 h thereafter). Calculation of the total AUC (e.g. from zero time to infinity) consists of adding the AUC from the time t_{last} at which the last measurable concentration C_{last} is obtained to infinity. The latter partial AUC requires estimation of the slope β of the terminal exponential phase of the plot of the logarithm of concentration versus time:

$$AUC - t_{last \to \infty} = C_{last}/\beta. \qquad (2.19)$$

The calculation of β is based on non-linear least-squares regression analysis, assuming that the terminal portion of the concentration–time curve is log-linear; the number of data points considered as part of this terminal phase can be automatically or interactively selected. In order to limit the contribution of this extrapolated AUC to the total AUC (e.g. < 10% is considered acceptable), the sampling protocol must be extended for at least three times the expected terminal half-life.

Compartmental analysis

Compartmental approaches require the specification of a pharmacokinetic model which is assumed to describe the distribution of the drug. Figure 2.5 shows a two-compartment model which is often sufficient to describe drug plasma concentration–time profiles after intravenous administration.

The two-compartment model is appropriate when the concentration–time data are properly fitted by the sum of two exponential terms [see Fig. 2.1(b)]:

$$C = A\exp(-\alpha t) + B\exp(-\beta t). \qquad (2.20)$$

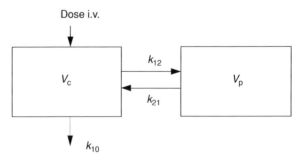

Figure 2.5. Schematic representation of the body as a two-compartment open model: V_c, central volume (containing the physiological plasma compartment where the drug was directly administered and drug concentrations were determined); V_p, peripheral volume; k_{12} and k_{21}, transfer rate constants. Drug elimination is restricted to the central compartment and has rate constant k_{10}. All constants are in units of reciprocal time.

The values of A, B, α and β are those that minimize the weighted sum-of-squares deviations of the calculated from the observed concentrations, and are obtained by computer-based iterative calculation; the choice of the algorithm and the weighting schemes is part of the model. Relationships exist between the exponential coefficients (e.g. α and β) allocated to the bi-exponential function and the rate constants of the compartment model. The term $A + B$ represents the initial concentration C_0 and hence dose/V_c. Integration of the eqn (2.20) from zero to infinity gives

$$\text{AUC} = A/\alpha + B/\beta. \qquad (2.21)$$

The value of CL obtained by dividing the administered intravenous dose by the AUC calculated as described above should be considered as a model-dependent parameter, in contrast with that obtained using the trapezoidal rule. Given adequate sampling times and the correct model the two values of AUC, and hence CL, will be similar.

The compartmental approach allows calculation of an additional volume parameter, the *volume of distribution at steady state (V_{ss})*:

$$V_{ss} = V_c(1 + k_{12}/k_{21}). \qquad (2.22)$$

The value of V_{ss} lies between the values of the initial dilution volume V_c and the volume of distribution V_{area}. V_{ss} is equal to $V_c + V_p$ and represents the volume in which a drug would appear to be distributed at steady state if the drug was present throughout that volume at the same concentration as in the plasma.

The *half-life $t_{1/2,\alpha}$* (where $t_{1/2,\alpha} = \ln2/\alpha$) corresponds to the distribution of the drug from the initial volume (i.e. the central volume V_c) into its 'final' volume (i.e. V_{ss}). The half-life $t_{1/2,\beta}$ (where $t_{1/2,\beta} = \ln2/\beta$) corresponds to the elimation process.

Pharmacokinetic models with more than two compartments may be required to fit the concentration–time data for some drugs. However, a model with too many compartments, and hence too many rate constants (e.g. k_{12}, k_{21}, k_{31}, k_{13}, and k_{10} in the case of a three-compartment model) relative to the amount of data available (e.g. plasma samples obtained during the initial phase of distribution) is adopted, the pharmacokinetic parameters may be unreliable. In such cases, large disparities in pharmacokinetic parameters among studied patients are the consequence not of a real interindividual variability in pharmacokinetic processes, but of overparametrization. The adequacy of models can be evaluated using a variety of criteria, including Akaike's information criteria, or by the magnitude of the standard errors of the estimated pharmacokinetic parameters.

Because of overparametrization, the two-compartment open model with first-order absorption often has parameter identification problems when it is used to fit concentration–time data after extravascular administration. Hence a single-compartment model is generally used (Fig. 2.6).

The *single-compartment model* is retained after extravascular administration when the concentration–time data are properly described by the difference between two exponentional terms:

$$C = \frac{(F \times \text{dose})k_a}{V(k_a - k)} \{\exp[-k(t - t_{lag})] - \exp[-k_a(t - t_{lag})]\} \quad (2.23)$$

where t_{lag} is the lag time for absorption and k and k_a are the rates of elimination and absorption, respectively. The concentration–time function is often expressed by the following equation, which is equivalent to eqn (2.23):

$$C = B\exp(-kt) - A\exp(-k_a t). \qquad (2.24)$$

B, A, k and k_a, and the corresponding half-lives ($t_{1/2,el} = \ln2/k$ for elimination, and $t_{1/2,abs} = \ln2/k_a$ for absorption), can be determined graphically (see Figure 2.3B)

Occasionally, the absorption half-life is much longer than the elimination half-life, such that the half-life of the decline of concentration corresponds to the

$F \times \text{dose}$

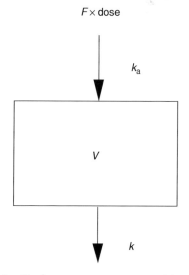

Figure 2.6. Single-compartment open model with extravascular administration: k_a and k, transfer rate constants corresponding to the first-order absorption and elimination processes, respectively; V, volume of distribution; $F \times \text{dose}$, bioavailable dose.

absorption half-life. This phenomenon is usually observed with controlled-release oral preparations.

Population approaches to pharmacokinetic analyses

The methods described above involve analysing the data from each patient individually. In some circumstances, it may be useful (or even necessary) to analyse the data from a patient either by taking into account the pharmacokinetics of the drug previously observed in persons like the patient (Bayesian analysis) or by simultaneously using the data from a whole-patient population.

Bayesian analysis

Individual analysis requires a large number of blood samples, especially as the pharmacokinetic model becomes more complicated (e.g. more than one compartment, extravascular administration). Sampling can be limited if missing individual information is compensated by using information about the drug accumulated within a patient population resembling the individual patient. This population information comprises the mean values of the pharmacokinetic parameters, their inter-individual variability (e.g. variance), and their covariance matrix. Analytical variability is also taken into account. The principle of the maximum *a posteriori* probability (MAP) Bayesian approach is used to balance the sparse concentration–time data of the individual patient against the information obtained previously from the population. Instead of minimizing only the weighted sum-of-squares deviations of the calculated from the observed concentrations, as in the case of individual patient analysis, the values derived for the pharmacokinetic parameters (the most likely values P_{pt}) are those that minimize the overall value of the MAP Bayesian objective function given by the expression

$$\sum_{i=1}^{n} \frac{(P_{pop} - P_{pt})^2}{SD^2 P_{pop}} + \sum_{i=1}^{m} \frac{(C_{obs} - C_{est})^2}{SD^2 C_{obs}} \qquad (2.25)$$

where P_{pop} (and $SD^2 P_{pop}$) are the mean values (and the squares of their standard deviations) of the population pharmacokinetic parameters (total number, n), C_{obs} and C_{est} are respectively the observed plasma concentrations (total number, m) and the estimates of these concentrations corresponding to the values of pharmacokinetic parameters (P_{pt}), and $SD^2 C_{obs}$ is the square of the standard deviation of each of the observed concentrations.

3.4.2 Population pharmacokinetic approach

The conventional method of testing the relationship between patient features and pharmacokinetics is the 'two-stage' approach. The first stage is the estimation of pharmacokinetic parameters through analysis of individual data. In the second stage, the descriptive summary statistics of the sample are calculated; typically, the mean and variance of each pharmacokinetic parameter are defined. Subsequently, classical statistical tests are used to analyse dependencies between pharmacokinetic parameters and covariates; for example, a multivariate regression analysis of relationships between pharmacokinetic parameters and patient covariates, or a Student *t*-test to compare pharmacokinetic parameters arising from two groups of patients differing by one characteristic.

The 'two stage' approach is still largely used during the clinical drug development; however, since it requires a large number of samples per individual, it is performed with small groups of volunteers or patients. Moreover, relatively homogeneous groups are needed in order to investigate the effect of a particular feature on drug pharmacokinetics. As a result, the groups studied are generally poorly representative of the target population for the drug.

In contrast, the population pharmacokinetic approach allows the population, rather than the individual, to be treated as the unit of analysis. This approach requires fewer data points per individual, but many more individuals. Importantly, data can be collected from patients receiving the drug in phase III trials and in the post-marketing period. The most commonly used computer program is NONMEM (NONMEM Project Group, University of California, San Francisco, CA), which stands for Non-linear Mixed Effects Model. By simultaneous analysis of concentration–time data from many individuals using to a relevant pharmacokinetic model, NONMEM allows determination of mean pharmacokinetic parameters and their inter-individual variability, and the magnitude of the residual variability which is composed mainly of the measurement errors. Moreover, quantitative relationships between pharmacokinetic parameters and physiopathological features (demographic, pathophysiological status, biochemical indices, concomitant drug therapy, etc) can be investigated in a single step. A Bayesian estimation of the pharmacokinetic parameters of each patient in the population can also be performed with NONMEM. A non-parametric maximum likelihood (NPML) approach has also been proposed as a method for analysing population pharmacokinetic data. This makes less stringent assumptions about parameter distributions than NONMEM, which assumes a normal or log-normal distribution of pharmacokinetic parameters.

Non-linear pharmacokinetics

So far in this chapter linearity of pharmacokinetics has been assumed. Indeed, in the majority of cases, drug transfer between compartments follows a first-order process. The amount of drug transferred per unit of time from a compartment is proportional of the amount A of drug within the compartment:

$$dA/dt = kA \tag{2.26}$$

where the proportionality constant k is known as the (first-order) rate constant. It corresponds to the terms previously considered, i.e. k_a, k, k_{12} and k_{21} for absorption, elimination and distribution processes, respectively. Indeed, eqn (2.4), which defines the concept of clearance, is derived from eqn (2.26). For a drug that follows first-order processes, pharmacokinetic parameters such as CL, volume of distribution and half-life do not vary with concentration, and as a consequence plasma concentrations or AUC increase linearly with the dose. Conversely, if the AUC (or C_{max}) versus dose relationship, as derived from pharmacokinetic data obtained from a phase I trial, shows a non-linear relationship, the drug is referred to as having *dose-dependent pharmacokinetics*.

Non-linearity is usually due to saturation of protein binding, hepatic metabolism or active renal transport of the drug.

Saturable protein binding occurs because there are a limited number of binding sites on plasma proteins. It causes V to increase because only the plasma unbound fraction is able to diffuse out of the plasma compartment. If the drug is metabolized by the liver, reduction in f_u will also cause hepatic clearance to increase unless intrinsic clearance (reflecting the metabolism activity) is already so high that dissociation of drug bound to plasma proteins is not a limiting factor. Metabolism of drugs is dependent on enzymatic reactions that are saturable processes described by the Michaelis–Menten equation:

$$\text{rate of metabolism} = V_{max}C/(K_m + C) \tag{2.27}$$

where C is the plasma concentration, V_{max} is the maximum rate of metabolism, and K_m is the Michaelis constant (i.e. the plasma concentration at which half the maximum rate of metabolism is reached). For a majority of drugs, therapeutic plasma concentrations are much lower than K_m ($C \ll K_m$) and hence their pharmacokinetics will appear to be linear with CL (= V_{max}/K_m), which is a constant independent of C and hence of administered dose. Alternatively, if the therapeutic plasma concentrations are of same order as K_m, non-linear kinetics are observed with CL decreasing with increasing plasma concentrations and administered dose.

Non-linearity may also result from a saturation of active renal transport. In this case, calculation of renal clearance (CL_{renal}) according to eqn (2.9), which requires determination of the cumulative amount of drug collected unchanged in urine, is not relevant because it will only indicate the 'mean value' of CL_{renal}. More 'instantaneous' values of CL_{renal} can be calculated from the amount of drug excreted unchanged within a given urine collection interval ($A_{e,t\to t+\Delta t}$) and the partial plasma AUC corresponding to the same interval ($AUC_{t\to t+\Delta t}$):

$$CL_{renal} = A_{e,t\to t+\Delta t}/AUC_{t\to t+\Delta t}. \tag{2.28}$$

The term 'non-linear pharmacokinetics' is also used when parameters such as CL, F, or V vary with time. *Time-dependent pharmacokinetics* is often due to modification of metabolism with time as a result of autoinduction or autoinhibition processes. For example, *autoinduction* (i.e. when a drug increases the synthesis of the enzymes responsible for its own metabolism) leads to a decrease of CL with time. In such a case, a pharmacodynamic effect (i.e. autoinduction) modifies the drug's pharmacokinetics. The opposite relationship is more usual: pharmacokinetic variability influences the intensity of the pharmacodynamic effects (see Chapter 4).

Bibliography

Benet LZ, Kroetz DL, Sheiner LB (2001) Pharmacokinetics. In Hardman JG, Limbird LE, Gilman AG (eds) *Goodman & Gilman's The Pharmacological Basis of Therapeutics* (9th edn). New York: McGraw-Hill, Chapter 1.

Gibaldi M, Perrier D (1982) *Pharmacokinetics* (2nd edn) New York: Marcel Dekker.

Rowland M, Tozer TN (1989) *Clinical Pharmacokinetics: Concept and Applications* (2nd edn). Philadelphia, PA: Lea & Febiger.

Sheiner LB, Beal S, Rosenberg B, Marathe VV (1979) Forecasting individual pharmacokinetics. *Clin Pharmacol Ther*, **26**, 294–305.

Whiting B, Kelman AW, Grevel J (1986) Population pharmacokinetics: theory and clinical application. *Clin Pharmacokinet*, **11**, 387–401.

3 | *Clinical implications and mechanisms of variability in the response to anticancer agents*

Jan H. M. Schellens

Introduction

Chemotherapeutic agents in general have a narrow therapeutic index, and as a result the exposure resulting in the required therapeutic effect (tumour cell kill) and that inducing significant side effects is relatively close. Exposure to anticancer agents is traditionally measured by the area under the plasma concentration–time curve (AUC). It is common practice in oncology to apply standard dosage regimens of anticancer drugs. However, this approach results in wide inter-patient variation in exposure (AUC), owing to variable absorption and elimination processes, and therefore the dose–exposure relationship is highly variable due to pharmacokinetic variation between patients. Pharmacokinetic variation is mainly caused by inter-patient differences in absorption after oral administration, renal elimination, and metabolic transformation. In addition, there are significant differences between patients in the relationship between the exposure to the drug and the biological effects (likelihood of tumour response, and pattern and severity of toxicity); this phenomenon is termed pharmacodynamic variability. At the level of the tumour response, variation may be the result of biological differences in the sensitivity of the tumour to the drug owing to diverse mechanisms of resistance, or pharmacological factors such as tissue perfusion in bulky tumours. With regard to side effects, variation may be the result of the intrinsic sensitivity of end-organs to the cytotoxic agent(s).

Pharmacokinetic and dynamic variability have major clinical consequences, and several methods have been developed to adapt doses to the individual and to iden-

tify patients at risk for over- and underdosing, or for severe toxicity, using clinical tests for end-organ function. For example, carboplatin is almost exclusively excreted by the kidneys and exposure is highly correlated with the dose-limiting thrombocytopenia. This understanding has resulted in the development of *dosing* algorithms minimizing inter-patient variation in exposure.[1–3] For other agents such as *6-mercaptopurine and azathioprine*, where there is genetically determined inter-patient variation in the formation of the active metabolite 6TGN, adaptive dosing using the white blood cell counts is feasible. Also, for more recently developed drugs, such as *topotecan*, there is a significant correlation between the exposure and the dose-limiting toxicity, i.e. leukocytopenia and granulocytopenia (Fig. 3.1). Variability in the exposure is particularly large when the drug is administered orally.[4] The coefficient of variation of the AUC after oral administration is approximately 50% higher than after intravenous administration. Despite this, simple clinical dosing algorithms can be applied, which limit the risk for over- and under dosing.

Application of pharmacological tools in the process of drug development is considered essential in order to be able to characterize concentration–response instead of dose–response relationships. Also, assessment of the pharmacokinetics of the drug(s) under investigation may enable a more optimal design and execution of phase I–III studies. In addition, in the case of drugs designed to interfere with well-defined molecular targets in cancer cells, it is important to develop clinical methods to measure the interaction between the drug and its molecular target.

Variability in pharmacokinetics

Compliance

An increasing number of anticancer agents are administered orally. This is a beneficial development because it

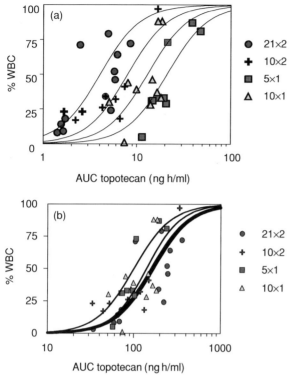

Figure 3.1. Relationship between the exposure (AUC) to topotecan and dose-limiting leukocytopenia (% WBC) when applied at different treatment schedules of 5, 10 and 21 days of continuous intake (modified from Kruijtzer *et al.*[26]). Topotecan was taken once daily (in the daily times 5 and 10 schedules, or twice daily in the daily times 10 and 21 schedules). (a) Relationship between AUC on day 1 of course 1 versus leukocytopenia, which shows clear differences between the four schedules. (b) Relationship between the AUC per treatment course of the same schedules as in (a) versus leukocytopenia, which reveals that the curves are almost completely overlapping (data from the first course were also used).

is more convenient and practical than parenteral administration. In addition, it enables development of chronic treatment schedules, which may be more effective for drugs where the biological effect largely depends on the time period of exposure. This is particularly the case for drugs that have a cell-cycle-specific cytotoxic effect and for agents that interfere with signal transduction pathways.

When drugs must be taken orally every day differences in exposure between patients may occur due to differences in compliance. Previous studies with non-anticancer agents, such as antihypertensives, have revealed that compliance is a major source of variability in the response. This factor is even more important in oncology because of the side effects associated with cytotoxic agents. In addition, compliance is known to be lower when drugs are to be taken frequently, for example more than twice daily. Careful instruction of patients and repeated motivation and monitoring of safety is important to optimize compliance.

Absorption

Constant and adequate systemic exposure to orally or rectally administered anticancer drugs is hampered by several factors, which are important to consider when drugs are given by these routes. The oral route is most often used for obvious reasons. Rectal administration is limited to drugs that are used to prevent or treat side effects of anticancer therapy or symptoms of the disease process itself, in particular nausea, vomiting, and pain. Also, the rectal route can be used for sedation and acute anticonvulsant therapy when the oral route is not appropriate.

A number of anticancer drugs cannot be applied orally because of instability in the acidic environment of the stomach, difficulties in pharmaceutical formulation resulting in inappropriate dissolution characteristics, or unacceptable toxicity upon oral administration. Such drugs include cisplatin, carboplatin, and doxorubicin. The oral absorption of *etoposide* is non-linear (Fig. 3.2), although the mechanism has not yet been fully identified.[5]

The gastrointestinal (GI) tract also has natural defence mechanisms which can result in very low bioavailability upon oral administration. For example, *5-fluorouracil (5FU)* is rapidly and extensively degradated presystemically by the catabolic enzyme dihydropyrimidine-dehydrogenase (DPD), which is expressed at high levels in the GI tract and liver.[6] Recently, 5FU prodrugs, such as capecitabine, UFT, and S1, have become available for oral administration. *Capecitabine*, which is activated by a cascade of three enzymes, is a prodrug of 5FU. It has a good bioavailability, limited oral toxicity and efficient conversion to 5FU in tumour tissue. The drug has recently been approved for clinical use in colorectal cancer. *UFT* is composed of *1-(2-tetrahydrofuryl)-fluorouracil (Ftorafur* or Tegafur) and *uracil* in a molar ratio of 1:4. Ftorafur is converted to 5FU *in vivo* in the liver, thereby behaving as a prodrug. *Uracil* inhibits the degradation of 5FU. Both drugs are well absorbed after oral administration. UFT is currently being investigated in trials in combination with leucovorin (LV) in advanced gastric cancer and other malignancies. Preliminary clinical data reveal good safety after oral administration.

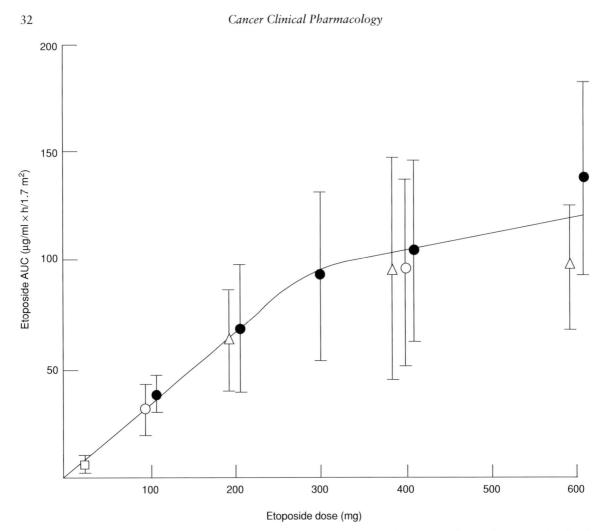

Figure 3.2. Non-linear oral absorption of etoposide. Data were obtained from four independent studies. Reproduced with permission[5].

S1 is a combination of 3 drugs: Ftorafur, 5-chloro-2,4-dihydroxypyrimidine (CDHP) and potassium oxonate (Oxo) in a molar ratio of 1:0.4:1. CDHP inhibits the degradation of 5FU and is about 200 times more active than uracil. Oxo inhibits 5FU phosphorylation by inhibition of the enzyme pyrimidine phosphorybosyl transferase. After oral administration S1 has the potential to reduce the 5FU-induced GI side effects. Overall, oral S1 administration is well tolerated, but it can result in pronounced diarrhoea and myelosuppression, which necessitates careful monitoring of the patient. These symptoms appear to be dose dependent.

Other recent approaches to the oral administration of 5FU include combining it with a DPD inhibitor. Another natural defence mechanism, which operates in the gut, is the expression of the drug efflux protein P-glycoprotein (P-gp).[7] P-gp is a membrane-bound ATP-dependent protein, which has a high affinity for a large number of natural products. Presumably P-gp has an important physiological function in protecting the body against exposure to toxic food constituents. Several currently used anticancer agents, including the taxanes, anthracyclines, vinca alkaloids, and epipodophyllotoxines, are natural products which have moderate to high affinity for P-gp. However, other drugs, such as the topoisomerase I (topo I) inhibitor topotecan which is a synthetic derivative of the natural product camptothecin originating from the Chinese tree *Camptotheca accuminata*, have a relatively low affinity for P-gp.

The prototypic taxane paclitaxel has a high affinity for P-gp and an associated very low oral bioavailability of <5%. In a novel approach, oral paclitaxel was com-

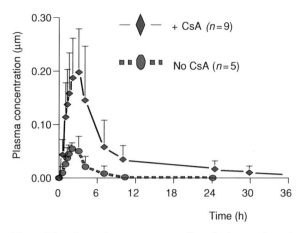

Figure 3.3. Systemic exposure to paclitaxel when paclitaxel was administered orally without and in combination with a single oral dose of the P-gp blocker cyclosporin A (CsA). Reproduced with permission from Meerum Terwogt *et al.* (1998) *Lancet*, **352**, 285.

bined with *cyclosporin A*, which blocks P-gp, and this resulted in a substantially increased apparent bioavailability of approximately 42% (Fig. 3.3). The safety of the oral route was acceptable.[8] If this approach is successful, combined treatment with a P-gp blocker may be useful for other anticancer drugs or drugs from different therapeutic areas. Other candidate drugs which could be combined with a P-gp blocker are docetaxel and etoposide.

There are several other candidate drug efflux pumps which have recently been cloned, such as the multidrug resistance proteins (MRPs) 1–7. However, an assessment of their tissue expression and characterization of their physiological function is needed. For oral pharmacokinetics and uptake of drugs from the GI tract, epithelial apical expression of the ABC transporters

P-gp, ABCG2 (BCRP) and MRP2 is most important (Fig. 3.4).

The coefficient of variation of systemic exposure after oral administration is on average 50–200% higher than after intravenous administration. This level of variation may necessitate careful monitoring of orally administered drugs in order to achieve a maximum likelihood of response combined with acceptable and manageable toxicity. An example is oral *topotecan*.[9] Numerous preclinical studies illustrate that the exposure and in particular the time period of the exposure can be a major determinant of anticancer activity. The oral bioavailability of topotecan is approximately 35% with a range of 20–45%.[4] The coefficient of variation of systemic exposure in patients after intravenous administration of a standard dosage regimen is approximately 30%, but after oral administration it is as high as 50%. This may result in over- or underdosing, and consequently increased myelosuppression or reduced activity. A simple algorithm for oral dosing is proposed as follows. Start oral topotecan at the recommended daily times 5 schedule and a dose of 2.3 mg/m². If there is no or almost no leukocytopenia after the first course, increase the dose for the second course by 25%. Make further increases to subsequent courses, if the second course proceeds uneventfully. If there is unacceptable myelosuppression, reduce the dose by 25%.

Presystemic drug metabolism can result in low systemic exposure and/or the formation of toxic metabolites, which make oral dosing unfavourable. An example is the high incidence of neurotoxicity following oral ifosfamide (see Chapter 7).

As indicated above, *rectal* administration is not used for anticancer agents. A number of agents that are used for palliative care, such as metoclopramide, domperidon, ondansetron, morphine, diazepam, temazepam, etc., can be administered rectally. In general, systemic exposure upon rectal administration is more variable than after oral administration and, in contrast to oral administration, the rectal route partially bypasses first-pass elimination. For drugs with very high presystemic elimination the rectal dose should be (much) lower than the oral dose. However, the agents listed above do not fall into this category, and the rectal doses are the same as or higher than the oral doses because of less complete dissolution or absorption. Therefore inadequate pharmacological response may be determined by pharmaceutical factors or by factors related to absorption kinetics.

GI transit time may be a factor contributing to interpatient variation in exposure for orally applied anti-

Selected transport mechanisms in the intestinal epithelium

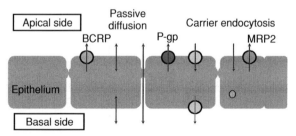

Figure 3.4. Schematic representation of transport mechanisms in the GI tract. Apical side indicates the luminal or epithelial side of the GI tract. BCRP (ABCG2), P-gp, and MRP2 indicate the three main ABC transporters expressed in the epithelial membrane of the GI tract.

cancer agents. For example, methotrexate absorption profiles may be protracted, resulting in prolonged exposure and potentially increased toxicity. Furthermore, there are incidental observations with oral topotecan in patients with a delayed transit time due to large abdominal masses, resulting in increased exposure and myelosuppression.

Distribution

Once a drug becomes systemically available it distributes both centrally and to tissues. The extent and kinetics of tissue distribution vary substantially between drugs and may also depend on the clinical condition of the patient. Tissue distribution depends on the extent of protein binding and accumulation in red blood cells in the blood compartment and the affinity of the drug for tissue binding sites. Overall distribution is reflected in a pharmacokinetic parameter, the volume of distribution V. Depending upon the distribution kinetics, V can be defined in terms of one, two, or more theoretical compartments including the central compartment (V_c) and one or more (deep) tissue compartments (V_p). The kinetics of distribution are important for certain anticancer drugs (see below). In addition, *protein binding* is important because the extent of binding determines the unbound, i.e. pharmacologically active, concentration of the drug in the blood compartment. Protein binding is generally rapidly reversible. However, *cisplatin* binds irreversibly to plasma (and tissue) proteins; the elimination half-life of unbound cisplatin is approximately 40 min, which is largely determined by protein binding.

Protein binding may also be important for drug–drug interactions. Methotrexate can be displaced from its binding to albumin by sulphonamides, tetracycline, chloramphenicol, phenytoin and non-steroidal anti-inflammatory drugs (NSAIDs), thereby increasing its pharmacologically active plasma concentration. This increase may result in myelosuppression and mucositis. However, the most important interaction between these drugs and methotrexate appears to be at the renal level (see below). Overall, inter-patient variation in the extent of protein binding is not very important clinically, except for competition for binding discussed above.

The volume of distribution for methotrexate is also very important clinically. This drug distributes rapidly in 'third-space' volumes, such as ascites and pleural fluid. Slow diffusion from this reservoir back to the plasma (and thereby to other tissues) can result in pronounced life-threatening toxicity.[10]

The kinetics of tissue distribution are also important in the case of drugs where the maximum plasma concentration is a major determinant of its toxicity. For example, the anthracyclines *doxorubicin and daunorubicin* have a very rapid distribution (or alpha) half-life of the order of a few minutes. Following a rapid bolus administration, the plasma concentration has dropped approximately 100-fold after 10–15 min. Slow infusions of doxorubicin result in substantially lower maximum plasma concentrations and are consequently less cardiotoxic. Weekly low-dose doxorubicin (doses of 15–20 mg/week) is also less cardiotoxic, most likely because of the lower plasma concentrations achieved. The acceptable cumulative dose of such a schedule is very much higher than of the traditional 3-weekly schedule. Similarly, the maximum plasma concentration of *cisplatin* is an important determinant of toxicity. Slow infusions over 3–4 h are clearly less acutely toxic than a bolus administration or short duration infusions.

Currently, novel *liposomal* drug formulations that dramatically change the volume of distribution and tissue distribution of anticancer drugs are becoming available for clinical testing. These formulations result in high drug availability at sites of tumour tissue and low availability in normal tissue. This selectivity depends on the greater integrity of the blood vasculature in normal versus tumour tissue. *Doxorubicin* (Doxil® or Caelyx®) is one example, and a Stealth® liposomal formulation has also been used to formulate cisplatin.

Body composition and age may also influence tissue distribution. Although these factors have been investigated for a number of anticancer agents, differences in fat-to-water ratio or age are not routinely taken into account in dosing of anticancer agents, with the exception of the very young. In the newborn and very young children dosing based on the body surface area (BSA) can result in higher exposure compared with adults.[11] However, BSA is superior to body weight for most clinical situations.

Metabolism

Biotransformation takes place mostly through metabolic oxidation (phase I reactions) and conjugation (phase II reactions). Some drugs (prodrugs) must undergo biotransformation, through oxidation or de-esterification, to generate the active metabolite which may then be further metabolized to inactive products. In patients, drug elimination by metabolic transformation is usually characterized by wide inter-patient variation. Total plasma clearance, the main pharmacokinetic parameter, may vary by more than 10-fold between patients after administration of the same dose. This variation is due to wide inter-patient differences in the activity of drug-metabolizing enzyme systems, which are mainly localized in the liver. The cytochrome P450 (CYP) system, consisting of a number of enzyme families, is the most important drug-oxidizing enzyme system. The most important enzyme families for oxidation of anticancer agents are CYP1A, 2B, 2C, 2D and 3A. These enzyme families comprise several isozymes; for example, within the *3A family isozymes* 3A4 and 3A5 are among the most important enzymes involved in drug oxidation. It is estimated that the 3A family metabolizes up to 60% of all xenobiotics, including a number of anticancer drugs such as cyclophosphamide, ifosfamide, the taxanes docetaxel and paclitaxel, the anthracyclines, etc.

Extreme variations in *clearance* may arise when one of the drug-metabolizing enzymes is not expressed. Clearance of affected drugs is then extremely slow [poor metabolizers (PM)] compared with the average clearance in normal metabolizers [extensive metabolizers (EM)]. The best-documented polymorphisms are CYP2D6 (sparteine/debrisoquine) and CYP2C9 (mephenytoin).[12]

The incidences of the 2D6 PM and 2C9 PM phenotypes in Caucasian populations are 7–8% and 2–3%, respectively. However, ethnic differences may be pronounced; for example, the incidence of the 2C9 PM phenotype in Oriental populations is around 20%. The clinical implications for anticancer agents are limited, because the major groups of anticancer drugs are not metabolized by these enzymes.

It is important to recognize the potential for drug–drug interactions at the level of drug metabolism, because some are clinically important (see also below). Co-administration of *doxorubicin and paclitaxel*, both substrates for CYP3A4, results in greater toxicity than expected, owing to the decreased metabolism of doxorubicin. Co-administration of other non-anticancer agents that inhibit CYP3A4 or other enzyme families may seriously affect metabolic oxidation and result in increased toxicity. A well-known interaction occurs between the P-gp inhibitor cyclosporin A, administered in clinical trials to augment tumour tissue exposure to anticancer agents with a high affinity for P-gp, and these anticancer agents at the level of biotransformation. *Cyclosporin A* is an effective inhibitor of CYP3A4 and inhibits the oxidation of doxorubicin and other

agents, resulting in increased toxicity. Cimetidine has a moderate but definite inhibitory effect on P450-mediated metabolism and may induce toxicity when co-administered with a number of anticancer agents. The antiviral agent ritonavir is also a strong inhibitor of 3A4.[13] In addition, it is a strong inhibitor of 2D6 and a moderate inhibitor of 2C19, resulting in clinically important drug–drug interactions. Of interest, *ritonavir* is a potent inducer of P450-related hydroxylation reactions and of glucuronidation, which is important for the metabolism and dosing of methadone and other agents. *Ketoconazole* is another well-known inhibitor of drug metabolism. In addition, induction of drug metabolism may also take place. For example, barbiturates induce the activity of several P450 enzyme families (e.g. CYP3A4 and CYP3A5) which results in increased metabolism of cyclophosphamide and ifosfamide; however, the clinical importance of the induction is not clear.

A number of non-invasive and invasive tests have been developed to characterize drug-metabolizing enzyme activity with a view to individualizing anticancer drug therapy. Although these methods are scientifically of interest, none are used on a routine basis in the clinic. Based on the clinical experience that elevated transaminases and elevated bilirubin are correlated with decreased inactivation of *anthracyclines*, doses are often reduced by 25–75% depending on the severity of the liver dysfunction. Doses can be increased during subsequent courses if the first course was uneventful and/or when the liver function improves. More recently, an elegant population analysis of docetaxel pharmacokinetics and dynamics revealed that liver dysfunction parameters were independent covariates in the relationship with toxicity, which resulted in a simple algorithm for docetaxel dose reduction in patients with liver dysfunction.[14]

Several other enzyme systems are important for inactivation or activation of anticancer agents, such as conjugation by glucuronidation (SN38, anthracyclines, epipodophyllotoxines, etc.), dehydrogenation (5FU), xanthine oxidation (degradation of 6-mercaptopurine and azathioprine), thiopurine methyltransferase (TPMT) (degradation of 6-mercaptopurine and azathioprine), hypoxanthine phosphoribosyltransferase [bioactivation of 6-mercaptopurine and azathioprine resulting in the active compound *6-thioguanine nucleotide (6TGN)*], glutathione conjugation (nitrosoureas, cisplatin, carboplatin, epipodophyllotoxines), and some others. Several of these metabolic pathways are characterized by wide inter-patient variation in activity, resulting in significant differences between patients in exposure to parent drug and/or metabolite(s). For example, variability in SN38 conjugation results in clinically important variability in the development of (severe) diarrhoea.[15] Co-administration of *allopurinol* and oral 6-mercaptupurine or azathioprine can result in pronounced myelosuppression due to a reduced degradation of these anticancer agents.

Some of the enzymatic pathways involved in the metabolism of anticancer drugs are subject to polymorphisms, which are clinically relevant.[16] Polymorphism in TPMT occurs in one in 200–300 patients, and results in significantly reduced catabolism and hence indirectly increased conversion of *6-mercaptopurine* and *azathioprine* to the active metabolite 6TGN. Such patients are at risk for severe myelosuppression. Also, heterozygotes are affected and are characterized by above average 6TGN levels. Currently, in selected clinical centres, genotyping is being used in order to individualize the dose. An alternative clinical approach is to adjust doses on the basis of white blood cell (WBC) cell counts. In view of the highly correlated relationship between the exposure to *6TGN*, doses of 6-mercaptopurine and azathioprine can be safely increased to ensure adequate exposure until a moderate reduction is achieved in WBC counts.

Deficiency in expression of *DPD* also occurs at a low frequency of one to two in 300 patients. Homozygous poor metabolizers and also heterozygotes may suffer from extreme *5FU* toxicity owing to an almost absent or very low rate of degradation of the drug.[6]

Detailed information about the metabolic fate of an anticancer agent is essential for two main reasons: to support bioanalysis and pharmacokinetics, and to identify metabolites with pharmacological anticancer activity or toxicity. *Bioanalysis* determines quantitatively total and unbound levels of the anticancer compound in plasma and drug levels in excreta after parenteral or oral administration of the compound. The data are used to assess the pharmacokinetic profile of the compound. This information is important in investigation of the disposition of the compound and the characteristics of the dose–exposure relationship, to quantify inter- and intra-patient variation in exposure in clearance, and to determine the mass balance of the drug. These data are particularly important when drugs are given orally. Variability in pharmacokinetics after oral administration is generally 50–200% higher than after intravenous administration. This increased variation may be due to variable dissolution, variable absorption because of transport by the membrane transport mech-

anisms in the gut, or variable first-pass metabolism in the gut wall or liver. Regardless of the route of administration, the identification of the metabolic profile is essential to obtain a complete picture of the bioanalytical and pharmacokinetic profile of the anticancer agent. In particular, it is important to identify metabolites with pharmacological activity which may contribute to the anticancer activity and/or the toxicity pattern of the novel compound. Quantitative assessment of metabolic products during drug development can help to explain inter-patient variation in toxicity patterns in early clinical studies (phases I–II) and variability in tumour response during later clinical studies (phases II–III).

Hitherto most anticancer drugs have been taken into clinical trials with only limited prior pharmacokinetic data. Excellent examples of such drugs are *cyclophosphamide and ifosfamide* (both are prodrugs with widely variable bioactivation that generate the severely uro-toxic metabolite acrolein), *mitoxantrone* (approximately 50% of the elimination is still unidentified), and more recently *paclitaxel* (non-linear and complex biotransformation). Mass balance studies of the registered topoisomerase I inhibitors *irinotecan and topotecan* have either not been performed (irinotecan) or have revealed that recovery was far from complete (topotecan[17]). The biotransformation of irinotecan is also complex. A clinically important and highly variable major route of elimination for the active metabolite *SN38* has only been identified during the late phase of clinical development. Similarly, two new routes of metabolic transformation for topotecan have been identified, of which one (N-demethylation) results in the formation of a metabolite with anticancer activity equal to that of the parent drug.[17] The other pathway is O-glucuronidation. The clinical implications of these novel findings have yet to be determined.

Renal elimination

Variability due to inter-patient differences in the rate and extent of renal elimination of a number of anticancer agents has important clinical consequences. A number of drugs (e.g. carboplatin, methotrexate, bleomycin, topotecan, and etoposide) are primarily eliminated by renal excretion. Variability in renal function is often defined in terms of differences in glomerular filtration rate (GFR). The renal clearance and total plasma clearance of drugs that are primarily excreted by glomerular filtration are correlated with the GFR. The best example is carboplatin, which has very limited non-renal clearance, and this kinetic behaviour has resulted in the design of simple dosing algorithms for carboplatin as established by Calvert *et al.*,[1] Egorin *et al.*,[2] and Chatelut *et al.*[3] The Calvert formula, which is used most often, is as follows:

carboplatin dose (mg) = target AUC × (GFR + 25)

The target AUC is most frequently chosen to be around 7 if carboplatin is administered as a single agent in chemonaive patients and around 5 or 6 when given in combination with other potentially bone-marrow-toxic drugs. A drawback is that an invasive [^{51}Cr]EDTA test should be performed for an optimal estimation of the GFR. At present, many clinicians replace the GFR determined by the [^{51}Cr]EDTA method by the *creatinine clearance*, calculated by the Cockroft–Gault method[18] or a similar method, or by a measured clearance using 24-h urine collection. These methods result in a bias of approximately 10% in the estimated GFR, but this appears to be clinically acceptable.[19] An alternative approach is the *Chatelut formula*,[3] which is based on the serum creatinine level at steady state and demographic parameters such as age and gender. Several studies have demonstrated that inter-patient variability in exposure to carboplatin is much less when dosing formulas based on renal function are used, than when the drug is dosed on the basis of BSA. In addition, because of the high correlation between AUC and dose-limiting thrombocytopenia, there is less unpredicted severe thrombocytopenia.

Cisplatin is also excreted by the kidneys, but to a much lower extent than carboplatin. The average fraction of the total dose that is excreted in the urine during the first 24 h is around 30%. Moderate variability in renal function does not affect the exposure to unbound cisplatin to a clinically relevant extent.

Renal function is an important determinant of the pharmacokinetics of *methotrexate* which is eliminated by glomerular filtration and tubular secretion. Reduction in GFR substantially reduces methotrexate renal clearance and thereby the total plasma clearance of the drug. Increased and prolonged exposure to methotrexate may induce life-threatening myelosuppression and mucositis, which may necessitate high dose and prolonged administration of leucovorin rescue. Drugs that compete with the tubular secretion pathway for weak acids, such as penicillins, probenicid and sulphonamides, may also substantially reduce the clearance of methotrexate.[10] An important interaction between methotrexate and *omeprazole* at the renal level has recently been documented, and omeprazole should be discontinued during methotrexate therapy. NSAIDs may significantly reduce GFR and thereby the renal clearance of methotrexate, resulting in increased toxicity.

There is a significant correlation between total plasma clearance of *topotecan* and GFR, and doses of the drug should be lowered in case of moderate or severe renal dysfunction.[20] Anticancer drug–drug interactions at the renal level are also important. Cisplatin preceding methotrexate or topotecan significantly reduces the total plasma clearance of the co-administered drug, resulting in increased toxicity.

In general, correlation coefficients for the relationship between GFR and the total plasma clearance of drugs that are primarily eliminated by the kidney are much higher (of the order of 0.6) than the correlation between BSA and total plasma clearance (~0.2–0.3). Surprisingly, despite this, BSA is still commonly used instead of adaptive dosing using renal function for anticancer agents.[11]

Renal function declines with age and the reduction in GFR is approximately 10% per decade. This reduction should result in age-related adaptive dosing of drugs that are largely excreted by the kidneys, but in fact adaptive dosing is rarely used.

In very young children the GFR is still immature and may be as low as 40 ml/min/1.7 m^2. GFR reaches normal adult values between 6 and 12 months of age, and very young children need dose adjustments for drugs such as carboplatin and methotrexate. Dosing formulas have been established.[11]

Variability in pharmacodynamics

Variability in tumour responsiveness

Despite equal exposure of patients with the same tumour type to a given anticancer agent or combination of agents, there is still a wide inter-patient variation in the likelihood of tumour response. Similarly, time to progression and survival may differ substantially between patients. Variability under conditions of equal systemic exposure is due to differences in the sensitivity of the tumour to the drugs given, which can be multifactorial. For example, metastatic sites may behave as 'sanctuary sites' because they cannot be reached by the chemotherapeutic agents, as in the case of primary testicular tumours or microscopic metastases of small-cell lung cancer or breast cancer to the brain. Bulky tumours may have areas of poor blood perfusion resulting in very low and inadequate exposure of tumour areas to systemically administered anticancer agents. The activity of chemotherapeutic agents may be further reduced in such bulky tumours because of resistance due to hypoxia.

In addition to these drug delivery problems, there are also many intrinsic tumour-cell-related factors which cause variability in response to anticancer agents. These factors include those related to cellular membrane, cytoplasmatic, or nuclear defence mechanisms.

One of the best characterized cellular-membrane-related defence mechanisms is the membrane-bound drug efflux protein *P-gp*. P-gp (molecular weight, 170 kDa) is a member of the ATP-binding cassette family, which has high affinity for a large number of anticancer agents. These agents are natural products or semi-synthetic derivatives, such as anthracyclines, vinca alkaloids, epipodophylotoxins, taxanes, and topoisomerase 1 inhibitors. Increased ATP-dependent drug efflux results in low intracellular exposure and tumour cell protection from the agent.[21] P-gp overexpression has been observed in several tumour types, including breast cancer, colorectal cancer, multiple myeloma, etc. The clinical implications of P-gp overexpression are not yet completely clear. However, it is hoped that ongoing clinical trials with combinations of cytotoxic drugs and P-gp antagonists (e.g. PSC833) will clarify the situation.

Recently, other membrane-bound efflux mechanisms, such as the multidrug-related protein (MRP), have been identified. Seven members of the drug efflux pump family have now been cloned and studies are underway to unravel the physiological functions of these proteins. Other membrane-bound drug efflux mechanisms have now also been identified e.g. for topotecan and mitoxantrone, which has been denoted *breast cancer resistance protein (BCRP, ABCG2)*[25]. Lung resistance protein (LRP), a major vault protein, is overexpressed in several solid tumour types. *LRP* is an independent prognostic parameter for response to chemotherapy in ovarian cancer, although the mechanism of resistance and function of the protein are still poorly understood.[22]

Cytoplasm-related resistance mechanisms that have been suggested include detoxification of anticancer agents by overexpression of *glutathione and metallothionein*, which results in resistance to cisplatin in tumour cell lines. Again, however, the clinical relevance of these pathways is unclear.

At the DNA level a number of different mechanisms may impart resistance to chemotherapy. Inactivation of *p53* or overexpression of *bcl2* is correlated with drug resistance, and overexpression of *Her2/neu* significantly reduces the likelihood of response to chemotherapy in breast cancer. Increased DNA repair by O^6-*alkyl guanine alkyl transferase* overexpression results in resistance to nitrosoureas, DTIC, procarbazine, and temozolomide. Mutation in *topo I or topo II* is correlated with resistance to topo I and topo II inhibitors. Alteration in drug targets, such as dihydrofolate reductase or TS, results in resistance to 5FU and methotrexate, respectively. DNA mismatch repair is correlated with resistance to DNA alkylators.[23]

These and other mechanisms of drug resistance have been characterized *in vitro*; however, not all clinical implications are clear yet.

Variability in end-organ sensitivity and drug–disease interactions

It is important to recognize that patients may be at risk of (severe) toxicity because of the increased sensitivity of their normal tissues. Previous treatments, even many years ago, may have induced tissue damage resulting in decreased functional organ reserve. For example, prior treatment with bone-marrow-toxic chemotherapy may result in more severe and prolonged myelosuppression if the patients are subsequently retreated with cytotoxic drugs, even if this is many years later. Mitomycin C and nitrosoureas induce significant myelosuppression such that several cycles may result in permanently reduced leukocyte and platelet counts. Such patients are at an increased risk for myelosuppression during second-line chemotherapy.

Similarly, extensive radiotherapy to the skeleton reduces the regeneration potential of the bone marrow. Therefore extensive previous radiotherapy is a risk factor for pronounced myelosuppression after chemotherapy. Radiotherapy to the head–neck region may induce persistent mucosal damage, and mucositis induced by chemotherapy in these patients may be expectedly severe.[24] A well-documented toxicity of left-sided and mediastinal radiotherapy is cardiomyopathy. Anthracyclines given later (e.g. in the case of advanced breast cancer) may induce symptomatic congestive heart failure at much lower cumulative doses than in patients who have not received prior radiotherapy.

In the setting of moderate to pronounced liver dysfunction, clearance of a number of anticancer agents may be significantly reduced, which can result in severe side effects. Clinically important in this respect are the taxanes paclitaxel and docetaxel, the vinca alkaloids, and the anthracyclines.

A further clinically important example of the impact of organ toxicity on cytotoxic drug pharmacokinetics exists at the level of the kidneys. A well-documented side effect of cisplatin therapy is renal glomerular and tubular damage, resulting in a reduced creatinine clearance and electrolyte loss. The kidneys are particularly vulnerable when there is a reduced renal blood flow, and cisplatin may induce nausea and vomiting which results in insufficient fluid intake, reduced circulating volume, and reduced renal blood flow. Administration of cisplatin during a subsequent course may induce severe renal dysfunction, which is only slowly and partly reversible. Therefore adequate hydration is a prerequisite for cisplatin therapy. In addition, reduced fluid intake even 1–2 weeks after cisplatin can result in significant renal dysfunction.

In general, a poor overall clinical status (e.g. a WHO performance score ≥2) is associated with more pronounced side effects after chemotherapy.

Drug–drug interactions

There are many important drug–drug interactions in oncology, and some examples have already been given above. These interactions may occur between anticancer drugs given in combination, or between anticancer and non-anticancer drugs. There is a well-established pharmacokinetic or pharmacodynamic basis for most interactions, and they may be unwanted or beneficial.

Cisplatin induces renal damage, resulting in a reduction in the renal and total plasma clearance of methotrexate. Consequently, *methotrexate exposure* increases, resulting in more significant myelosuppression and mucositis. Similarly, exposure to *topotecan* is increased after treatment with cisplatin shortly before topotecan. The pharmacokinetic basis of these interactions is that the renal damage induced by cisplatin results in a reduction in the renal and total plasma clearance of topotecan and methotrexate.

As discussed above, several non-anticancer agents, such as penicillins, probenicid, sulfonamides and NSAIDs, reduce the renal clearance of methotrexate and thereby increase the risk of methotrexate-induced toxicity.

Drug–drug interactions between high-dose methotrexate and benzimidazole proton pump inhibitors can be severe and life threatening. The underlying mechanism is most likely the inhibition of ABCG2 (BCRP) mediated transport of methotrexate by benzimidazoles.[25] Other anticancer drug–drug interactions at the level of ABC transport proteins may also occur, as shown by the enhancement of the oral bioavailability of the taxanes docetaxel and paclitaxel by the P-gp inhibitor *cyclosporin A*, and of topotecan by the P-gp and BCRP inhibitor elacridar.[25–27]

As outlined above, at the metabolic level the interaction between *paclitaxel and doxorubicin* has clinical implications, and *allopurinol* significantly reduces the metabolic inactivation of *6-mercaptopurine*, thereby increasing the risk for increased toxicity. *Antiseizure* medication can induce the metabolic inactivation of the experimental topo I inhibitor 9-aminocamptothecin. Clearly, these pharmacokinetic interactions are unwanted.

At the pharmacodynamic level the increased neurotoxicity of the combination of *cisplatin and paclitaxel* is clinically important. In particular, the effect is significant when paclitaxel is administered as infusions of relatively long duration (e.g. 24 h). The interaction between *carboplatin and cisplatin and paclitaxel*, at the level of the bone marrow, is not very well understood. However, the interaction is beneficial and simultaneous administration results in much less myelosuppression than when the platinum agent precedes paclitaxel.[28]

Beneficial pharmacodynamic interactions also occur between 5FU and leucovorin at the level of thymidylate synthase, potentiating the pharmacological effect of 5FU. Leucovorin is also commonly used as an antidote for methotrexate.

These and other pharmacological interactions require further investigation and the reader is referred to other chapters for additional examples.

Conclusions

Pronounced inter-patient variability in dose–effect relationships for anticancer agents is common. In view of the narrow therapeutic window of current cytotoxic drug therapy, it is important to recognize the clinical, pharmacological, and biochemical factors that contribute to this variability. Intra-patient variability is usually less pronounced. An understanding of the pharmacokinetic and pharmacodynamic factors that contribute to inter-patient variability can help to individualize anticancer therapy, which in turn should result in achieving the optimal balance between anticancer activity and predictable and manageable toxicity.

References

1. Calvert AH, Newell DR, Gumbrell LA, *et al.* (1989). Carboplatin dosage: prospective evaluation of a simple formula based on renal function. *J Clin Oncol*, **11**, 1748–56.

2. Egorin MJ, Van Echo DA, Olman EA, Whitacre MY, Forrest A, Aisner J (1985) Prospective validation of a pharmacologically based dosing scheme for the *cis*-diamminedichloroplatinum (II) analogue diamminecyclobutanedicarboxylatoplatinum. *Cancer Res*, **45**, 6502–6.

3. Chatelut E, Canal P, Brunner V, *et al.* (1995) Prediction of carboplatin clearance form standard morphological and biological patient characteristics. *J Natl Cancer Inst*, **8**, 573–80.

4. Schellens JHM, Creemers GJ, Beijnen JH, *et al.* (1996) Bioavailability and pharmacokinetics of oral topotecan: a new topoisomerase I inhibitor. *Br J Cancer*, **73**, 1268–71.

5. McLeod HL, Evans WE (1998) Epipodophyllotoxins. In Grochow LB, Ames MM (eds) *A Clinician's Guide to Chemotherapy, Pharmacokinetics and Pharmacodynamics*. Baltimore, MD: Williams & Wilkins, 259–87.

6. Milano G, Etienne MC (1998) 5-Fluorouracil. In Grochow LB, Ames MM (eds) *A Clinician's Guide to Chemotherapy, Pharmacokinetics and Pharmacodynamics*. Baltimore, MD: Williams & Wilkins, 289–300.

7. Schinkel AH (1997) The physiological function of drug-transporting P-glycoproteins. *Semin Cancer Biol*, **8**, 161–70.

8. Meerum Terwogt JM, Beijnen JH, ten Bokkel Huinink WW, Rosing H, Schellens JHM (1998) Co-administration of cyclosporin enables oral therapy with paclitaxel. *Lancet*, **352**, 285.

9. Herben VMM, ten Bokkel Huinink WW, Beijnen JH (1996) Clinical pharmacokinetics of topotecan. *Clin Pharmacokinet*, **31**, 85–102.

10. Crom WR (1998) Methotrexate. In Grochow LB, Ames MM (eds) *A Clinician's Guide to Chemotherapy, Pharmacokinetics and Pharmacodynamics*. Baltimore, MD: Williams & Wilkins, 311–330.

11. Grochow LB, Baker SD (1998) The relationship of age to the disposition and effects of anticancer drugs. In Grochow LB, Ames MM (eds) *A Clinician's Guide to Chemotherapy, Pharmacokinetics and Pharmacodynamics*. Baltimore, MD: Williams & Wilkins, 35–53.

12. Crommentuyn KM, Schellens JHM, van den Berg JD, Beijnen JH (1998) *In-vitro* metabolism of anti-cancer drugs, methods and applications: paclitaxel, docetaxel, tamoxifen and ifosfamide. *Cancer Treat Rev*, **24**, 345–66.

13. Koudriakova T, Iarsimirskaia E, Utkin I, *et al.* (1998) Metabolism of the human immunodeficiency virus protease inhibitors indinavir and ritonavir by human intestinal microsomes and expressed cytochrome P450A4/3A5: mechanism-based inactivation of cytochrome P4503A by ritonavir. *Drug Metab Dispos*, **26**, 552–61.

14. Bruno R, Hille D, Riva A, *et al.* (1998) Population pharmacokinetics/pharmacodynamics of docetael in phase II studies in patients with cancer. *J Clin Oncol*, **16**, 187–96.

15. Gupta E, Wang X, Ramirez J, Ratain MJ (1997) Modulation of glucuronidation of SN-38, the active metabolite of irinotecan, by valproic acid and phenobarbital. *Cancer Chemother Pharmacol*, **39**, 440–4.

16. Weinshilboum R. (1998) Pharmacogenetics of anticancer drug metabolism. In Grochow LB, Ames MM (eds) *A Clinician's Guide to Chemotherapy, Pharmacokinetics and Pharmacodynamics*. Baltimore, MD: Williams & Wilkins, 17–33.

17. Herben VMM (1998) PhD Thesis, State University Utrecht.

18. Cockroft DW, Gault MH (1976) Prediction of creatinine clearance from serum creatinine. *Nephron*, **16**, 31–4.

19. Nannan Panday VR, van Warmerdam LJC, Huizing MT, *et al.* (1998) Carboplatin dosage formulae can generate inaccurate predictions of carboplatin exposure in carboplatin/paclitaxel combination regimens. *Clin Drug Invest*, **15**, 327–35.

20. O'Reilly S, Rowinsky EK, Slichenmyer W, *et al.* (1996) A phase I and pharmacologic study of topotecan in patients with impaired renal function. *J Clin Oncol*, **14**, 3062.

21. Schinkel AH, Borst P (1991) Multidrug resistance mediated by P-glycoproteins. *Semin Cancer Biol*, **2**, 213–26.

22. Izquierdo MA, van der Zee AGJ, Vermorken JB, *et al.* (1995) Drug resistance-associated marker LRP for prediction of response to chemotherapy and prognoses in advanced ovarium carcinoma. *J Natl Cancer Inst*, **87**, 1230–7.

23. Kaufman D, Chabner BA (1996) Clinical strategies for cancer treatment: the role of drugs. In Chabner BA, Longo DL (eds) *Cancer Chemotherapy and Biotherapy: Principles and Practice*. Philadelphia, PA: Lippincott–Raven, 1–16.

24. Doroshow, JH (1996) Anthracyclines and anthracenediones. In Chabner BA, Longo DL (eds) *Cancer Chemotherapy and Biotherapy: Principles and Practice*. Philadelphia, PA: Lippincott–Raven, 409–434.

25. Schellens JH, Malingre MM, Kruijtzer CM, *et al.* (2000) Modulation of oral bioavailability of anticancer drugs: from mouse to man. *Eur J Pharm Sci*, **12**, 103–10.

26. Kruijtzer CM, Beijnen JH, Schellens JH. (2002) Improvement of oral drug treatment by temporary inhibition of drug transporters and/or cytochrome P450 in the gastrointestinal tract and liver: an overview. *Oncologist*, **7**, 516–30.

27. Kruijtzer CM, Beijnen JH, Rosing H, *et al.* (2002) Increased oral bioavailability of topotecan in combination with the breast cancer resistance protein and P-glycoprotein inhibitor GF120918. *J Clin Oncol*, **20**, 2943–50

28. Gerrits GJ, Schellens JH, Burris H, *et al.* (1999) A comparison of clinical pharmacodynamics of different administration schedules of oral topotecan. *Clin Cancer Res*, **5**, 69–75.

4 | *Drug development and study design*

Jim Cassidy

Introduction

Drug development encompasses the entire process by which an idea in the mind of a scientist is converted into a therapeutic agent for the widespread benefit of mankind. The process of drug development in oncology is different from that employed in every other branch of medicine. These differences are often cited by our more traditional 'mainstream' clinical pharmacologist colleagues as the reasons why we have not been more successful in the quest for more effective therapies for this disease. Most of these differences can be easily explained by the very nature of neoplasia and the public reactions and perceptions which surround the disease. Thus traditional phase I trials in normal healthy volunteers are simply not possible in the case of cytotoxics with potentially lethal short-term toxicities and unknown long-term effects, particularly with respect to reproductive health.

Some of these differences also relate to our understandable desire to make better treatment available as soon as possible. This can lead to a frame of mind that 'we don't care how it works as long as it works', which implies that a degree of empiricism is acceptable in this field of pharmacology which would be entirely out of place in, for example, cardiovascular disease. However empirical, the methodologies that have evolved for clin- ical testing of cytotoxics have allowed the introduction of many novel agents over the last two decades. It does seem clear that we are entering a new era in cancer pharmacology; fuelled by the burgeoning understanding of cellular processes at a molecular level. Since new agents coming from this molecular approach have novel targets (other than damage to DNA and cell division apparatus), it should be no surprise that we will be faced with new problems and challenges in developing such drugs. Hence, we are entering a period when we are going to be forced to make some fundamental changes to our developmental strategies.

The purpose of this chapter is to review the current state of the art in cytotoxic development and to highlight areas in which novel strategies are required for novel compounds. Traditionally, drug discovery and development are thought of as a linear process, as shown below, but it should be stressed at the earliest opportunity that flexibility within the plan and a desire to answer the fundamental mechanistic questions about the new agent as soon as possible should be guiding forces. It is only through a fuller understanding of drug action at a cellular level that we will be able to leave behind the somewhat empirical ways of the past.

Preclinical phase

The steps in drug development can be summarized as follows:

drug discovery
↓
formulation
↓
animal toxicology
↓
choice of schedule
↓

starting dose
↓
patient selection
↓
dose escalation scheme
↓
modifications for toxicity
↓
definition of 'maximal tolerated dose'
↓
definition of dose and schedule for phase II
↓
phase II trials
↓
phase III trials
↓
marketing approval

Drug discovery

The direct translation of a research idea into a therapeutic entity has actually been quite rare in oncology. Serendipity has had a hand in many of the currently available cytotoxics on the market. Drug discovery in the past was primarily through random screening of compounds for a cytotoxic effect. This was pioneered by the US National Cancer Institute using a murine P388 leukaemia system. This system was reasonably effective at finding 'DNA-targeted poisons' but the clinical utility of this class of compounds has probably now been exhausted. Therefore a replacement system using a panel of 60 human tumour cell lines was initiated in 1990 in an attempt to broaden the scope of the screen and make it more relevant to human cancer. Sophisticated automated techniques of cell culture, cytotoxicity assays, and methods of analysis such as COMPARE[1] have been developed to operate alongside this screen with the major objective being to find compounds which display disease-specific activity, possibly indicating novel mechanisms of action. Figure 4.1 shows an example of a small section of a COMPARE printout (more detail on a selection of cytotoxics is available at http://www.ncifcrf.gov/DTP/dbs/stdagnt.html). The basic message of these tabulations is that if compounds show patterns of cytotoxicity which are novel and/or highly specific, then the compound merits further testing. On the other hand, if it looks like a known cytotoxic or is highly toxic to all lines, it is deemed to be of low interest. Such large-scale screening is obviously expensive and may not be the most efficient way of selecting new agents.

Most pharmaceutical companies have pursued an alternative, and perhaps more intellectually pleasing, strategy for drug discovery with a more directed mechanistic approach. Examples are the search for inhibitors of *ras* farnesylation and a variety of signal transduction inhibitors. In this context a mechanism-driven high throughput cellular or biochemical screen is developed and lead compounds generated from basic research clues are screened for activity against the target system. Those which show promise in the primary screen become the templates for further groups of chemical derivatizations to form a new set of compounds. The process continues in a stepwise fashion until it is possible to select the optimum compound for further *in vivo* experimentation.

Various modifications of the above scheme which involve generation of potential drug candidates using information about the potential target are also increasingly being used. A current example is the application of knowledge of the crystal structure of the protein of interest.[2] Our 'mainstream' colleagues will recognize that this is cancer pharmacology catching up on the receptor–ligand interaction paradigm which has proved so successful in other therapeutic areas. The future expansion of approaches such as genomics, proteomics, and serial analysis of gene expression promises many more exciting leads for new therapies.

It is not yet clear which of these strategies will be the most efficient or cost effective in the long run. However, it is logical to imply that a screen based on cytotoxicity, such as that operated by the National Cancer Institute, is not going to be a good way of selecting agents which are (for example) cytostatic, antimetastatic or anti-angiogenic. In these circumstances the mechanistic approach is to be preferred, but will be predicated by sufficient knowledge of the complex physiological controls which govern cell division, migration, and angiogenesis. Knowledge of these processes is increasing at an almost exponential rate, but it is still imperfect and this hampers the setting of design criteria for an ideal agent. History would also suggest that we should be on the lookout for the hand of serendipity!

Formulation

Consideration of this issue may seem a little out of place in a clinically orientated discussion of drug development. However, the potential for things to go astray at this stage is very high. Examples are agents which are not sufficiently soluble and thus crystallize out in

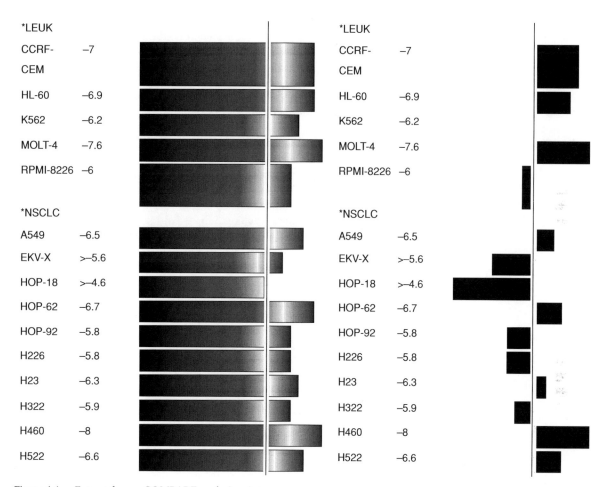

Figure 4.1. Extract from a COMPARE analysis printout.

the renal tubules, causing severe nephrotoxicity (CB3717), agents which cause haemolysis in high concentration and therefore need to be given into central venous access devices (gamma linoleic acid), agents which require complex and even toxic excipients (taxol), and agents which when given orally have very poor and highly variable bioavailability (5-fluorouracil). Due care should be taken to ensure that adequate solubility, stability, and quality control studies have been performed using the final version of the drug and for-

mulation. Even very simple issues such as bottling and storage requirements have been known to cause serious delays in trial initiation. As far as possible, it is wise to ensure from the outset that sufficient drug is available in the final formulated form to ensure supplies for all phase I and planned phase II trials as an absolute minimum. It is frustrating and even perhaps unethical to perform a phase I trial, find some anticancer activity, and then not be able to obtain drug supplies for the next steps in the development plan.

Animal toxicity

At first sight this area seems highly regulated, non-contentious, and simple to understand and perform, with multiple guidelines available from many drug regulatory authorities. The main aims are to define the types of toxicity likely to be observed in humans and the approximate dose range in which they may become problematic. The system is based on the belief that animal toxicology will be at least qualitatively similar to that in humans. This has largely held true for the group of DNA poisons that have gone before, but is less likely to continue into non-DNA-targeted agents.[3] A current example is the human toxicity seen with *matrix metalloproteinase inhibitors*. This group of drugs was designed as cytostatic and antimetastatic compounds, and therefore they will probably need to be administered for a prolonged period of time. In humans, one dose-limiting toxicity after prolonged administration is the development of painful stiff joints, sometimes associated with skin changes. These effects are mainly subjective and were not observed in animals. A similar problem was dose-limiting headache observed with mitoquidone.[4] The subjective nature of joint stiffness or headache indicates that no amount of animal testing could ever be expected to discover these problems. An alternative to ever more complex animal experimentation is to reduce it to a bare minimum. This may mean accepting a slightly higher risk in the setting of a safe starting dose, but it is worth noting that the problem with *mitoquidone* occurred at the start dose which had been defined in the usual way.[4] Cancer Research UK has adopted a policy of minimal animal toxicology.[5] So far, no compounds have been studied in which the starting dose was considered unsafe and no unpredicted toxicity has been observed in human subjects in the clinical trials.[3] It is important to stress that this toxicity testing is compound specific; the testing is done in a fashion as close as possible to the projected use in humans in terms of dose, schedule, and route of administration. The potential benefits of this approach in respect of resources and time are self-evident, but in addition the reduction of animal toxicology experimentation is perceived by society as a laudable goal in itself.

Phase I trials

Choice of schedule

In the past the dictation of schedule has been usually based on the average time for haematological recovery to occur, resulting in the traditional 21 day cycle for most intravenously administered cytotoxics. The advent of agents which do not have dose-limiting marrow toxicity has necessitated a rethink of this empirical approach. It is unusual to have compelling evidence of an optimum scheduling from animal experimentation, and even when this is the case (e.g. etoposide) it may not be deemed acceptable from a logistical point of view. The justification is usually that the proposed schedule might not be acceptable to patients (or, more likely, research staff). This attitude often results in testing schedules which are known to be suboptimal.[6] Theoretically, this could lead to the anticancer activity of the drug being under-estimated or missed completely, with the result that the agent would then be rejected for further human study. The counter-argument is that even if all current cytotoxics were administered in a suboptimal way, it is likely that some anticancer activity would be observed. This argument is, of course, circular, in that the only method of verification would be to reassess fully a number of agents which had already been in clinical study and had been subsequently rejected—it seems unlikely that such a strategy would be feasible.

Ideally, the choice of schedule should be informed by knowledge of the mechanism of action and supported by animal experimentation. In the absence of this knowledge a schedule should be selected which is practicable, and consideration should be given to performance of clinical trials with a variety of schedules. This may eventually lead to a need to compare schedules in randomized phase II studies. This will increase the resources required for these studies, but has the advantage that the drug schedule chosen for further development will have been at least partly 'optimized'. Whenever possible the use of 'surrogate markers' of activity against the drug target (see below) should be incorporated.

Starting dose

In general, one-tenth of the mouse equivalent LD_{10} ($MELD_{10}$), i.e. dose lethal in 10% of mice, is selected as a safe starting dose in humans. This is usually verified as safe in at least one other species. If the other species is more sensitive, then it will be used for starting dose selection. This is based on the historical observation that the maximal tolerated dose (MTD) in humans and the LD_{10} in mice were similar for most drugs.[7] It is important to carry out the toxicity testing in an appropriate species, avoiding known or suspected inter-species differences in drug handling or effect; a good example is the avoidance of rodents in testing of thymidylate synthase inhibitors because of differences in extracellular thymidine levels. This approach has recently been reviewed and does appear to at least offer safety.[8] The fundamental issue in selecting the starting dose is the dichotomy between safety and the desire to reach the top dose (and presumably more likely effective dose) in as few escalation steps as possible. Patients express concerns at both ends of the spectrum; those in the early dose steps are worried that the dose they receive will be little better than placebo, whilst those at the top doses with attendant toxicity are worried that they may be exposed to excessive toxicity. Oncologists share these concerns and are also keen to progress trials in as short a timescale as possible. It has been observed that those responses which do occur in phase I trials tend to occur at doses that are 80% of the MTD.[3] A recent review of 100 drugs tested in Europe concluded that one-tenth $MELD_{10}$ was safe but very conservative. The author recommended that a starting dose of 20–40% of rodent LD_{10} would be more acceptable.[9] We would be better able to select a starting dose (and many other aspects of the trial design) if we could assess the drug activity at the intracellular level in the tumour tissue. Unfortunately, this is not yet possible but should be an aim for all involved in anticancer drug development in the future.

Patient selection

The standard phase I design calls for inclusion of patients with advanced cancer which is intractable or resistant to standard therapy. Simultaneously, the patients must have normal or near-normal renal, hepatic, and marrow function. Such patients tend to be relatively rare, since both the manifestations of cancer and its prior treatment will often result in end-organ dysfunction. Therefore the trial will inevitably define the drug effect and tolerability in an unrepresentative subset of patients. The rationale for this selection is to avoid problems of aberrant drug metabolism or clearance which might result in excessive toxicity. It is usually well into the phase II or even phase III evaluation of a drug before specific studies are commissioned to examine the effects in patients with organ dysfunction who are more representative of the usual population of patients with the disease in question. This superselection slows down study recruitment, and it is a viable alternative to conduct studies in patients more like the standard population with stratification for variables such as hepatic function and/or liver metastases.

It has been commonplace to enrol an unselected tumour population into phase I trials. The balance of tumour types usually reflects the underlying clinical practice of the principal investigators. However, with the introduction of disease-specific (see COMPARE above) or mechanism-specific agents, it may be more logical to concentrate recruitment on patients with tumours which are considered more likely to respond. This will also slow recruitment but perhaps maximize the individual patient's chance of benefit. It also does not preclude the future investigation of the compound in diseases which were not picked out in the COMPARE analysis, but it would take a good deal of persuasion to continue to pursue a drugs development if it had 'failed' in its target tumour. It is also important to recall that the primary end-point of a phase I is the maximal tolerated dose (not response), and there is no a priori reason why the MTD should be significantly different between patients with a variety of tumour types.

Most commonly patients are enrolled in multiples of three for each dose cohort. This is entirely arbitrary and for some agents may not be necessary.

Dose escalation

Traditionally, dose escalation has been performed using a 'modified' Fibonacci scheme: if the starting dose at level 1 is x_1, at level 2 it is $x_1 + 100\%$, at level 3 it is $x_2 + 67\%$, at level 4 it is $x_3 + 50\%$, and at level $n \geq 5$ it is $x_{n-1} + 30$–35%. This method, which was introduced in the early 1970s for nitrosourea and the epipodophyllotoxin drugs, has a number of problems. The 'modified' part is usually the number of dose-doubling steps that are allowed at the start. This is often decided in an arbitrary fashion and can have a profound effect on the number of dose escalations required in total. If the starting dose is set low, very many steps will be required to reach the MTD as there is no clear mechanism for reversion to larger dose increments in the absence of expected toxicities. A widely practised method is to maintain dose doublings until the first sign of toxicity becomes apparent and then return to the Fibonacci scheme. This also has limitations; the types of patients in phase I trials almost invariably have systemic manifestations of the underlying cancer, and therefore some subjective types of toxicity (malaise, nausea, pain, anorexia, fatigue) can be difficult to attribute correctly as drug or cancer effects. The tendency is to err on the side of caution, enter the Fibonacci phase, and then find that these 'toxicities' are absent in the subsequent cohorts.

Dose escalation usually takes place with each new cohort. Intra-patient dose escalation is less common.

The argument against it is that if cumulative toxicities occur, it will be more complex to attribute them correctly if intra-patient escalation is performed. However, if an adequate wash-out period is allowed, it may be reasonable to allow patients to have a higher dose with more expectation of therapeutic benefit.

Two innovations in the area of dose escalation strategies are worth discussing in more detail: pharmacokinetically guided dose escalation (PGDE) and the continuous reassessment method (CRM).

PGDE was proposed in 1986–1987[10] and is based on the hypothesis that the area under the plasma concentration time curve (AUC) at the LD_{10} in mice is similar to that at the MTD in humans. In this way a target AUC can be defined from animal work; patient AUCs are measured in the trial and the next dose step is determined with the knowledge of how close to the target the dose has been in humans. Thus if the AUCs are far apart the dose escalation is aggressive, and conversely it is cautious as the AUCs converge.[11] This methodology has not been widely adopted, partly because of organizational issues in ensuring pharmacokinetic results are available in time to make dose escalation decisions and partly because of problems in interpretation of results which may indicate non-linearity in pharmacokinetic behaviour.[12] Various adaptations to this methodology have been suggested; one is to use a percentage cut-off of the target AUC and then to escalate beyond that point in a Fibonacci scheme.[13]

The continuous reassessment method uses all available data to provide an estimate of the human MTD. Initially, all the data will be preclinical and the confidence in the predicted MTD will be small. As each individual patient is treated in the trial, the estimated MTD is updated based on a probability distribution for the MTD and a dose toxic-response model. The statistical rationale for this method is complex, but the practicalities are somewhat simpler than for PGDE.[14] This method allows for even single patients at each dose level, thus reducing the numbers treated at low (inactive) doses. The method may not actually reduce the time to reach MTD, which is a crucial determinant in the success of a phase I study. This method has been used in very few trials as yet, and it remains to be seen if it represents a step forward. As with PGDE, efforts continue to refine the methodology.[15]

The escalation scheme also has to be modified for agents in which the expectation is that some form of *cumulative toxicity* may occur with chronic dosing. This has been a particular concern in recent clinical studies of oral variants of the fluoropyrimidines (e.g. capecitabine, Xeloda™, OGT-719). In this instance it was necessary to design dose escalation steps and recruitment of cohorts that overlapped each other, so that later cohorts would have information about the chronic toxicities experienced at lower doses.[16] This would then allow investigators the opportunity to stop dosing in the higher-level cohort if serious (life-threatening) problems were observed in the groups with lower dose but longer duration.

Modifications for toxicity

In the past, with DNA-targeted agents, it was possible to set an arbitrary limit on haematological parameters and institute dose delay and/or reduction when these parameters were met or exceeded. In the era of non-DNA drugs with unpredictable toxicities, the challenge is to pick up the toxicities at a stage when they can be easily handled and are still reversible. The limitations of rodent toxicology studies, as detailed above, make it difficult to be sure that we are monitoring the correct target tissues in the human subjects. The usual way around this problem is to monitor intensively a standard battery of haematological and biochemical parameters, urine analysis, electrocardiography, and clinical examination. It is likely that the new generation of agents which are not DNA targeted will produce novel toxicity patterns and we will be forced to introduce ad hoc monitoring for these adverse events. It is incumbent upon early clinical trial investigators to be vigilant for unexpected problems that may be drug related. It is also essential that all untoward events are investigated as fully as possible. It is this aspect of phase I that makes it advisable to have investigators who are experienced in this early phase of development and to have as small a number of centres as possible involved in the execution of the study, thus allowing communication between the centres/sponsor to be sufficiently frequent and detailed to pick up even subtle toxicities which may be the forerunners of more serious problems ahead.

Definition of maximal tolerated dose

Oncologists are usually trained to expect maximal benefit at the maximal dose. This does seem to hold true for our current battery of 'anti-DNA' drugs and therefore it is not surprising that it has remained unchallenged. It was also convenient that most of these agents have haematological toxic effects which eventually limit dosing in humans. Thus the definition of

MTD has most often been expressed as a function of *myelosuppression*. This allowed the application of very simple numerical rules to define the end-point of the study. The simplest and most widely applied rule is that the end-point is reached when more than 30% of any cohort experience grade 4 neutropenia or thrombocytopenia (usually at least two of six patients).

Application of the same rules to agents which are not myelotoxic may be a grave error. For example, if we are dealing with an inhibitor of a critical step in signal transduction, would it not be more appropriate to measure this effect in the target tissue (tumour)? The dose escalation would then cease when the maximal inhibition was observed. This is even more important if one recalls the 'bell-shaped' response curve of many agents in biology. In other words, increase in dose resulting in concentrations of drug beyond a certain level will result in diminution of the biological effect. If we simply continue dose escalation until toxicity in humans, we may well miss the desired dose range for effect. It is also evident to clinical investigators that the serial biopsy of tumour lesions necessary to fulfil this ideal will never be a practical proposition in routine practice. Therefore we need to make a major effort to develop 'surrogate markers' of activity which will be assessable in a serial fashion. Since the ideal matrix is blood, this will mean more effort in early trials in the correlation of pharmacokinetics and pharmacodynamics, or for intracellular processes perhaps the serial analysis of leukocyte effects (although this may not be a good surrogate for tumour cells). Newer non-invasive approaches to the problem of trying to assess drug effects within a human tumour are nuclear magnetic resonance or positron-emission tomography-labelled drug imaging. It is in the field of antifolates that we are perhaps currently closest to approaching this ideal, mainly because there are already a number of known (somewhat imperfect) blood markers of intracellular folate status.[17]

In fact, even the seemingly simple haematological end-points have now also been subverted by the introduction of a range of agents which support marrow function, such as haematological growth factors. It is now commonplace to define an MTD with and without such support. As the range and efficacy of these 'support' molecules expands, it is more than likely that we will have to revisit the maximal dosing of many established cytotoxics and combination regimens.

One further limitation of the current methodology is that we tend to place some arbitrary time limit on both the time for toxicity to develop and for antitumour effect to be observed. Thus MTD may be defined by dose-limiting toxicities observed in the first 6 weeks of therapy. Tumour response may be assessed every two cycles (e.g. 2×21 days). Since most patients will show evidence of progression of the underlying tumour at formal assessment, the numbers who then go on to receive more than two cycles are small. The phase I trial then concludes with an MTD over just two cycles, and with little or no experience of cumulative dosing or cumulative side-effect profile. It would be ethically difficult *not* to assess the underlying tumour response and thus the problem is inevitable. This is yet another area in which 'surrogate markers' would be useful.

Definition of dose and schedule for phase II

When the MTD is defined it is usual to step back one dose level (assuming that it is not a large incremental drop) and expand experience into a larger cohort. This is an attempt to reduce the confidence intervals around the selected dose, to explore more protracted dosing, and to define 'good'- and 'poor'-risk patients for certain toxicities (this usually means those who have had light or heavy exposure, respectively, to previous marrow-toxic therapy). It is not unusual to be left with a degree of uncertainty at this stage as to the tolerability of protracted dosing with the new agent. This can usually be adequately dealt with in the phase II study design and should not delay progress at this stage.

There is also an understandable desire to look more closely for anticancer effect in these cohorts. The precise patient accrual to such expanded cohorts should be defined prior to the start of phase I. The desire to see antitumour effect should not lead to continued enlargement of the phase I population, thereby subverting the next step of the development process.

The other major advantage of expansion of cohort size at this juncture is that these patients tend to be the most informative in terms of developing a pharmacokinetic–pharmacodynamic model, since they are receiving a dose which many more will also be given and they also have a fair chance of both activity and toxicity.

Phase II trials

In this phase of development the emphasis changes from toxicology to anticancer activity. The dose and schedule (or a variety of them) selected from phase I is now administered to groups of patients with the same tumour. The most commonly used design is a two step-procedure,[16] whereby 14 patients are enrolled in the first instance. If objective anticancer activity is demonstrated by serial disease assessment, then a further 11 patients are entered. The statistics behind this technique are such that by adopting this methodology when no responses are identified the drug has a 95% chance of having a true response rate below 20%. The probability of erroneously rejecting an effective drug will be ≤0.05. The advantage of a two-stage scheme is that it allows early rejection of an ineffective drug. The disadvantage is that in many clinical situations a response rate even below 20% would be potentially very interesting. Once more these patients tend to be selected as resistant or refractory to at least one prior standard therapy, so a 20% response in breast cancer may not be exciting whereas a 20% response rate in colorectal cancer would be quite an achievement.

The selection of which disease types to test is often contentious. The preclinical data may point to certain tumour types, or hints of activity in phase I may serve as encouragement to study one or two particular tumour types. Commercial considerations also have a bearing, since a drug active in one of the three common solid cancers (breast, colon, lung) will have a larger potential market. For this reason, it is exceedingly unusual to see pharmaceutical company trials carried out in the rarer malignancies. The compromise is to test in some common tumours, some directed by science and some by commerce. The limitation on the total number of different tumour types or schedules tested is usually financial.

Care should be exercised in the *dosing* recommendations for phase II, since more patients will tend to receive the drug for a longer time than in phase I. Dose delay and/or reduction criteria need to be agreed at the stage of protocol design. Occasionally provision is made for dose increase if there is concern that the phase I MTD was inaccurate.

Patients in phase II often share eligibility criteria with those in phase I, as they must if we are to extrapolate tolerance from one group to the next, and so again we are dealing with an unrepresentative group. The patients also tend to be younger, fitter, and more motivated than the general 'off-study' population. This often leads to an over-estimation of true response rate at this stage, which is then subject to imprudent over-reporting, leading to the 'wonder drug' claims so often made in the lay press. Adoption of standardized objective response criteria, independent review of response,

and randomization (occasionally against placebo) can all help to minimize this problem. The true value of a new agent is impossible to assess until properly conducted randomized large-scale phase III studies have been completed and an adequate follow-up period observed.

In the hiatus between phases II and III much remains to be done with novel compounds. This is the usual time to explore in small-scale trials the influence of organ dysfunction, age, sex, ethnicity, potential drug interactions and many other important pharmacological issues if the compound is to supplant the current standard of care.

Phase III trials

Of necessity, these trials are usually large multicentre studies which almost always involve infrastructural and financial support from pharmaceutical companies. The aim is now to conduct studies which will allow the compound to be successfully licensed for use in a particular disease setting. The new treatment must be *compared with the current 'gold standard'* for the disease in question. The definition of the standard is often a major stumbling block. There are differences of opinion and practice for all common cancers. These become even more stark when comparing the United States with Europe, or even Southern with Northern Europe. In actual fact, it is very unusual to reach consensus amongst all potential investigators. The relatively long timescale of such studies also presents a problem. Will the 'standard' now be regarded as inadequate by the time that the trial reports? The *end-points* chosen can also be crucial. Survival is regarded as a solid end-point by clinicians, regulatory authorities, and patients, but will take a long time to define. Response rates are regarded as somewhat 'softer', but can be reported much earlier. There is also a groundswell of opinion that quality of life should be included in all such studies. Dialogue with the relevant regulatory authorities at this stage is vital if the studies are going to lead to product registration.

Unfortunately, many phase III studies, although large, are simply not large enough to demonstrate benefit convincingly. This may be because the statistical assumptions used in defining sample size were ill founded. The phase II response rate will usually be an over-estimate (see above) or the magnitude of difference between treatments may be unrealistically large. This can lead to inconclusive results, with disastrous consequences for all concerned. The drug does not receive a license, the company have a huge financial liability, and patients may miss out on improved therapy. Many large companies now commission at least two phase III studies simultaneously with a global perspective in an attempt to develop contemporaneous supportive data for regulatory approval. Investigators in these studies should maintain vigilance of the patients under their care as occasionally side effects only come to light with larger patient numbers and longer follow-up.

General and ethical issues

If the above schema is not to flounder, all the steps have to be performed meticulously and published good laboratory and good clinical practice guidelines must be adhered to. In essence, these rules exist not only to protect us from overtly fraudulent claims, but also in a more subtle way to prevent us from being carried away on a wave of enthusiasm for our own projects. The sharp end of this is a sea of paperwork and source document verification. The time and effort taken to complete case record forms is the part of the process which most investigators like least. However, it is a necessary evil, since regulatory authorities scrutinize this documentation very thoroughly and will reject drugs in which there are doubts about the validity of trial results. This is precisely why monitors and auditors arrive at frequent intervals to review progress and ensure that all study procedures are being followed.

All the *patients taking part* in the development process must be fully informed volunteers. The definition of 'fully' informed is not clear, but at the very least the individual should have had a copy of the study-specific information sheet and had sufficient time to digest the information and formulate any questions for the research team. Ideally, patients should have had adequate time with the research staff to talk through all of their questions and anxieties. The involvement of an independent patient advocate is often recommended in this process. It should be recognized by all concerned that patients with cancer are by definition a 'vulnerable' group, and their psychological well-being is also an important consideration.

The studies must all be reviewed and approved by local and/or national *ethical review boards (ERBs)*. Significant new information that becomes available during the study should be discussed with the ERB and the patients. Reporting of serious adverse events and thorough investigation are particularly important. A two-way flow of information between the investigators and the sponsor company is particularly crucial in the development of new anticancer drugs, since this allows us to share our experience and expertise for the good of patients.

Conclusions

The development of new anticancer agents has always been challenging. The new generation of compounds designed to interfere with intracellular processes, angiogenesis, and the metastatic phenotype will provide even more challenges in the future. Our guiding principle should be the desire to understand the drug action at the most fundamental level, as it is this knowledge that will enable us to face these new challenges.

Refereances

1. Paull KD, Shoemaker RH, Hodes L, *et al.* (1989). Display and analysis of patterns of differential activity of drugs against human tumor cell lines: development of mean graph and COMPARE algorithm. *J Natl Cancer Inst*, **81**, 1088–92.
2. Jackson RC (1997) Contributions of protein structure-based drug design to cancer chemotherapy. *Semin Oncol*, **24**, 164–72.
3. Burtles SS, Jodrell DI, Newell DR (1998) Evaluation of 'rodent only' preclinical toxicology for phase I trials of new cancer treatments—the Cancer Research Campaign experience. *Proc AACR*, **39**, 363.
4. Cassidy J, Bissett D, Kerr DJ (1992) Methodological aspects of phase I studies of novel anticancer agents. *Int J Oncol*, **1**, 195–9.
5. Burtles SS, Newell DR, Henrar REC, Connors TA (1995) Revisions of general guidelines for the preclinical toxicology of new cytotoxic anticancer agents in Europe. *Eur J Cancer*, **31**, 408–10.
6. Cassidy J (1994) Chemotherapy administration: doses, infusions and choice of schedule. *Ann Oncol*, **5**, S25–30.
7. Collins JM, Grieshaber CK, Chabner BA (1990) Pharmacologically guided phase I clinical trials based on preclinical development. *J Natl Cancer Inst*, **82**, 1321–6.
8. Dent SF, Eisenhauer EA (1996) Phase I trial design: are new methodologies being put into practice? *Ann Oncol*, **7**, 561–6.
9. Verweij J (1996) Starting dose levels for phase I studies. *Ann Oncol*, **7**, 16–22.
10. Collins JM, Zaharko DM, Dedrick R, Chabner BA (1986) Potential roles for preclinical pharmacology in phase I clinical trials. *Cancer Treat Rep*, **70**, 73–80.
11. EORTC Pharmacokinetics and Metabolism Group (1987) Pharmacokinetically guided dose escalation in phase I clinical trials. *Eur J Cancer Clin Oncol*, **23**, 1083–7.

12. Graham MA, Workman P (1992) The impact of pharma-cokinetically guided dose escalation strategies in phase I clinical trials: critical evaluation and recommendations for future studies. *Ann Oncol*, **3**, 339–47.

13. Judson I, Briasoulis E, Raynaud F, Hanwell J, Berry C, Lacey H (1997) Phase I trial and pharmacokinetics of the tubulin inhibitor 1069C85—a synthetic agent binding at the colchicine site designed to overcome drug resistance. *Br J Cancer*, **75**, 608–13.

14. O'Quigley J, Pepe M, Fisher L (1990) Continual reassessment method: a practical design for phase I clinical trials in cancer. *Biometrics*, **46**, 33–48.

15. O'Quigley J, Shen LZ (1996) Continual reassessment method: a likelihood approach. *Biometrics*, **52**, 673–84.

16. Cassidy J, McLeod HL (1995) Is it possible to design a logical development plan for an anti-cancer drug? *Pharm Med*, **9**, 95–103.

17. Rafi I, Taylor GA, Calvette JA, *et al.* (1995). Clinical pharmacokinetic and pharmacodynamic studies with the nonclassical antifolate thymidylate synthase inhibitor 3, 4-dihydro-2-amino-6-methyl-4-oxo-5-(4-pyridylthio)-quinazolone dihydrochloride (AG337) given by 24-hour continuous intravenous infusion. *Clin Cancer Res*, **1**, 1275–84.

5 | *Pyrimidine antimetabolites*

Gérard Milano and Jan H. M. Schellens

Summary

	5-Fluorouracil	Capecitabine	Cytosine arabinoside
Generic names	5-Fluorouracil	Capecitabine	Cytosine arabinoside, cytarabine
Commercial names	Fluorouracil, Adrucil, Éfudix	Xeloda	Cytosar-U, Cytarbel
Molecular weight	130	359.55	243
Mechanism of action	Inhibition of thymidylate synthase activity; incorporation into RNA, DNA	Same as 5FU	Inhibition of DNA polymerase; incorporation into DNA
Cell-cycle specificity	S-phase	Same as 5FU	S-phase
Route of administration	Intravenous	Oral	Intravenous
Protein binding (%)	30	50–60	20
Metabolism	Three steps; rate-controlling step, conversion to dihydrofluorouracil	Pre-prodrug of 5FU	Deamination
Elimination	Biotransformation, 80%; renal, 20%	Biotransformation, >90%; 95% of dose via urine; renal for parent drug, 3%	Biotransformation in ara-U and renal elimination (70%)
Terminal half-life	15 min	<1 h	20 min
Toxicities	Bone marrow, gastrointestinal mucosa	Bone narrow, hand–foot syndrome	Bone marrow
Unique features	10-fold variability in total body clearance between patients	Practical and convenient because of oral therapy	Drug acts by causing cell kill or by inducing differentiation

Introduction

Antimetabolites have structural similarities with intermediates of normal metabolism and they interact with the synthesis of RNA and DNA precursors.[1] In the majority of cases antimetabolites are enzyme substrates and act by inhibiting enzymes which are essential for RNA and DNA synthesis. Alternatively, antimetabolites may be cytotoxic because of their incorporation into nucleic acids; this is well characterized for 5-fluorouracil for instance. The mechanism of action of antimetabolites implies that these compounds affect not only cancer cells but also normal cells of the organism which are dividing rapidly.

Therefore antimetabolites may cause significant toxicity, mainly at the haematological and gastrointestinal levels. Understanding of the plasma pharmacokinetics of antimetabolites has accumulated in the last decade, with interesting relationships shown between pharmacokinetic parameters (mostly plasma drug AUC) and pharmacodynamic events (host toxicity and tumour response)

5-Fluorouracil (5FU)

Clinical use

Although 5FU is one of the oldest anticancer drugs, its use in cancer chemotherapy is still increasing. 5FU is not only considered as the standard drug for the treatment of advanced colorectal cancer, but is also one of the major drugs in the treatment of carcinoma of the oral cavity and breast. Most of the current clinical protocols incorporating 5FU include one or more of the so-called 5FU biomodulators, of which *folinic acid* is the most frequently used.[2]

5FU is commercially available for intravenous injections in NaOH 20% (pH 9.4) and for cutaneous applications as 5% cream. 5FU is slightly soluble in methanol and acetonitrile. Storage of 5FU intravenous formulations at 4°C is not recommended as precipitates may form.

Mechanisms of action

There are at least two mechanisms by which 5FU may cause cell lethality: inhibition of the enzyme thymidylate synthase (TS), and fraudulent incorporation into RNA.[3] TS inhibition proceeds through the generation of FdUMP. The presence of a reduced-folate cofactor ($5,10\text{-}CH_2FH_4$) is required for the tight binding of FdUMP to TS. The molecular characteristic of optimal TS inhibition by FdUMP is the rationale which justifies the modulation of 5FU by folinic acid. The second mechanism results from the incorporation of FUTP into RNA and the subsequent effects on RNA function. There are experimental arguments indicating that short-term exposures to high concentrations of 5FU kill cells by an RNA-mediated effect, while prolonged exposure to low doses is cytotoxic via inhibition of TS and consequently DNA synthesis.[4] 5FU acts primarily against cells in the S-phase.

Mechanisms of resistance

The complexity of the mechanism of action of 5FU inevitably leads to the existence of a variety of resistance mechanisms. We will focus on those mechanisms which have been identified at both the experimental and the clinical level. When examining preclinical models, it is not obvious that over-expression of TS is always a determining factor with respect to 5FU resistance.[5,6] Similarly, at the clinical level, there are many reports showing that an elevated expression of tumoral TS at a pretherapeutic stage is an indicator of resistance to 5FU-based treatment for colorectal cancer,[7] but there are also recent data showing that over-expression of TS is linked to improved efficacy of 5FU-based chemotherapy in patients with breast cancer.[8] In addition to TS, there are other enzymatic pathways which have been identified as possible sources for 5FU resistance. The enzyme *dihydropyrimidine dehydrogenase (DPD)* is the *rate-limiting* step for the catabolism of 5FU. Experimental data indicate that an increase in DPD activity may be responsible for a relative loss of 5FU efficacy;[9] the role of DPD in 5FU resistance was confirmed at the clinical level in patients with cancer of the head and neck.[10] The cellular retention of reduced folates is optimal when these compounds are in a polyglutamated form. The formation of polyglutamates is under the control of the enzyme *folylpolyglutamate synthetase (FPGS)*. Recent experimental data suggest that a lack of FPGS activity may be linked to a loss of 5FU cytotoxicity.[11,12] This possible role of tumoral FPGS as a factor of 5FU resistance was recently confirmed at the clinical level in patients with colorectal cancer treated by 5FU-based chemotherapy.[13]

Chemistry

5FU is uracil in which the hydrogen in position 5 is substituted by a fluorine atom. The molecular weight of 5FU is 130.

Analytical methodology

Unchanged 5FU in biological fluid can be measured by high-pressure liquid chromatography (HPLC) with UV detection after extraction from the biological fluid with an organic solvent. The limit of detection is at about 50 ng/ml. An HPLC method as been recently described which allows the separation and quantification of 5FU and its main metabolites from plasma.[14] Interestingly, concentrations of 5FU and metabolites can be measured in tumoral tissue using ^{19}F NMR spectrometry.[15]

Pharmacokinetics

Absorption

Oral administration of 5FU gives rise to erratic plasma concentrations because of great variability in bioavailability.[16] Because bioavailability increases with higher 5FU doses,[17] one can suspect saturable first-pass metabolism in the liver as the main explanation for the low and variable 5FU bioavailability. The bioavailability and feasibility of subcutaneous 5FU have recently been studied.[18] Patients with advanced cancer received 250 mg 5FU as an infusion over 90 min either intravenously or subcutaneously into the abdominal wall. The mean bioavailability of subcutaneous 5FU was 0.89 ± 0.23. No local side effects were observed. Further work is needed to show the practical and clinical interest of subcutaneous FU infusion. Absorption of 5FU through the intact skin has been reported to be less than 10%.[19] Interestingly, the use of DPD blocking agents, such as *ethynyl uracil*, has altered the bioavailability of oral 5FU, with 100% bioavailability reported.[20]

Distribution

Reports concerning the pharmacokinetics of 5FU in the central nervous system are rare. The plasma and cerebrospinal fluid (CSF) pharmacokinetics of 5FU were examined in a primate model.[21] Following intravenous bolus administration, the AUC ratio between CSF and plasma was 48%. When the duration of administration was extended to 4 h, this ratio reached a value of 10–20%.

Metabolism

More than 80% of an administered dose of 5FU is eliminated in the liver by catabolism through DPD, the rate-limiting enzyme that catabolizes 5FU to dihydrofluorouracil.[22] DPD is a saturable enzyme with a K_m for 5FU of approximately 5 μM.[22] This characteristic explains, to some extent, the non-linearity of 5FU pharmacokinetics during intravenous bolus injections: at conventional doses, 5FU blood concentrations may equal or exceed the K_m value of DPD. After the initial step of 5FU catabolism involving DPD, dihydrofluorouracil is transformed into α-fluoro-β-ureidopropionic acid (FUPA) via dihydropyrimidinase, and then FUPA is transformed into α-fluoro-β-alanine via the β-ureidopropionase.

Elimination

5FU is primarily eliminated through the liver by a saturable metabolic process.[22] 5FU is very rapidly cleared from plasma with an elimination half-life of 15 min. This leads to a non-linear relationship between dosage and circulating drug concentrations. This is evident during bolus intravenous injections where dosage escalations are followed by disproportionate increases in 5FU concentrations. Therefore, from a practical point of view, it is impossible to predict the change in blood concentration after a given dose modification administered as an intravenous bolus. In contrast, when 5FU is administered by continuous venous infusion (CVI) in the usual clinical dose range, 5FU disposition is linear with dose. During 5-day CVI of 5FU with doses ranging from 1.25 to 2.25 g/m^2/day, 5FU clearance remains constant at around 2 l/min/m^2 (Table 5.1) A practical consequence is that during CVI, 5FU blood concentrations can be predicted after a dose

Table 5.1 5FU pharmacokinetic characteristics following intravenous bolus or continuous intravenous administration

Administration schedule	Total body clearance	$T_{1/2}$ (min)	V_d (l/m^2)
Intravenous bolus			
700–1000 mg total dose	0.39–1.47 l/min		
11 mg/kg	0.55–2.67 l/min	11 ± 2	
500 mg/m^2	0.38–1.01 l/min/m^2	13 ± 7	9 ± 4
Continuous intravenous administration			
750–1000 mg (over 8 h)	5.41–57.9 l/min	4–12	
1.25–2.25 g/m^2/day × 5	1.79–2.41 l/min/m^2		
550–1000 mg/m^2/day × 5	0.79–7.77 l/min/m^2		

$T_{1/2}$, half-life of the apparent elimination phase; V_d, apparent volume of distribution.[71]

modification. Accordingly, when given by CVI, individual dose adaptation for targeting an optimal 5FU exposure is feasible.

A circadian rhythm in the plasma clearance of FU was demonstrated in patients receiving the drug as a CVI at a constant rate for 5 days.[23] This circadian rhythm was characterized by a double amplitude (total extent of variation) of 50% of the 24 h mean and an acrophase located at 1 a.m. (estimated time of the peak) The existence of this circadian rhythm was confirmed by Harris *et al.*[24] Interestingly, these authors demonstrated a close association between the *circadian variability of DPD* activity measured in peripheral blood molecular cells and that of FU plasma concentration. Confirmatory evidence of a correlation between 5FU clearance during 5-day CVI and lymphocytic DPD activity was reported by Fleming *et al.*[25]

Interactions

The sustained interest in 5FU can be explained to a great extent by the co-administration of so-called 5FU biochemical modulators which potentiate 5FU through its different routes or metabolism. One can wonder about the possible pharmacokinetic interaction between these so-called modulators and 5FU. There is no evidence for a modification of 5FU disposition when co-administered with *FA*. A dose-dependent decrease in 5FU clearance when α-interferon (α-IFN) is co-administered with 5FU has been reported.[26] Some authors have confirmed the reduction in 5FU clearance produced by the *α-IFN* treatment,[27] whereas others have not found such an effect.[28]

Ethynyluracil (EU, GW 776C85) is a potent mechanism-based irreversible inhibitor of DPD *in vitro* and *in vivo* that improves the efficacy, therapeutic index, and bioavailability of 5FU in preclinical and clinical settings. The pharmacokinetics of 5FU is dramatically modified when it is combined with EU.[29] Bioavailability of 5FU becomes complete, with a mean ± SD of 122 ± 40%. The terminal half-life declines to 4.5 ± 1.6 h and $V_{d\,ss}$ is unchanged at 21.4 l/m². The change in the clearance is most dramatic, declining to 57 ± 16 ml/min/m². In the presence of EU, renal clearance becomes predominant, with a high correlation between 5FU clearance and creatinine clearance. The maximal tolerated dose of 5FU with EU drops to 10 mg/m² twice daily.[20]

Alterations with disease or age

Renal elimination of unchanged 5FU accounts for only 10% of the injected dose; thus renal abnormalities

have, a priori, a minimal effect on 5FU pharmacokinetics. The majority of 5FU elimination occurs via metabolism by DPD in the liver and other tissues.[29] Several authors[30,31] have followed 5FU pharmacokinetics in patients with liver dysfunction, but it was unclear whether 5FU pharmacokinetics were altered and whether these alterations required dose reduction. It is known that the pharmacokinetics of several drugs are modified in patients with poor nutritional status, which is prevalent in cancer patients, especially those who have cancers of the head and neck and of the digestive system. Because the therapeutic range of 5FU is narrow, alteration in its pharmacokinetics caused by poor nutritional status may cause increased toxicity.

The possible influence of hepatic function and nutritional status on the pharmacokinetics of 5FU given by CVI has been studied in 187 patients with head and neck cancer.[32] Weak linear correlations ($r < 0.25$) between log 5FU clearance and the hepatic parameters (AST, ALT, Alk Phos, GGT, LDH, bili) were observed. Likewise, the log 5FU clearance was poorly correlated with the serum concentration of various measures of nutritional status (albumin, prealbumin, transferrin). Because only 12% of patients with *head and neck* cancer develop distant metastases to organs, including the liver, the study group was not particularly well suited to testing the effects of severe liver dysfunction on 5FU disposition. Clearly, additional studies in large groups of advanced colorectal cancer patients with extensive liver metastases are still necessary to determine the influence of liver dysfunction on 5FU pharmacokinetics and pharmacodynamics.

Age and sex are among the factors that have been implicated in the variability of drug disposition. A retrospective analysis was recently performed on a series of 380 patients to investigate the influence of *age and sex* on 5FU clearance.[33] Clearance showed a wide dispersion for both men and women, and was found to be 15% lower in women than in men ($p = 0.0005$) There was no evidence that age (range 25–91 years) modified the 5FU clearance when adjusted for sex and dose. It would be of interest for future studies to know whether the sex-related difference is relevant, by considering both toxicity and tumour response. A preliminary answer has been provided by a recent study showing that older age, female sex, and higher 5FU AUC are associated with lower nadir counts and/or increased mucositis.[34]

DPD determination in blood lymphocytes allows identification of a low proportion (1–3%) of patients at risk of developing more or less severe FU-related toxicity.[22] The practical interest of this routine investigation must be carefully weighed in terms of cost–benefit balance. An indirect approach consisting of plasma uracil : digydrouracil ratio determination seems much more rele-vant for a large-scale identification of DPD-deficient patients. There is not a close link between mutations in the DPD gene and the toxicity to 5FU.

Pharmacodynamics

Bearing in mind that 5FU is a prodrug which needs intracellular activation to exert its effects, an appreciable discrepancy exists between 5FU blood concentrations and effect site concentrations of the active metabolite for tumoral or normal host cells. Theoretically, this renders it difficult to make a direct association between blood drug concentrations and cell toxicity. However, data from the literature have proved the existence of such relationships.[35] Dose adaptation based on 5FU pharmacokinetics has proved to be feasible and clinically useful.[36]

The relationships between 5FU pharmacokinetics and response have been less extensively explored. We studied 186 patients receiving induction chemotherapy, including cisplatin and 5-day CVI of 5FU.[37] The 5FU AUC over the duration of pharmacokinetic follow-up ($AUC_{0-105 h}$) was calculated for each cycle. The averaged $AUC_{0-105 h}$ and the averaged total dose administered for the three cycles was analysed for each patient. Obtaining a tumour response (30% CR, 47% PR) was significantly linked to initial tumour staging ($p < 0.001$) and averaged AUC ($p = 0.05$), but not to averaged dose. Similar observations have been made more recently.[38] Remarkably, the 5FU AUC was a significant predictor for overall survival in a multivariate analysis including tumour staging: the greater the 5FU systemic exposure, the longer the survival. In a study of 34 cases (colorectal, pancreas, and breast carcinoma), a relationship was reported between clinical response and intra-tumoral 5FU pharmacokinetics determined using ^{19}F NMR spectroscopy.[39]

Capecitabine

Clinical use

Capecitabine (Xeloda®) is currently registered for three indications.[40] First, it is indicated for use as monotherapy in the first line of treatment of advanced and metastatic colorectal cancer. Secondly, it is indicated as combination therapy with docetaxel in the treatment of locally advanced or metastatic breast cancer after

failure of previous cytotoxic chemotherapy. The previous treatment should have included an anthracycline. Thirdly, capecitabine is indicated as monotherapy in locally advanced or metastatic breast cancer after failure of a taxane and an anthracycline-containing chemotherapy regimen, or for patients for whom anthracycline therapy is not indicated.[40]

Capecitabine is becoming increasingly popular in oncology. It has rapidly replaced 5FU in a number of indications and combination therapies, as treatment with capecitabine is considered more practical and convenient than intravenous 5FU. In addition, clinical efficacy and survival is equal to 5FU, as has been demonstrated in a number of large clinical trials.[41]

Capecitabine is available in tablets of strength 150 and 500 mg. The recommended dose as monotherapy is 1250 mg/m² twice daily for 14 days. Retreatment is indicated after a week of rest. Capecitabine tablets should be swallowed with water within approximately 30 min after a meal. The recommended dose of capecitabine in *combination with docetaxel*, which is dosed at 75 mg/m² in a 1 h infusion once every 3 weeks, is also 1250 mg/m² twice daily for 14 days. In the combination therapy of capecitabine and docetaxel, treatment should be preceded by dexamethasone according to standard practice for docetaxel treatment.

Dosing of capecitabine is based on the body surface area (BSA), although proof of the usefulness of this practice has never been provided.[41]

Although capecitabine is generally well tolerated, it can induce significant and disabling toxicity. However, this is mostly reversible. Typical signs and symptoms of toxicity include crampy diarrhoea, sometimes with rectal blood loss, nausea, mucositis of the upper gastrointestinal tract, bone marrow suppression, and the hand–foot syndrome. Diarrhoea has been observed in up to 50% of patients, to whom standard antidiarrhoeal treatment (e.g. loperamide) can be given.[40,42]

The hand–foot syndrome, or palmar–plantar erythrodysaesthesia, usually presents with numbness, dysaesthesia, paraesthesia, erythema, and swelling. It can become severe with desquamation, ulceration, and blistering of the hands and/or feet, which has an adverse effect on the patient's daily life activities. Hyperpigmentation of the palms and soles can occur in black patients.[43]

Angina-like chest pain can occasionally occur with capecitabine, as with continuous intravenous 5FU.[44] Other cardiac toxicities, such as arrhythmias and myocardial infarction, are rare events but may complicate capecitabine therapy.

Mechanisms of action

Capecitabine is a pre-prodrug of 5FU and is preferentially converted to 5FU in tumour tissue.[45] Bioactivation of capecitabine to the active metabolite 5FU is a three-step process (Fig. 5.1). As it has been explained for 5FU, inhibition of the enzyme thymidylate synthase is one of the main mechanisms of action of capecitabine. Activation of 5FU in the anabolic pathway blocks the methylation reaction of deoxyuridylic acid to thymidylic acid, which results in interference with the synthesis of DNA. Incorporation of 5FU results in inhibition of RNA and therefore inhibition of protein synthesis.

Mechanisms of resistance

As capecitabine is a pre-prodrug of 5FU, the same mechanisms of resistance that apply to 5FU also apply to capecitabine. The ratio of dihydropyrimidine reductase, which inactivates 5FU in tumour tissue, to DPD, which catabolizes 5FU, seems to be a relevant determinant for antitumour activity in preclinical models. Clinical implications of this observation are not yet clear. In addition, the activation processes of capecitabine to 5FU in patients are subject to wide inter-patient variation, which may at least in theory contribute to clinical drug resistance.

Chemistry

Capecitabine is a fluoropyrimidine carbamate with the chemical name 5'-deoxy-5-fluoro-N-[(pentyloxy)-carbonyl]-cytidine. The molecular formula is $C_{15}H_{22}FN_3O_6$. The molecular weight is 359.55.

Analytical methodology

The measurement of capecitabine and its active and inactive metabolites is a challenging enterprise. HPLC with UV detection and gas chromatography coupled to mass spectrometry (GC–MS) have been used for detec-

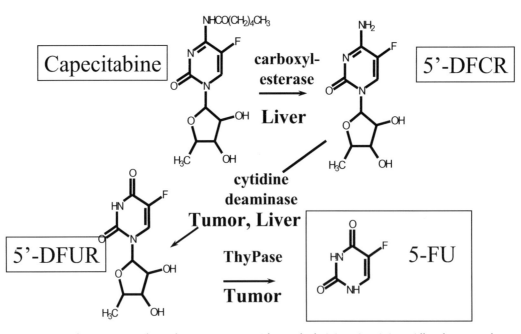

Figure 5.1. Capecitabine is activated in a three-step process. After oral administration, it is rapidly taken up and extensively converted in the liver by carboxylesterase to 5'-deoxy-5-fluorocytidine (5'-DFCR), which is further converted in the liver and in tumour tissue by cytidine deaminase to 5'-deoxy-5-fluorouridine (5'-DFUR). This metabolite is preferentially converted in tumour tissue to 5-fluorouracil (5FU) by thymidine phosphorylase (ThyPase). 5FU is catabolized by dihydropyrimidine dehydrogenase (DPD) to inactive metabolites.

tion. In addition, liquid chromatography coupled to MS has been used for analysis of capecitabine and its metabolites in plasma.[46]

Recently, *in vivo* monitoring of capecitabine metabolism in human liver by [19]fluorine NMR spectroscopy has been described as a useful non-invasive method for the prediction of the activity and toxicity of capecitabine.[47]

Pharmacokinetics

Absorption

After oral administration, capecitabine is rapidly and extensively taken up from the gut and converted to its main metabolites 5'-DFCR and 5'-DFUR.[42,45,48] Systemic 5FU levels are low after capecitabine intake.[45] Intake of food has significant consequences for the oral pharmacokinetics of capecitabine.[49] The before-food versus after-food intake ratios of the maximal plasma concentration (C_{max}) were 2.5 for capecitabine and 1.6 for 5FU. The ratios for the AUCs were 1.5 for capecitabine and 1.1 for 5FU. Although there is a profound effect of food intake on the pharmacokinetics of capecitabine, the effect on the disposition of its main metabolite 5FU seems to be limited. It is recommended that capecitabine is administered shortly after a meal (within ~30 min) as this was the procedure in the clinical trials.[45] After food intake, the time T_{max} to reach the maximal plasma concentration is 1.5 h for capecitabine and 2 h for 5FU.

Oral pharmacokinetics were found to be linear over the dose range studied (502–3514 mg/m²/day). The pharmacokinetics were also linear in preclinical *in vivo* studies in mice, rats, and monkeys.

The absolute bioavailability is estimated to be 40–45%.[50]

Protein binding

In human plasma *in vitro* the protein binding of capecitabine is 54%; that of the metabolites 5'-DFCR, 5'-DFUR, and 5FU is 10%, 62%, and 10%, respectively.[42,45] Binding is mainly to albumin.

Metabolism

After oral uptake, capecitabine is first metabolized to 5'-DFCR in the liver by hepatic carboxylesterase. Subsequently, 5'-DFCR is converted by cytidine deaminase to 5'-DFUR in the liver and in tumour tissue, which is then converted in tumour tissue to 5FU by thymidine phosphorylase. In patients with colorectal cancer treated with capecitabine the ratio of 5FU in tumour to that in normal tissue is 24, whereas the ratio of 5FU in adjacent normal tissue to that in plasma is 9.[42,45] Tumour expression of thymidine phosphorylase was found to be four times higher in colon cancer tissue than in normal colon tissue.

Catalytic inactivation of 5FU to the inactive metabolites dihydro-5FU (FUH2), 5-fluoro-ureidopropionic acid (FUPA) and α-fluoro-β-alanine (FBAL) occurs by DPD.

Elimination

Capecitabine is eliminated largely as metabolites. The terminal half-life of capecitabine is short, of the order of 1 h in plasma.[45,51] The terminal half-life of the metabolites 5'-DFCR, 5'-DFUR, and 5FU in plasma is also of the order of 1 h, or less (see discussion of 5FU above). Excretion of capecitabine and its metabolites proceeds mainly via urine. More than 95% of the dose is recovered in urine and only 3% in faeces. Approximately 3% of the dose is excreted in the urine as the parent drug.[42,45]

Population pharmacokinetic analysis revealed statistically significant effects of gender, BSA and total bilirubin on the plasma clearance of 5'-DFUR. However, this does not have clinical consequences.[51] No clinically relevant differences between Japanese and Caucasian breast cancer patients were found in the pharmacokinetics of capecitabine and its main metabolites.[52]

Interactions

Interactions between capecitabine and a range of other drugs have been reported.

Coumarin-derived anticoagulants
The interaction between capecitabine and the coumarins is clinically its most important interaction with other drugs. The mechanism behind the interaction is inhibition of cytochrome P450 (CYP) isozyme 2C9, which is the main oxidizing enzyme for coumarins in humans. In an interaction study in patients a single dose of capecitabine increased the AUC of S-warfarin by 60% and the international normalized ratio (INR) by 90%.[45] Patients on coumarin therapy should be monitored frequently, or changed to low-molecular-weight heparin anticoagulation therapy during period of treatment with capecitabine.

Phenytoin

Phenytoin plasma levels can increase during treatment with capecitabine. Phenytoin plasma concentrations should be monitored more frequently during capecitabine therapy to prevent intoxications.[40]

Soruvidine and analogs

Lethal interactions between 5FU and the antiviral drug sorivudine have been described.[53,54] The mechanism is inhibition of DPD by sorivudine [1-β-D-arabino-furanosyl-(E)-5-(2-bromovinyl)uracil]. Sorivudine is converted into (E)-5-(2-bromovinyl)uracil by the gut flora. This compound forms a reactive intermediate in the presence of NADPH, which irreversibly inhibits DPD. As capecitabine is converted to 5FU, this interaction may also be clinically significant and therefore should be avoided.[40]

DPD inhibitors

The example of sorivudine illustrates the risks of combination therapy of capecitabine and DPD inhibitors. In an alternative strategy capecitabine has been combined with tumour-activated prodrugs of inhibitors of DPD in an attempt to increase the activity and tumour selectivity of capecitabine.[55] In this preclinical research only slightly elevated levels of 5FU were found, whereas tumour levels of 5FU were substantially increased compared with administration of capecitabine alone.

Alterations with disease or age

The pharmacokinetic parameters of capecitabine and its main metabolites were changed to a clinically relevant extent in patients with mild to moderate liver insufficiency.[50] The absolute bioavailability in patients with mild to moderate liver dysfunction was 62%, whereas it was 42% in patients without liver dysfunction.

Renal impairment has significant consequences for the safety of capecitabine, as has been demonstrated in patients with mild, moderate, and severe renal dysfunction.[56] The patients with moderate and severe renal dysfunction developed severe drug-related serious adverse events (SAEs). In patients with moderate renal dysfunction (creatinine clearance 30–50 ml/min) the dose of capecitabine should be reduced to 75% of the recommended dose in patients without renal dysfunction. Capecitabine should not be used in patients with severe renal dysfunction (creatinine clearance <30 ml/min).[40,49]

In a population pharmacokinetic analysis of a large population of 234 patients with an age range of 27–86 years the pharmacokinetics of 5'-DFUR and 5FU was not affected by age.[51,57] However, wide inter-patient variability in the pharmacokinetics of capecitabine and its metabolites was found. Systemic exposure to capecitabine was poorly predictive for efficacy and toxicity in this large population of colorectal cancer patients. No validated algorithm is available that helps to individualize dosing using significant patient covariates and DPD status. Development of an individualized dosing strategy should be further explored in future clinical trials.

Combination therapy

Capecitabine has been investigated in combination with a range of other anticancer agents, including docetaxel, paclitaxel and cisplatin.[42,58,59] The recommended dose of capecitabine in combination with *docetaxel* is 1250 mg/m^2 twice daily, which is the same as when given as monotherapy. The recommended dose of docetaxel in this combination is 75 mg/m^2. In a phase III trial in metastatic breast cancer pretreated with anthracycline, the combination of capecitabine and docetaxel was found to be superior to docetaxel monotherapy of 100 mg/m^2 in terms of survival and time to progression.[60] However, despite initial reports of good safety, patients often develop severe toxicity, especially bone marrow suppression and hand–foot syndrome.[61]

This is in line with the experience with the combination of capecitabine and *paclitaxel* in patients with advanced *breast cancer*.[59] In this combination the total daily dose of capecitabine was 1650 mg/m^2 for 14 days plus paclitaxel 175 mg/m^2 in a 3-h intravenous infusion every 3 weeks. The dose-limiting toxicities seen were myelosuppression and hand–foot syndrome.[59]

In combination with *cisplatin* in patients with *head and neck cancer*, the advised dose is capecitabine 1000 mg/m^2 twice daily for 14 days and cisplatin 100 mg/m^2 on a three-weekly schedule.[58] The combination was found to be feasible and active.

Pharmacodynamics

Relationships between capecitabine dose and response, or between capecitabine pharmacokinetics, and response are difficult to assess in patients and have not been extensively explored. In preclinical models the expression of the key enzyme *thymidylate synthase* is correlated with 5FU activity and therefore probably also with the activity of capecitabine. In the clinic such relationships are difficult to demonstrate. Population analysis in a large population of patients with colorectal cancer did not show a significant relationship between capecitabine pharmacokinetics and likelihood of clinical activity.[57] In addition, as outlined above, there are no algorithms for adaptive dosing based on demographic or biochemical parameters to protect patients from development of significant toxicity.[57]

Analysis of results of the combined data of 1207 patients from two combined large randomized phase III studies in chemo-naive metastatic colorectal cancer revealed that capecitabine is as effective as bolus 5FU–leucovorin according to the Mayo Clinic regimen.[41] The response rate of capecitabine was significantly higher than with 5FU–leucovorin (26% versus 17%, $p < 0.0002$). However, this did not translate into a longer time to progression or survival.

Cytosine arabinoside (ara-C)

Clinical use

Ara-C is used primarily in combination with anthracyclines for remission induction or for consolidation in acute myelocytic leukaemia. It is also used in combination therapy for large-cell lymphoma and as secondary therapy for childhood acute lymphocytic leukaemia.[62]

Ara-C is commercially available for intravenous, subcutaneous, and intrathecal administrations. Ara-C is available as lyophylisates (100, 500, 1000 and 2000 mg) or intravenous formulations (2% or 5% solutions). Ara-C is highly soluble in aqueous solutions (0.9% NaCl and 5% dextrose). Ara-C is less soluble in alcohol. Ara-C is stable in solution for 48 h at room temperature.

Mechanisms of action

Ara-C acts as an analogue of deoxycytidine and has multiple effects on DNA synthesis. It is not active in the nucleoside form and must be activated into ara-CTP to exert its cytotoxicity. The cytotoxicity of ara-C correlates closely with the level of ara-CTP incorporation into DNA.[2] Ara-C acts primarily against cells in the S-phase.

Mechanisms of resistance

Resistance to ara-C has been studied both experimentally and in patients.[7] Leukaemic blasts were preferentially used for the clinical studies, as this is a clinical material which is more easy to obtain than tumoral biopsies. Most causes of clinical resistance to ara-C concern the mechanisms which can modulate the intracellular level of ara-CTP.[7] Interestingly, it has been proposed that in leukaemic cells the ratio between the deaminase and the kinase may be a determinant factor for the efficacy of ara-C.[63]

Chemistry

The chemical name of ara-C is β-D-arabinofuranosyl-1-amino-4 [1*H*] pyrimidone-2, and it has a molecular weight of 243.

Analytical methodology

Analytical methods for measuring the concentrations of antimetabolites in biological fluids are numerous and HPLC is used in the majority of cases. By using HPLC with UV detection it is possible to quantify both ara-C and ara-U in the same sample;[63] in this case the limit of detection for these compounds is 15 ng/ml. Ara-C concentrations can also be determined by GC–MS with the limit of detection lowered to 1 ng/ml.

Pharmacokinetics

Absorption

Gastrointestinal mucosa and liver tissue contain a high activity of cytidine deaminase which deactivates ara-C. Therefore oral doses of ara-C have a bioequivalence of 0.1–0.3 and the oral route is not clinically used for this anticancer agent.[64]

Distribution

Owing to the high water solubility of ara-C, this drug is rapidly distributed after parenteral administration into a volume equivalent to total body water. The CSF concentration is approximately 10% of plasma concentration.[65]

Metabolism

Ara-C is not active in the nucleoside form and must be activated to its triphosphate anabolite ara-CTP to exert its cytotoxicity. The rate-limiting step in the cascade of activation of ara-C to ara-CTP is dCk, the enzyme that activates the nucleoside to the monophosphate anabolite ara-CMP. The key step in determining the cellular concentrations of ara-CTP lies with the dCk of the target cell. The accumulation of ara-CTP in leukaemic cells is a saturable process, most apparent after high-dose ara-C therapy.[66] Ara-C in plasma or whole blood readily undergoes deamination to ara-U in a reaction that is catalyzed by cytidine deaminase. The enzyme activity is highly expressed in the liver; K_m is in the range $(1.2–1.6) \times 10^{-4}$ M.[64]

Elimination

After intravenous bolus administration, ara-C is rapidly cleared with biphasic elimination; the initial half-life is approximately 12 min and the terminal half-life is around 2 h[67] Ara-U has a half-life of 3–6 h and is excreted predominantly in the urine, with some biliary excretion.[68] Within 24 h, 78% of a bolus dose is excreted in urine (71% as ara-U and 7% as ara-C). During continuous intravenous infusion, steady-state plasma levels of ara-C increase linearly to 5–10 µM and the clearance is around 100 ml/min/m². Thereafter, deamination is saturated and plasma levels can increase unpredictably.

Interactions

Based on experimental models, it has been shown that ara-C has synergistic antitumour activity with other antitumour agents, including alkylating agents, cisplatin, purine analogues, methotrexate, and etoposide.[61] The most frequently used association in the clinic is ara-C combined with *6-thioguanine (6TG)* in the treatment of acute leukaemia. Ara-C, as an inhibitor of DNA synthesis, blocks the incorporation of 6TG into DNA; when ara-C is given 12 h before 6TG, enhanced incorporation of the purine analogue is obtained. There is also evidence that 6TG enhances ara-C incorporation into DNA by blocking repair exonuclease inherent in DNA polymerase.[61]

Alterations with disease or age

On the basis of studies of plasma ratios of ara-U/ara-C, the phenotype for ara-C deamination was analysed and followed in 56 subjects treated with high-dose ara-C.[69] The authors found two phenotypes for ara-C deamination corresponding to a ratio of distribution for 'slow' (ratio <14) and 'fast' (ratio <14) deaminators of 70% and 30%. In a subgroup of 36 patients with leukaemia, the ara-U/ara-C pattern was similar to that observed for all 56 subjects. In these leukaemia patients, a tendency towards a positive response (complete remission plus partial remission) was found in those showing low ara-U/ara-C ratios. The outcome of patients with acute leukaemia showing different phenotypic profiles of deamination needs to be evaluated prospectively.

Pharmacodynamics

There is no correlation between ara-C pharmacokinetics in plasma and ara-CTP pharmacokinetics in circulating leukaemia cells. Most of the pharmacokinetic-pharmacodynamic studies related to ara-C have concentrated on the behaviour of ara-CTP in leukaemia cells. Strong correlations were found between the extent of accumulation and the subsequent retention of ara-CTP by blasts *in vitro* and the duration of clinical response to ara-C treatment.[68] Other investigators also reported strong correlations between the likelihood of achieving complete remission and the ability to accumulate and retain ara-CTP.[70]

References

1. Peters GJ, Schornagel JH, Milano GA (1993) The clinical pharmacokinetics of anti-metabolites. In Workman P, Graham MA (eds) *Cancer Survey. Pharmacokinetics and Cancer Chemotherapy*. Cold Spring Harbor, NY: Cold Spring Harbor Laboratory Press, 123–57.
2. Poon MA, O'Connell MJ, Weiland HS, *et al.* (1991) Biochemical modulation of fluorouracil with leucovorin. Confirmatory evidence of improved therapeutic efficacy in advanced colorectal cancer. *J Clin Oncol*, 9, 1967–72.
3. Grem JL (1996) 5-Fluoropyrimidines. In Chabner BA, Longo, DL (eds) *Cancer Chemotherapy and Biotherapy* (2nd edn). Philadelphia, PA: Lippincott–Raven, 149–211.
4. Aschele C, Sobrero A, Faderan MA, Bertino JR (1992) Novel mechanism(s) of resistance to 5-fluorouracil in human colon cancer (HCT-8) sublines following exposure to two different clinically relevant dose schedules. *Cancer Res*, 52, 1855–64.
5. Peters GS, Laurensse E, Leyra A, *et al.* (1986) Sensitivity of human murine and rat cell to 5-fluorouracil and 5-deoxy-5-fluorouridine in relation to drug-metabolizing enzymes. *Cancer Res*, 46, 20–8.
6. Aiba K, Allegra C, Park J, Chabner B (1990) Multifactorial resistance of 5-fluorouracil in human colon cancer cell lines. *Proc AACR*, 31, 424.
7. Peters GJ, Jansen G (1996) Resistance to antimetabolites. In Schilsky RL, Milano GA, Ratain MJ (eds) *Principles of Antineoplastic Drug Development and Pharmacology*. New York: Marcel Dekker, 543–85.
8. Pestalozzi BC, Peterson HF, Gelber RP, *et al.* (1997) Prognostic importance of thymidylate synthase expression in early breast cancer. *J Clin Oncol*, 15, 1923–31.

9. Beck A, Etienne MC, Cheradame S, *et al.* (1994) A role for dihydropyrimidine dehydrogenase and thymidylate synthase in tumor sensitivity to fluorouracil. *Eur J Cancer*, 30, 1517–22.

10. Etienne MC, Cheradame S, Fischel JL, *et al.* (1995) Response to fluorouracil therapy in cancer patients: the role of tumoral dihydropyrimidine dehydrogenase activity. *J Clin Oncol*, 13, 1663–70.

11. Wang FS, Aschele C, Sobrero A, *et al.* (1993) Decreased folylpolyglutamate synthetase expression: a novel mechanism of fluorouracil resistance. *Cancer Res*, 53, 3677–80.

12. Cheradame S, Etienne MC, Chazal M, *et al.* (1997) Relevance of tumoral folylpolyglutamate synthetase and reduced folates for optimal 5-fluorouracil efficacy: experimental data. *Eur J Cancer*, 33, 950–9.

13. Chazal M, Cheradame S, Formento JL, *et al.* (1997) Decreased folylpolyglutamate synthetase activity in tumors resistant to fluorouracil–folinic acid treatment: clinical data. *Clin Cancer Res*, 3, 553–7.

14. Barberi-Heyob M, Weber B, Merlin JL, *et al.* (1995) Evaluation of plasma 5-fluorouracil nucleoside levels in patients with metastatic cancer: relationships with toxicities. *Cancer Chemother Pharmacol*, 37, 110–16.

15. Wolf W, Presant CA, Sernis KL, *et al.* (1990) Tumor trapping of 5-fluorouracil: *in vivo* ^{19}F NMR spectroscopic pharmacokinetics in tumor-bearing humans and rabbits. *Proc Natl Acad Sci USA*, 87, 492–6.

16. Fraile RJ, Baker LH, Buroker TR, *et al.* (1980) Pharmacokinetics of 5-fluorouracil administered orally, by rapid intravenous and by slow infusion. *Cancer Res*, 40, 2223–8.

17. Almersjo CE, Gustavsson BG, Regardh CG, *et al.* (1980) Pharmacokinetic studies of 5-fluorouracil after oral and intravenous administration in man. *Acta Pharmacol Toxicol*, 46, 329–36.

18. Borner MM, Kneer J, Crevoisier C, *et al.* (1993) Bioavailability and feasibility of subcutaneous 5-fluorouracil. *Br J Cancer*, 68, 537–9.

19. Erlanger M, Martz G, Ott F, *et al.* (1970) Cutaneous absorption and urinary excretion of 6-^{14}C-5-fluorouracil ointment applied to healthy and diseased human skin. *Dermatology*, 140 (Suppl.1), 7–14.

20. Baker SD, Khor SP, Adjei AA, *et al.* (1996) Pharmacokinetic, oral availability, and safety study of 5-fluorouracil in patients treated with 776C85, an inactivator of dihydropyrimidine dehydrogenase. *J Clin Oncol*, 14, 3085–96.

21. Kerr IG, Zimm S, Collins JM, *et al.* (1984) Effect of intravenous dose and schedule on cerebrospinal fluid pharmacokinetics of 5-fluorouracil in the monkey. *Cancer Res*, 44, 4929–32.

22. Milano G, Etienne MC (1994) Potential importance of dihydropyrimidine dehydrogenase in cancer chemotherapy. *Pharmacogenetics*, 4, 301–6.

23. Petit E, Milano G, Levi F, *et al.* (1988) Circadian rhythm—varying plasma concentration of 5-fluorouracil during a five-day continuous venous infusion at a constant rate in cancer patients. *Cancer Res*, 48, 1676–9.

24. Harris BE, Song R, Soong S, *et al.* (1991) Relationship between dihydropyrimidine dehydrogenase activity and plasma 5-fluorouracil with evidence for circadian variation of enzyme activity and plasma drug levels in cancer patients receiving 5-fluorouracil by protracted continuous infusion. *Cancer Res*, 50, 197–201.

25. Fleming RA, Milano G, Thyss A, *et al.* (1992) Correlation between dihydropyrimidine dehydrogenase activity in peripheral mononuclear cells and systemic clearance of fluorouracil in cancer patients. *Cancer Res*, 52, 2899–902.

26. Grem JL, McAtee N, Murphy RF, *et al.* (1991) A pilot study of interferon α-2a in combination with fluorouracil plus high-dose leucovorin in metastatic gastrointestinal carcinoma. *J Clin Oncol*, 9, 1811–20.

27. Danhauser LL, Freinman JL, Gilchrist TL, *et al.* (1993) Phase I and plasma pharmacokinetic study of infusional fluorouracil combined with recombinant interferon α-2b in patients with advanced cancer. *J Clin Oncol*, 11, 751–61.

28. Seymour MT, Patel N, Johnston A, *et al.* (1994) Lack of effect of interferon α-2a upon fluorouracil pharmacokinetics. *Br J Cancer*, 70, 724–8.

29. Naguib FN, El Kouni MH, Cha S (1985) Enzymes of uracil catabolism in normal and neoplastic tissues. *Cancer Res*, 45, 5405–10.

30. Ensminger WD, Rosowsky A, Raso V, *et al.* (1978) A clinical–pharmacological evaluation of hepatic arterial infusions of 5-fluorouracil 2′-deoxyuridine and 5-fluorouracil. *Cancer Res*, 38, 3784–92.

31. Nowakowska-Dulawa, E (1990) Circadian rhythm of 5-fluorouracil and pharmacokinetics and tolerance. *Chronobiologia*, 17, 27–30.

32. Fleming RA, Milano G, Etienne MC, *et al.* (1992) No effect of dose, hepatic function, or nutritional status on 5FU clearance following continuous (5-day), 5-FU infusion. *Br J Cancer*, 66, 668–72.

33. Milano G, Etienne MC, Cassuto-Viguier E, *et al.* (1992) Influence of sex and age on fluorouracil clearance. *J Clin Oncol*, 10, 1171–5.

34. Vokes EE, Ratain MJ, Mick R, *et al.* (1993) Cisplatin, fluorouracil and leucovorin augmented by interferon alfa-2b in head and neck cancer, a clinical and pharmacologic analysis. *J Clin Oncol*, 11, 360–8.

35. Milano G, Etienne MC (1998) 5-Fluorouracil. In Grochow LB, Ames MM (eds) *A Clinican's Guide to Chemotherapy, Pharmacokinetics and Pharmacodynamics*. Baltimore, MD: Williams & Wilkins, 289–300.

36. Santini J, Milano G, Thyss A, Renée N, Viens P, Ayela P (1989) 5FU therapeutic monitoring with dose adjustment leads to an improved therapeutic index in head and neck cancer. *Br J Cancer*, 59, 287–90.

37. Milano G, Etienne MC, Renée N, *et al.* (1994) Relationship between fluorouracil systemic exposure and tumor response and patient survival. *J Clin Oncol*, 12, 1291–5.

38. Vokes EE, Mick R, Kies MS, *et al.* (1996) Pharmacodynamics of fluorouracil-based induction chemotherapy in advanced head and neck cancer. *J Clin Oncol*, 14, 1663–71.

39. Presant CA, Wolf W, Walunch V, *et al.* (1994) Association of intratumoral pharmacokinetics of fluorouracil with clinical response. *Lancet*, 343, 1184–7.

40. http://www.emea.eu.int/index/indexh1.htm. Main index: Xeloda.

41. van Cutsem E, Hoff PM, Harper P, *et al.* (2004) Oral capecitabine vs intravenous 5-fluorouracil and leucovorin: integrated efficacy data and novel analyses from two large, randomised, phase III trials. *Br J Cancer*, **90**, 1190–7.

42. de Bono JS, Twelves CJ (2001) The oral fluorinated pyrimidines. *Invest New Drugs*, **19**, 41–59.

43. Narasimhan P, Narasimhan S, Hitti IF, Rachita M (2004) Serious hand-and-foot syndrome in black patients treated with capecitabine: report of 3 cases and review of the literature. *Cutis*, **73**, 101–6.

44. Kuppens IE, Boot H, Beijnen JH, Schellens JH, Labadie J (2004) Capecitabine induces severe angina-like chest pain. *Ann Intern Med*, **140**, 494–5.

45. Reigner B, Blesch K, Weidekamm E (2001) Clinical pharmacokinetics of capecitabine. *Clin Pharmacokinet*, **40**, 85–104.

46. Xu Y, Grem JL (2003) Liquid chromatography–mass spectrometry method for the analysis of the anti-cancer agent capecitabine and its nucleoside metabolites in human plasma. *J Chromatogr B Biomed Appl*, **783**, 273–85.

47. van Laarhoven HW, Klomp DW, Kamm YJ, Punt CJ, Heerschap A (2003) *In vivo* monitoring of capecitabine metabolism in human liver by 19 fluorine magnetic resonance spectroscopy at 1.5 and 3 Tesla field strength. *Cancer Res*, **63**, 7609–12.

48. Mackean M, Planting A, Twelves C, *et al.* (1998) Phase I and pharmacologic study of intermittent twice-daily oral therapy with capecitabine in patients with advanced and/or metastatic cancer. *J Clin Oncol*, **16**, 2977–85.

49. Reigner B, Verweij J, Dirix L, *et al.* (1998) Effect of food on the pharmacokinetics of capecitabine and its metabolites following oral administration in cancer patients. *Clin Cancer Res*, **4**, 941–8.

50. Twelves C, Glynne-Jones R, Cassidy J, *et al.* (1999) Effect of hepatic dysfunction due to liver metastases on the pharmacokinetics of capecitabine and its metabolites. *Clin Cancer Res*, **5**, 1696–1702.

51. Gieschke R, Reigner B, Blesch KS, Steimer JL (2002) Population pharmacokinetic analysis of the major metabolites of capecitabine. *J Pharmacokinet Pharmacodyn*, **29**, 25–47.

52. Reigner B, Watanabe T, Schuller J, *et al.* (2003) Pharmacokinetics of capecitabine (Xeloda) in Japanese and Caucasian patients with breast cancer. *Cancer Chemother Pharmacol*, **52**, 193–201.

53. Okuda H, Nishiyama T, Ogura Y, *et al.* (1997) Lethal drug interactions of sorivudine, a new antiviral drug, with oral 5-fluorouracil prodrugs. *Drug Metab Dispos*, **25**, 270–3.

54. Beijnen JH, Schellens JHM (2004) Drug interactions in oncology. *Lancet Oncol*, **5**, 689–96.

55. Hattori K, Kohchi Y, Oikawa N, *et al.* (2003) Design and synthesis of the tumour-activated prodrug of dihydropyrimidine dehydrogenase (DPD) inhibitor, RO0094889 for combination therapy with capecitabine. *Bioorg Med Chem Lett*, **13**, 867–72.

56. Poole C, Gardiner J, Twelves C, *et al.* (2002) Effect of renal impairment on the pharmacokinetics and tolerability of capecitabine (Xeloda) in cancer patients. *Cancer Chemother Pharmacol*, **49**, 225–34.

57. Gieschke R, Burger HU, Reigner B, Blesch KS, Steimer JL (2003) Population pharmacokinetics and concentration-effect relationships of capecitabine metabolites in colorectal cancer patients. *Br J Clin Pharmacol*, **55**, 252–63.

58. Pivot X, Chamorey E, Guardiola E, *et al.* (2003) Phase I and pharmacokinetic study of the association of capecitabine–cisplatin in head and neck cancer patients. *Ann Oncol*, **14**, 1578–86.

59. Villalona-Calero MA, Blum JL, Jones SE, *et al.* (2001) A phase I and pharmacologic study of capecitabine and paclitaxel in breast cancer patients. *Ann Oncol*, **12**, 605–14.

60. O'Shaughnessy J, Miles D, Vukelja S, *et al.* (2002) Superior survival with capecitabine plus docetaxel combination therapy in anthracycline-pretreated patients with advanced breast cancer: phase III trial results. *J Clin Oncol*, **20**, 2812–23.

61. Park YH, Ryoo BY, Lee HJ, Kim SA, Chung JH (2003) High incidence of severe hand–foot syndrome during capecitabine–docetaxel combination chemotherapy. *Ann Oncol*, **14**, 1691–2.

62. Chabner BA (1996) Cytidine analogues. In Chabner BA, Longo DL (eds) *Cancer Chemotherapy and Biotherapy* (2nd edn). Philadelphia: Lippincott–Raven, 213–34.

63. Plunkett W, Gandhi V (1992) Pharmacokinetics of arabinosylcytosine. *J Infus Chem*, **2**, 169–76

64. Avramis VI (1998) Cytosine arabinoside (ara-C). Efficacy, cytotoxicity and resistance: biochemical, molecular and clinical aspects. In Grochow LB, Ames MM (eds) *A Clinician's Guide to Chemotherapy, Pharmacokinetics and Pharmacodynamics*. Baltimore, MD: Williams & Wilkins, 209–227

65. Donehower RC, Karp JE, Burke PJ (1986) Pharmacology and toxicity of high-dose cytarabine by 72-hour continuous infusion. *Cancer Treat Rep*, **70**, 1059–64.

66. Plunkett W, Liliemark JO, Adams TM, *et al.* (1987) Saturation of 1-α-D-arabinofuranosylcytosine 5′-triphosphate accumulation in leukemia cells during high-dose 1-α-D-arabinofuranosylcytosine therapy. *Cancer Res*, **47**, 3005–11.

67. Ho DHW, Frei E III (1971) Clinical pharmacology of 1-α-D-arabinofuranosylcytosine. *Clin Pharmacol Ther*, **12**, 944–50.

68. Rustum YM, Riva C, Preisler HD (1987) Pharmacokinetic parameters of 1-α-D-arabinofuranosylcytosine (ara-C) and their relationship to intracellular metabolism of ara-C, toxicity, and response of patients with acute non lymphocytic leukemia treated with conventional and high-dose ara-C. *Semin Oncol*, **14** (Suppl 1), 141–7.

69. Kreis W, Lesser M, Budman DR, *et al.* (1992) Phenotypic analysis of 1-α-D-arabinofuranosylcytosine deamination in patients treated with high doses and correlation with response. *Cancer Chemother Pharmacol*, **30**, 126–30.

70. Estey EH, Keating MJ, McCredie KB, Freireich EJ, Plunkett W (1990) Cellular ARA-CTP pharmacokinetics, response, and karyotype in newly diagnosed acute myelogenous leukemia. *Leukemia*, **4**, 95–9.

6 | *Purine analogs and antifolates*

Jan Liliemark and Curt Peterson

Purine nucleoside analogues

Background

Cladribine

The first report on the synthesis and antileukaemic effect of cladribine [2-chloro-2'-dioxyadenosine (CdA)] (Fig. 6.1) was published in 1972.[1] Owing to the absence of a confirmed patent, the development of the drug for clinical use was very slow. Thanks to the efforts of Dennis Carson and Ernest Beutler at Scripps Clinic, La Jolla, California, cladribine was eventually taken through preclinical and early clinical testing phases.[2-4] Through the Orphan Drug Act, cladribine was licensed as Leustatin® in 1994 and has become an important drugs in the therapeutic armament against lymphoproliferative disorders.[5] The use of cladribine in children was investigated independently at St Jude Children's Hospital, Memphis, Tennessee.[6] Although

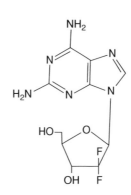

Figure 6.2. Chemical structure of fludarabine (6-amino-9-β-D-arabinofluranosyl-2-fluoro-purine).

the metabolism and mechanism of action of cladribine was elucidated early, the clinical pharmacokinetics have only recently been established.

Fludarabine

The potency and successful introduction of cytarabine as a chemotherapeutic agent triggered the development of purine arabinose analogues. However, the adenosine analogue ara-A (vidarabine) is subject to rapid degradation by adenosine deaminase (ADA) and therefore is not useful. Halogenated analogues are resistant to ADA, and fludarabine (Fig. 6.2) which was first synthesized by Montgomery and coworkers[7]

Clinical use

Cladribine

Cladribine is the drug of choice for the treatment of hairy cell leukaemia.[8,9] It is active against chronic lymphocytic leukaemia[10-13] and low-grade non-Hodgkin's lymphoma,[13-16] particularly the lymphoplasmacytoid type,[13,17,18] although its exact role in the treatment of these diseases is still a matter of some controversy. The use of purine analogues in the treatment of

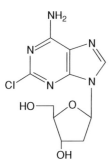

Figure 6.1. Chemical structures of cladribine (CdA; 2-chloro-2-dioxyadenosine) and F-ara-A.

low-grade lymphoproliferative disorders has recently been reviewed.[19] Responses are also seen in acute myelogenous leukaemia in children[20] and in psoriatic arthritis.[21] A randomized double-blind crossover trial showed impressive activity in chronic progressive multiple sclerosis,[22,23] and the role of cladribine in this disease has recently been reviewed.[24] In experimental systems, cladribine potentiates the immunosuppressive effect of cyclosporin A and has a potential in the treatment of transplant rejection.[25,26]

Fludarabine

In phase I trials, complete responses were seen in acute leukaemias at doses > 100 mg/m^2.[27,28] However, neurological side effects were dramatic, and in some cases lethal, and the drug development programme was temporarily abandoned. However, the effect of fludarabine at much lower doses (< 25 mg/m^2 five times daily) in chronic lymphatic leukaemia[29,30] revived interest in the drug. Today fludarabine is one of the most active and well-characterized drugs in the treatment of chronic lymphocytic leukaemia.[31] In first-line treatment it has been shown to be more effective than intensive combination therapies.[32]

The other major indication for fludarabine is follicular lymphoma, where the combination with mitoxantrone and dexamethasone is of particular interest.[33]

The respective roles of the two purine nucleoside analogues in the treatment of lymphoproliferative disorders is still of matter of controversy.[34]

Bioactivation

Both cladribine and fludarabine are phosphorylated to their 5′-monophosphate by deoxycytidine kinase (dCK)[35] Cladribine is also phosphorylated by deoxyguanosine kinase.[36] This enzyme is found in mitochondria and a high activity is present in samples from brain tumours and melanomas;[36] thus it may be of importance with respect to the therapeutic effect in these tumours.[37] However, deoxyguanosine kinase is a mitochondrial enzyme and it is unclear whether the phosphorylation of cladribine in mitochondria induces the same cytotoxic effects as phosphorylation in the cytoplasm by dCK (or in the nucleus as has recently been suggested[38]) dCK phosphorylates a number of nucleoside analogues and is the rate-limiting enzyme in the bioactivation of ara-C and fludarabine. However, cladribine seems to be readily phosphorylated to the monophosphate, and the concentrations of the di- and triphosphate nucleotides are approximately seven and three times lower, respectively, than that of the monophosphate.[6,39,40]

Mechanism of action

Cladribine

In 1992 it was discovered that severe immunodeficiency in some children was due to deficient adenosine deaminase (ADA)[41] Deoxyadenosine accumulates in plasma and *dATP* accumulates in cells with high dCK activity. Such perturbations of the deoxyribonucleotide pools leads to DNA strand breaks, poly(ADP) ribosyl transferase activation, consumption of NAD, ATP depletion, and loss of viability.[42] Cladribine 5′-triphosphate, with similar toxic effects to dATP, accumulates in dCK-rich tissues and therefore treatment with cladribine can mimic ADA deficiency. It is also an inhibitor of ribonucleotide reductase.[43] Therefore, like fludarabine or gemcitabine, cladribine can self-potentiate its effect by decreasing the intracellular concentration of dCTP, the nucleotide which inhibits the phosphorylation of cladribine by dCK and also competes with CdATP for incorporation by DNA polymerase. This is also the mechanism underlying the interaction between cytarabine and cladribine/fludarabine.

It has also been shown that CdA interacts with lipid metabolism and could interfere with synthesis of plasma membrane structures.[44] As the leukaemic cell in hairy cell leukaemia often has pseudopodes ('hairs'), and thus more cell membrane than other lymphatic cells, it could be more vulnerable to inhibition of lipoprotein synthesis. This could explain why hairy cell leukaemia is the most sensitive to cladribine of all tumours. Recently it has been suggested that cladribine also interferes with mitochondrial function.[45] The relevance of this finding to the action of cladribine is as yet unknown.

Fludarabine

The triphosphate of fludarabine is an effective inhibitor of *ribonucleotide reductase*.[43] As with gemcitabine and cladribine, this may provide a self-potentiating effect as it results in a decrease of dCTP which inhibits the phosphorylation of fludarabine to the 5′-monophosphate (the rate-limiting step) and competes with F-araATP for incorporation into DNA.

Fludarabine is a very strong terminator of DNA chain elongation.[46] This may in part be due to the poor affinity of fludarabine for the exonuclease activity of polymerase-epsilon.[47] Consequently, incorporation of the triphosphate has been shown to correlate with the loss of clonogenesity.[46]

Mechanism of resistance

In view of the above discussion, it is not surprising that an impaired activity of dCK has been postulated as the most important mechanism for resistance of cladribine and fludarabine *in vitro*.[48,49] It has been suggested that this impaired activity is due to hypermethylation of the *dCK* gene.[50]

However, it has not been shown clinically that this is an important mechanism for acquired resistance. Furthermore, both *in vitro* studies[49] and clinical observations[51] have indicated that resistance to one purine nucleoside analogue does not confer resistance to the other. The activity of *5'-nucleotidase*, which dephosphorylates the nucleotide metabolites of cladribine, has also been shown to play a role in the clinical resistance towards cladribine.[52] This enzyme seems to be a specific resistance factor for cladribine in contrast with other nucleoside analogues.[53] Therefore mechanisms other than simple deletion of dCK probably play a role in the acquired resistance to fludarabine and cladribine.

Both cladribine and fludarabine induce apoptosis in chronic lymphocytic leukaemia cells *in vitro*.[54] It has been shown that induction of the anti-apoptotic oncogene Bcl-2 *in vitro* confers resistance to nucleoside analogues. However, it could not be shown that there was a relationship between Bcl-2, bax, or p53 expression and sensitivity to fludarabine in cells from patients.[55]

Chemistry
Cladribine

Cladribine is a purine (deoxyadenosine) analogue with a hydrogen substituted for a chlorine at C-2. Cladribine and other C-2-halogenated purines (e.g. fludarabine) are resistant to ADA due to protonation at N-7 instead of N-6,[56] which prevents hydroxylation and deamination at N-6. The molecular weight is 286 Da, the molar extinction coefficient is 15.0×10^{-3} at pH 7.0, pK is 1.8, and the octanol–water partition coefficient is 2.265 (log P = 0.025).[57] The cladribine used in the first clinical trials was synthesized by ribose–deoxyribose substitution using thymidine as the substrate. Today cladribine is produced by variants of

the sodium salt glycosylation procedure first described by Kazimierczuk *et al.*[58]

Fludarabine

Since fludarabine is insoluble in aqueous solutions, it is provided for infusion as its 5'-monophosphate nucleotide, which has a molecular weight of 365.2 Da. However, this molecule is rapidly cleaved by phosphatases in plasma, and within a few minutes of intravenous infusion only the nucleoside is recovered in patients.[59] Thus all pharmacokinetic studies describe the kinetics of the nucleoside.

Analytical methodology
Cladribine

The plasma pharmacokinetics of cladribine has been studied during continuous infusion and after short intravenous infusion, subcutaneous injection, oral administration, and rectal administration. The concentration of cladribine has been determined using liquid chromatography [60,61] and radio-immunoassay.[20,62] Liquid chromatography has the advantage of identifying the catabolite 2-chloroadenine, while radio-immunoassay can be rather more sensitive (detection limits, 1 nm versus 0.2 nM). A high-pressure liquid chromatography–mass spectrometry (HPLC–MS) method has also been used.[63] Although this method is claimed to be sensitive, a validation has never been published. Comparison of pharmacokinetic data for cladribine between investigators is obscured by differences in the extinction coefficient (15.0×10^3 m^{-1})[1,64] (used for determination of the cladribine concentration in standards).[2] In the early clinical and pharmacokinetic studies (before 1993) the extinction coefficient for chloroadenine (12.6×10^3 m^{-1}) was used. Therefore the dose and plasma concentration in these studies were over-estimated by 15%.

Fludarabine

Two methods for the determination of plasma fludarabine concentrations have been presented. Early investigators used a fairly simple and less sensitive method based upon ultrafiltration of plasma and measurement of the free fludarabine concentration in the ultrafiltrates by reversed phase HPLC.[59,63,65,66] The limit of detection was 53 nM. In 1991, Kemena *et al.*[67] developed a solid phase extraction method which measures the total plasma concentration of fludarabine with reversed phase HPLC, with a detection limit of 2 nM.

Intracellular concentrations of the active metabolite *F-ara-ATP* is determined after $HClO_4$ acid extraction using anion-exchange HPLC.[66] The detection limit is approximately 1 µM.

Pharmacokinetics

Cladribine

Oral administration

There are four reports on the oral bioavailability of cladribine.[63,68–70] The oral bioavailability in these trials varies between 37% and 51% when the saline solution for intravenous administration is given to patients to drink.[63,68,69] Thus, when cladibrine is administered orally at about twice the intravenous dose, the AUCs are similar (Fig. 6.3).

When compared with intravenous infusion for 2 h (0.12 mg/kg ≈ 5 mg/m²) the maximum concentration was slightly higher, but the peak was narrower, than after oral administration (0.24 mg/kg ≈ 10 mg/m²) or subcutaneous administration (0.12 mg/kg) (142 nM versus 165 and 268 nM).[69] For some other anti-metabolites (i.e. cytarabine and 6-mercaptopurine[71,72]) bioactivation is impaired when the drug concentrations achieved are above the K_m of the bioactivating enzymes. However, the plasma concentration of cladribine achieved by subcutaneous or oral administration is at least one logarithmic unit lower than the K_m of the dCK.[73] Thus the drug concentrations achieved with a standard dose are far from saturating the bioactivation, which is sometimes a problem with other antimetabolites like cytarabine[72] or 6-mercaptopurine.[71]

The inter-individual variability of the bioavailability is considerable (CV, 28%) but the variability of the AUC after oral administration is no greater than that after intravenous administration (CV, 38% versus 36%).[69]

Cladribine is not stable at low pH (pH <2) However, neither attempts to increase the pH in the stomach with omeprazole before oral administration of cladribine[68] nor the use of enteric-coated capsules[69] have improved the bioavailability significantly. Concomitant food intake slowed and reduced the uptake of cladribine to some extent.[68] However, despite somewhat limited bioavailability, oral administration of cladribine has been used successfully in the treatment of previously untreatable chronic lymphocytic leukaemia[74,75] and psoriatic arthritis.[21]

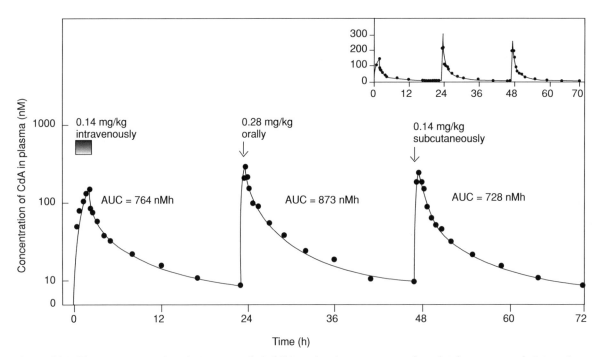

Figure 6.3. Plasma concentration–time curves of cladribine after intravenous, oral, and subcutaneous administration. Reproduced from Liliemark *et al.* (1992) *J Clin Oncol*, **10**, 1514–18.

Subcutaneous administration

Cladribine has no local tissue toxicity, and when given subcutaneously the bioavailability is 100%.[69] Subcutaneously administered cladribine was used in one large trial for the treatment of hairy cell leukaemia. The therapeutic results seem to be equivalent to those obtained after continuous intravenous infusion.[8]

Rectal administration

Based on the impressive improvement of the bioavailability of 6-mercaptopurine with rectal administration compared with oral dosing,[76] an attempt has been made to improve the bioavailability of cladribine by administering it rectally. However, cladribine is degraded by bacterial enzymes and the bioavailability by the rectal route is poor (only 20%).[77]

Protein binding

The protein binding of cladribine is low (<15%) and of no clinical importance.[78]

Distribution

During continuous infusion (5–10 mg/m^2 per 24 h, which corresponds to a dose of 0.12–0.24 mg/kg per 24 h),[79] the concentration of cladribine in plasma is 10–50 nM,[3,20,80] while during a 2 h infusion at a dose of 5 mg/m^2 it is 100–400 nM.[62,80–82] There appears to be a linear dose–concentration relationship for cladribine in this dose range (0.2–2.5 mg/m^2/h), although Marks *et al.*[81,82] report a dose-dependent clearance decreasing from 878–442 ml/min/m^2 with increasing dose to 3.5–10.5 mg/m^2. The plasma elimination follows a two- or three-compartment open model depending on sampling procedure. The terminal half-life $t_{1/2}$ is relatively long (7–19 h).

Fludarabine

All pharmacokinetic studies of fludarabine describe the kinetics of the nucleoside. A number of investigators have studied the plasma pharmacokinetics of fludarabine after intravenous bolus injection, short intravenous infusion, and continuous infusion.[59,65,66,83,84] All the investigators except Kemena *et al.*[84] measured the drug concentration in deproteinized samples; thus only the free unbound fraction was determined.

Protein binding

There are no published data on the degree of protein binding of fludarabine, but one investigator states that <15% of the total drug is lost with the deproteiniza-

tion procedure.[66] Thus data from all these studies can probably be compared.

Oral administration

The oral bioavailability of fludarabine has been studied in dogs and humans. The bioavailability is good in both species, being 78–100% at different doses in dogs[85] and 75% in man.[84] Fludarabine was administered as gelatin capsules to dogs, and the human patients were given the intravenous solution to drink. Studies evaluating the oral bioavailability of fludarabine tablets are ongoing. However, the oral route has not yet been used in therapeutic trials.

Distribution

Most investigators report a biphasic plasma decay curve although some have also detected a short initial distribution phase. In most studies the terminal half-life $t_{1/2}$ of fludarabine is about 10 h Kemena *et al.*[84] report a much longer elimination phase with $t_{1/2} = 33$ h. This difference is probably because their assay was much more sensitive (detection limit of 2 versus 53 nM) and they monitored the plasma concentration for 72 h compared with 24 h in the other investigations. Avramis *et al.*[83] showed that the clearance of fludarabine is much lower in children (0.7 l/h/m^2) than in adults (4–15 l/h/m^2). This is an important finding, although it is not yet confirmed.

Central nervous system penetration

Cladribine

The concentration of cladribine in the cerebrospinal fluid (CSF) is approximately 25% of the plasma concentration at intravenous dose rates between 0.17 and 2.5 mg/m^2/h in patients without known meningeal disease.[37,86,87] The kinetics of the CSF concentration roughly follows that of the plasma kinetics.[87] The CSF concentration increases linearly with dose.[37,87] No data are available on the penetration of cladribine into cerebral tissues. However, several responses have been noted in patients with astrocytomas, indicating that the drug is distributed to the brain, at least when the blood–brain barrier is damaged. Furthermore, cerebral toxicity was noted in patients treated with higher doses of cladribine than commonly used (0.4–0.5 mg/kg daily for 7–14 days).[62] In two papers it has been reported that cladribine can indeed have an effect on meningeal disease when administered intravenously.[88,89] In one patient with a meningeal involvement of Waldenström's macroglobulinemia, the concentration of cladribine in the CSF exceeded that in plasma, which suggests that meningeal involvement increases the penetration of cladribine into the CSF.[88]

Fludarabine

There are no published data on concentrations of fludarabine in the CSF.

Metabolism (catabolism)

Cladribine

2-Chloroadenine (CAde) is the major metabolite in plasma.[90] The higher plasma concentration of this catabolite after oral administration of cladribine (Fig. 6.4) is probably due to degradation of cladribine by gastric acid, and subsequent absorption of the metabolite, or by the hepatic or intestinal first-pass effect. CAde has no cytotoxic or antitumoral effect at the concentrations achieved.

Excretion

About 21–32% of cladribine administered intravenously is excreted unchanged in the urine in the first 24 h,[81,82,90] and the renal clearance is 51% of the total systemic cladribine clearance.[11,86] After oral administration, $(25 \pm 21)\%$ of the dose (corrected for bioavailability) was excreted unchanged in the urine and $(3.8 \pm 1.9)\%$ as CAde. A small amount of CAde is also found in plasma after intravenous administration, and $(1.5 \pm 1.6)\%$ of the dose is excreted renally as CAde in the first 24 h (Lindemalm *et al.*, unpublished data).

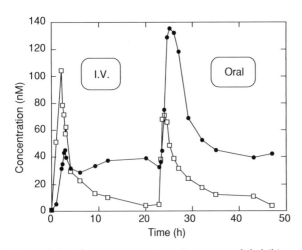

Figure 6.4. Plasma concentration–time curves of cladribine (closed circles) and its metabolite 2-chloroadenine (CAde) (open squares) after intravenous and oral administration of cladribine.

Since most trial protocols require that patients have normal hepatic and renal function, there are few pharmacokinetic or toxicity data on the significance of impaired organ functions. Therefore it is not possible to make any recommendations on dose modifications in such situations.

Pharmacokinetic interaction

Both cladribine and fludarabine interact in a similar fashion with the intracellular bioactivation of ara-C. Pretreatment of patients with cladribine increases the intracellular accumulation of ara-CTP, the active metabolite of cytarabine, by 36–40%,[91,92] and after fludarabine there is an 80% increase.[91–93] This effect might be due to inhibition of ribonucleotide reductase, decreasing deoxyribonucleotide pools, in particular dCTP which is an inhibitor of ara-C (and cladribine) phosphorylation by dCK. Although there are no data, it is likely that other nucleoside analogues which are bioactivated by dCK (e.g. fludarabine and gemcitabine) may be the subject of a similar interaction with cladribine.[91–93]

Alterations with disease or age

A population pharmacokinetic study of 340 cladribine administrations has shown that there is no relation between pharmacokinetic parameters and age, body weight, hepatic function (the majority of patients have no impairment), or age (adult patients between 30 and 87 years). An impaired creatinine clearance did increase the AUC, but only to a limited and clinically unimportant extent (Lindemalm *et al.*, unpublished data).

Pharmacodynamics

Intracellular pharmacokinetics

Cladribine

The intracellular pharmacokinetics of the total cladribine nucleotide pool has been described in hairy cell, chronic lymphocytic, and acute myelogenous leukaemias after intravenous, oral, and subcutaneous administration.[70] The intracellular concentration of the cladribine nucleotides is several hundredfold higher than the plasma concentration of the parent drug (Fig. 6.5). Furthermore, the cladribine nucleotides are well retained in leukaemia cells in patients with chronic lymphocytic leukaemia with a terminal half-life $t_{1/2}$ of around 30 h when the cellular concentration is moni-

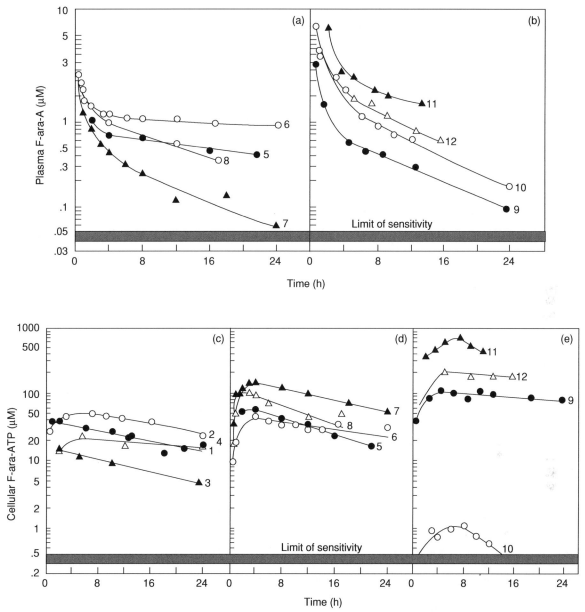

Figure 6.5. Concentration–time curves of cladribine in (a and b) plasma and in (c–e) leukemia tumor cells, showing approximately 100-fold higher levels of cladribine in plasma.

tored for 3–7 days. These data support the use of intermittent administration, which has recently been becoming widely used.[94–96]

However, the retention of cladribine nucleotides *in vivo* in leukaemia cells from patients with acute myelogenous leukaemia appears to be somewhat lower. In the first 24 h after administration the $t_{1/2}$ is 9.0 h in patients with acute myelogenous leukaemia compared

with 12.9 h and 15.1 h in patients with chronic lymphocytic leukaemia and hairy cell leukaemia, respectively.[70] Therefore twice daily administration of cladribine in acute myelogenous leukaemia might be worthwhile.

A new method allowing a specific determination of cladribine mono- and triphosphate in leukaemia cells *in vivo* has recently been developed. Preliminary data show that the kinetics of the mono- and triphosphate are similar. However, the relation between the two intracellular nucleotides seems to vary.[39]

Fludarabine

Fludarabine enters the cell via a facilitated transport mechanism. As discussed above, the active metabolite of fludarabine is its 5′-triphosphate (*F-ara-ATP*) The intracellular phosphorylation to the 5′-monophosphate, which is mediated by dCK, is the rate-limiting step in the bioactivation of fludarabine.

Apparently there is no saturability of the rate-limiting step of the bioactivation of fludarabine at the plasma levels (<10 μM) achieved at the doses currently used.

The pharmacokinetics of F-ara-ATP are very different from the plasma pharmacokinetics of the parent compound. The kinetics of F-ara-ATP has been studied mainly in tumour cells from patients with acute leukaemia, lymphoblastic lymphoma, and chronic lymphocytic leukaemia. There seems to be a monophasic elimination of F-ara-ATP from leukaemia cells and $t_{1/2}$ is very long. In patients with acute leukaemias the median $t_{1/2}$ was 15.0 h with four of 16 patients having a $t_{1/2}$ >24 h.[66] In patients with chronic lymphocytic leukaemia, the rate of elimination of F-ara-ATP from leukaemia cells is even longer (median, 23 h).[97] This difference in the rate of elimination of the nucleotide from leukaemic cells in different diseases seems to be a general phenomenon. Leukaemia cells from patients with chronic lymphocytic leukaemia eliminate ara-CTP,[72] F-ara-ATP,[97] and cladribine nucleotides[70] more slowly than leukaemic cells from patients with acute leukaemias.[66,70,72] These studies indicate that intermittent dosing of fludarabine once daily is sufficient to maintain the intracellular level of F-ara-ATP. Therefore continuous infusion or bolus loading injection is no improvement from a pharmacokinetic point of view. Furthermore, employing such modes of administration in clinical trials has not improved the therapeutic outcome.[98]

Plasma–cell concentration relationship

Cladribine

The inter-individual differences in the intracellular metabolism of cladribine are important since there seems to be no direct relationship between plasma AUC and intracellular cladribine nucleotide AUC. Thus the concentration of the active metabolites on the target site, i.e. the malignant cell, cannot be predicted

from plasma concentrations in the individual patient. In contrast, the intracellular concentration of cladribine nucleotides appears to depend on both the plasma cladribine concentration and the activity of dCK in the leukaemia cells.[99]

Fludarabine

In contrast with cytarabine[100] and cladribine,[99] the amount of F-ara-ATP formed in the leukaemic cells of an individual seems to depend on the plasma levels and time of exposure.[97] However, it is important to emphasize that the inter-individual variability of the cellular pharmacokinetics of F-ara-ATP is pronounced compared with the plasma pharmacokinetics (Fig. 6.3).

Pharmacodynamic relationships

Cladribine

It was recognized early that the action of cladribine is highly schedule dependent.[40,101] Therefore continuous infusion for 7 days was chosen as the preferred mode of administration in the early clinical trials.[2] However, several investigators have shown that intermittent dosing of cladribine works just as well in both hairy cell leukaemia[8] and chronic lymphocytic leukaemia.[11,12]

In vitro data suggest that there is no simple relationship between the formation of cladribine triphosphate intracellularly and antileukaemic effect.[102] Nor is there any correlation between the AUC of the total cladribine nucleotide pool or plasma cladribine concentration and the response to treatment in chronic lymphocytic leukaemia.[99]

On the other hand, a weak ($p = 0.028$) relationship was found between the plasma cladribine area under the curve and the response in hairy cell leukaemia.[8] However, considering the lack of correlation between plasma and cellular drug concentrations mentioned above, this finding needs to be assessed critically and confirmed before its clinical relevance can be determined.

A weak but significant relationship between the activity of dCK in leukaemia cells and response was also found by two independent groups.[52,103]

Thus the available data indicate that there are indeed unknown factor(s) beyond the bioactivation of cladribine which determine the final response and do not allow any conclusions to be drawn at present on the usefulness of the clinical pharmacokinetics for individualization of the treatment. However, the intracellular pharmacokinetics of cladribine provides important information on the effect of route and mode of administration for distribution, bioactivation, and retention of the drug at the site of action—the tumour cell. Thus intracellular pharmacokinetics is an important tool in deciding on routes and intervals of administration in treatment protocols.

Fludarabine

The most important indication for fludarabine is chronic lymphocytic leukaemia. In this disease there is no correlation between the peak concentration, AUC, or $t_{1/2}$ of F-ara-ATP in the leukaemic cells and therapeutic response.[93] The situation is similar for cytarabine,[104] but there is a good correlation between the ara-CTP levels in leukaemic cells in acute leukaemias and the therapeutic response.[105]

Thiopurines

Background

The pioneering work of Hitchings and Elion in the 1950s on the biochemical and biological properties of analogues of natural purine bases, nucleosides, and nucleotides led to the introduction of the thiopurines 6-mercaptopurine (6-MP), 6-thioguanine (6-TG), and azathioprine (AZA) in cancer chemotherapy.[106] In addition, a number of important antiviral drugs were also introduced. The hypoxanthine analogue *allopurinol*, a potent inhibitor of xanthine oxidase, was developed as a by-product. Recent advances in understanding the complicated intracellular metabolism of thiopurines and the interaction of these metabolites with normal cellular biochemical reactions have led to a reappraisal of these old drugs.

Clinical use

6-MP was originally used as a remission-inducing therapy for acute lymphoblastic leukaemia (ALL) in children.[107] Currently, it is a cornerstone in remission maintenance therapy. It is occasionally used in adult lympoblastic leukaemia. 6-TG is a second- or third-line agent in the treatment of acute myeloblastic leukaemia (AML), particularly in the elderly.

The dose of 6-MP in the daily oral long-term maintenance therapy of ALL is of the order of 50–100 mg/m². In AML, 6-TG is used in oral doses of 100–200 mg/m² for periods of 5–10 days. AZA is preferentially used when immunosuppression is the aim of the treatment, for example to prevent rejection after organ transplantation and in autoimmune diseases (e.g. Crohn's

disease, rheumatoid arthritis). The daily dose is 1–4 mg/kg orally.

The mechanistic background to these differences in clinical use is not fully clear. A small study in kidney-transplanted dogs in the early days of organ transplantation proved that AZA prevented rejection slightly better than 6-MP.[108] Randomized clinical studies are currently ongoing in the United Kingdom and Germany to compare the effects of 6-MP and 6-TG in the maintenance therapy of ALL. In the German study,[109] the event-free survival rates in the two arms were equal after a median observation period of 27 months. However, interesting differences in the concentrations of metabolites were found (see below).

Mechanism of action

6-MP and 6-TG have similar effects on cellular biochemistry. They inhibit the purine *de novo* synthesis and they are metabolized to 6-TG nucleotide metabolites, which are incorporated into nucleic acids and interfere with replication, transcription, and possibly also DNA repair. In addition, certain methylated metabolites seem to be of importance via mechanisms that are not yet fully elucidated. The relative contribution of these two major reactions to the cytotoxicity of thiopurines is unclear.

The drugs are metabolized to their respective ribonucleotide monophosphate by hypoxanthine-guanine phosphoribosyl transferase (HGPRT). Thioinosine monophosphate formed from 6-MP is further metabolized to thioguanosine monophophate. The mononucleotides inhibit the first step of the purine *de novo* synthesis, leading to an accumulation of phosphoribosyl pyrophosphate (PRPP), which facilitates the activation of 6-MP and 6-TG by HGPRT. Ribonucleotide reductase converts the ribonucleotide thiopurines to deoxyribonucleotide metabolites, which can be incorporated into DNA. Incorporation of 6-MP and 6-TG correlates with cytotoxicity in experimental systems.[110]

Mechanism of resistance

Biochemical resistance to thiopurines in cell lines results from a defective HGPRT, leading to decreased ability to form active nucleotide metabolites.[111] Interestingly, ongoing studies have shown that a MOLT-4 cell line made resistant to 6-TG is as sensitive as the wild-type cell line to methylated thioinosine monophosphate, but is resistant to other metabolites tested including non-methylated thioinosine monophosphate.[112]

Chemistry

6-MP and 6-TG are analogues of the natural purine bases hypoxanthine and guanine, respectively, in which the keto group on C-6 is replaced by a sulphur atom (Fig. 6.6). AZA is a methyl-nitro-imidazolyl derivative of 6-MP and was designed as a prodrug. The drugs have a low solubility in water and are commercially available only as tablets.

Analytical methodology

Several HPLC methods have been described for determination of thiopurine concentrations in human plasma. However, the plasma half-lives are short (around 1 h) and most methods can only detect the parent drug for 4–6 h following dose intake. For monitoring purposes, methods have been developed to determine concentrations of thiopurine nucleotides in erythrocytes.[113] This level is much more stable than the plasma concentration of the parent drugs.

The activity of the methylating enzyme thiopurine methyltransferase (TPMT) (see below) can be determined by incubating concentrated erythrocytes with 6-MP and a radioactive methyl donor followed by quantitation[114] of the [^{14}C]methyl-6-MP formed. Non-radioactive HPLC methods have also been described.

Pharmacokinetics

All three thiopurines have low and variable oral bioavailability. For 6-MP, a mean value of 16% has been reported at a dose of 75 mg/m^2, with a large inter-individual variability.[115] There is also a large intra-individual variability in plasma concentrations after oral 6-MP.[116] In some studies, food intake reduces the plasma concentrations of 6-MP,[117] but in others no effect was seen on the area under the plasma concentration versus time curve.[118] However, drug intake with food shortened the time to peak concentration. The differences found with regard to the effect of food intake can be explained by the type of food ingested. The plasma half-life of 6-MP is less than 1 h.

6-MP is metabolized by three major pathways (Fig. 6.7). The major catabolic pathway is oxidation by *xanthine oxidase* to form 6-thiouric acid, which is rapidly excreted in the urine. Therefore concomitant administration of *allopurinol*, an inhibitor of xanthine oxidase, requires dose reduction of 6-MP (75%). Another metabolic route is methylation by the polymorphic regulated enzyme *TPMT*, giving 6-methyl-MP and also methylated phosphorylated metabolites. This can be regarded as a mixed catabolic and anabolic route. The physiological function and the endogenous substrate(s) for TPMT have not been identified. The methylated metabolites occur in plasma in much higher concentrations than non-methylated metabolites. The

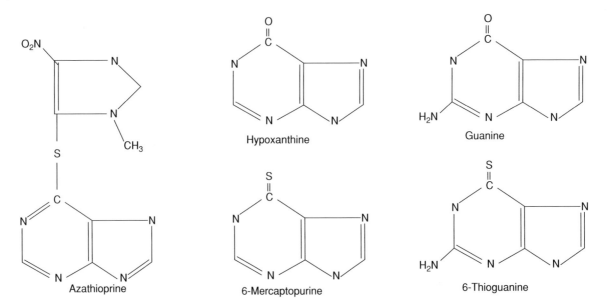

Figure 6.6. Chemical structures of hypoxanthine, guanine, and their thiopurine analogues.

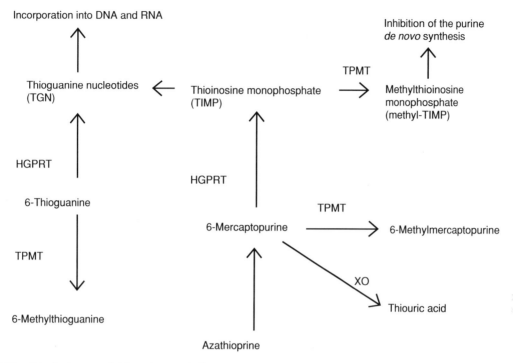

Figure 6.7. Principal routes of thiopurine metabolism.

third major metabolic pathway is intracellular phosphorylation to various nucleotides which can ultimately be incorporated into DNA. A substantial amount of the thiopurines is desulphurated, and part of the ingested sulphur can be recovered as inorganic sulphate in urine.

6-TG is not a substrate for xanthine oxidase but is converted to thioinosine by the enzyme *guanase* and has a higher oral bioavailability (14–46%). Concomitant administration of 6-TG and *allopurinol* does not require dose reduction of 6-TG as is the case for 6-MP. Methylation of 6-TG by TPMT is more extensive than the methylation of 6-MP. At about equitoxic doses of 6-MP (75 mg/m²) and 6-TG (40 mg/m²) the concentrations of thioguanine nucleotides in red blood cells were more than five times higher after 6-TG than after 6-MP.[119] Erb *et al.*[120] found that the concentration of methylated thioguanine nucleotides reached about 40% of that of non-methylated thioguanine nucleotides after 6-TG. In contrast, the methylated thiogunaine nucleotides reached several-fold higher concentrations than non-methylated metabolites after 6-MP.

AZA is non-enzymatically cleaved to 6-MP.

Studies by Weinshilboum[121] and others on red blood cells have shown that 10–15% of Caucasians have low

TPMT activity and that about one in 300 individuals completely lack enzyme activity. The trimodal distribution of TPMT activity is due to genetic polymorphism; the enzyme activity is controlled by a single gene locus with one active wild-type allele and several mutant alleles coding for enzymatically inactive protein. At least four mutant alleles responsible for the low enzyme activity have been identified. There is a substantial inter-individual variability in the group of individuals with high enzyme activity. Figure 6.8 shows the distribution of TPMT activity in 213 healthy Swedish blood donors. Males had a higher activity than females.

There seem to be pronounced ethnic differences in TPMT activity, probably as a result of differences in allele frequencies. Thus, it has been reported that black Americans have a lower TPMT activity than whites.[122] The Saami population in northern Scandinavia has a higher enzyme activity than Caucasians living in the same area.[123] Oriental populations do not show this trimodal distribution.[124]

TPMT activity in erythrocytes correlates with enzyme activity in other tissues such as lymphocytes, kidney and liver.[125]

On thiopurine therapy, there seems to be an induction of TPMT activity since patients with chronic

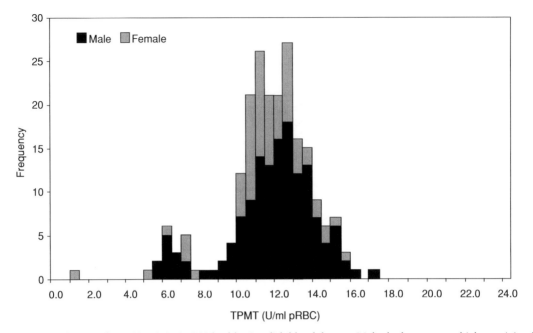

Figure 6.8. Distribution of TPMT activity in 213 healthy Swedish blood donors. Males had on average higher activity than females.

inflammatory bowel disease exhibit about 20% higher enzyme activity than healthy blood donors.

The variability in bioavailability of oral thiopurines may be an important determinant for the therapeutic outcome because low plasma levels of 6-MP have been correlated with a poor outcome in maintenance therapy of ALL of childhood.[126,127]

About 30% of 6-MP is bound to plasma proteins. The drug is well distributed in most organs with the exception of the central nervous system (CNS). However, 6-MP can be detected in the CSF after oral drug intake.[128]

Pharmacodynamics

It is believed that incorporation of the 2′-deoxyribonucleotide triphosphate of 6-TG into DNA, thus interfering with replication, is a common mechanism of action for the thiopurines. Several studies of both 6-MP in maintenance therapy of childhood leukaemia and AZA to prevent rejection after organ transplantation have shown correlations between the concentration of thioguanine nucleotides (mono-, di- and triphosphates together) and clinical outcome.[113]

AZA inhibits T-lymphocyte activity to a greater extent than B-lymphocyte activity. It interferes with the synthesis of interleukins. When AZA yields 6-MP *in vivo*, the imidazolyl group reacts with SH groups on

glutathione and cysteine. Reaction with lymphocyte thiol groups may be important in AZA immunosuppression.

Clinical toxicity

The major dose-related toxicities of 6-MP are myelosuppression and gastrointestinal toxicity. Hepatotoxicity with elevation of plasma transaminases is very common and generally reversible. Bone marrow suppression is dose limiting for 6-TG and gives more pronounced thrombocytopenia than 6-MP by an unknown mechanism.

Methylation of thiopurines can be regarded as a competing pathway to phosphorylation, which would lead to lower nucleotide concentrations. A pronounced toxicity is also seen in individuals lacking TPMT activity. Lennard *et al.*[129] have indeed found an inverse correlation between erythrocyte TPMT activity and nucleotide concentration, but others have not been able to confirm this correlation.[130] However, after large dose reduction in patients homozygous for deficient TPMT activity, so that they tolerate continued treatment, these patients still have higher nucleotide levels than individuals with high TPMT activity.[131] This indicates that certain methylated metabolites are of importance for the cytotoxicity.

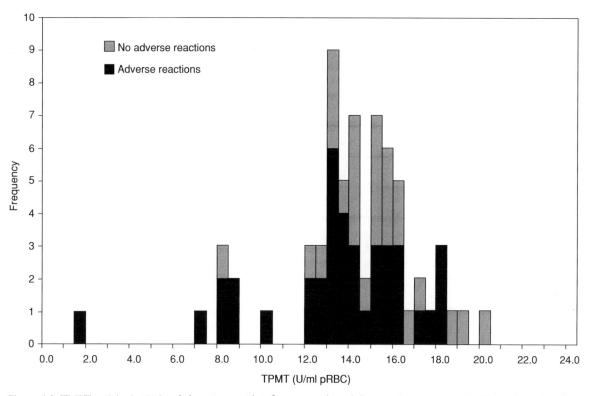

Figure 6.9. TMPT activity in 65 Swedish patients with inflammatory bowel disease who were treated with azathioprine. One patient lacking TPMT activity and six of seven patients heterozygous for TPMT activity had adverse reactions from treatment. Several patients with high TPMT activity also encountered adverse reactions to treatment.

We have studied the TPMT activity in 65 Swedish patients with inflammatory bowel disease who have been treated with AZA. One patient lacking TPMT activity and six of seven patients who were most probably heterozygous with regard to the TPMT locus had adverse reaction from treatment. In addition, several patients with high TPMT activity also had adverse drug reactions (Fig. 6.9).

Antifolates

Background

Antifolates have played a historic role in cancer chemotherapy since 4-amino folic acid (aminopterin) was the first antimetabolite to demonstrate significant activity in patients with malignant diseases. In the late 1940s, temporary remissions were induced in children with ALL.[132] Aminopterin was later replaced by 4-amino-10-methyl folic acid [methopterin or methotrexate (MTX)], which induced the first cures of solid tumours (choriocarcinoma).[133]

Antifolates represent the best characterized and most versatile of all antineoplastic drugs in current clinical use. Originally the effect of MTX was solely attributed to its inhibition of dihydrofolate reductase (DHFR), thus depleting the cellular stores of reduced folates. However, it is now evident that other mechanisms also contribute.[134] The interest in folate antagonism as a mechanism of cancer chemotherapy increased further with the introduction of high-dose regimens followed by the administration of the reduced folate analogue, leucovorin, as a rescue principle. This approach has two potential benefits. One is the circumvention of resistance at a modest level, resistance being a quantitative phenomenon. The second is an improved drug penetration into the CSF, allowing treatment of CNS leukaemia, and other pharmacological sanctuaries (e.g. the testes).

Clinical use

MTX has a broad spectrum of antitumour activity and is used in both hematopoietic malignancies, (e.g. ALLs and Hodgkin's lymphoma) and solid tumours (e.g.

breast cancer, head and neck cancer, and osteosarcomas). In the treatment of osteogenic sarcoma and to consolidate remission of childhood ALL, MTX is given in high-dose regimens of several grams per square metre. Borsi and Moe[135] reported the safe use of a dose of 33.6 g/m^2, provided that careful attention is paid to fluid hydration, urinary alkalinization, and adequate administration of leucovorin guided by monitoring the plasma MTX level.

The schedule for plasma level monitoring is dependent on the treatment regimen. In the current Nordic protocol for childhood ALL, MTX 5 g/m^2 is administered to standard risk patients as an infusion for 24 h.[136] Blood samples for the determination of plasma MTX concentrations are taken 1 h before the end of the infusion (steady-state concentration usually around 100 µM) and then every 6 h starting 36 h after the beginning of the infusion. Leucovorin administration at a dose of 15 mg/m^2 begins 36 h after the start of the MTX infusion and it is given every 6 h until the plasma MTX concentration has fallen below 0.2 µM. The leucovorin dose is increased if the plasma concentration at 42 h exceeds 1 µM.

In other solid tumours, conventional dose therapy of 40–200 mg/m^2 is used in combination chemotherapy protocols. To prevent relapses in the CNS in leukaemias and lymphomas, intra-tecal therapy of MTX 12 mg is used. Weekly oral therapy of 20 mg/m^2 is used in the maintenance of remission in childhood ALL.

In addition, MTX is increasingly being used in autoimmune diseases such as rheumatoid arthritis and severe psoriasis. It is most often used in oral doses of 10–15 mg once weekly, but also as injections. In the past, MTX was only used in arthritis after all other therapeutic alternatives had failed and excessive joint destruction had occurred. A shift of paradigm has now occurred, with the aim of inducing remission by early onset of cytotoxic therapy.

Mechanism of action

Fully reduced folates are important cofactors in single-carbon transfer reactions. One key reaction is the methylation of 2′-deoxyuridylate to thymidylate catalysed by thymidylated synthase. Production of thymidylate is necessary for the formation of DNA. This reaction utilizes 5,10-methylenetetrahydrofolate as the methyl donor and results in the oxidation of the reduced folate to dihydrofolate. This activity creates the requirement for DHFR to maintain the reduced folate pool needed for single-carbon transfer reactions.

Another reduced folate, 10-formyltetrahydrofolate, is used by the enzymes glycinamide ribonucleotide (GAR) transformylase and aminoimidazole carboxamid ribonucleotide (AICAR) transformylase in purine *de novo* synthesis. However, it has been demonstrated that the depletion of intracellular reduced folates is insufficient to account for the observed inhibition of DNA synthesis.[137] Additional metabolic effects of MTX result from its transformation to polyglutamates formed by folylpolyglutamyl synthetase, which adds up to six glutamyl groups. Up to 80% of MTX found in malignant tissues is in the polyglutamated form.[138] MTX is a weak inhibitor of the enzyme thymidylate synthase and the inhibition is increased several hundred times following polyglutamation. Polyglutamation seems to occur to a higher extent in tumour cells than in normal cells.[139] Another mechanism of selectivity could be that tumour cells seem to rely more than normal cells on purine *de novo* synthesis as opposed to salvage.[140]

As with most antimetabolites, MTX is also toxic to normal dividing cells, especially in the bone marrow and the gastrointestinal epithelium. MTX preferentially kills cells in the S phase.

The mechanisms of the anti-inflammatory effect of MTX as used in the treatment of autoimmune diseases remain unclear. MTX has multiple *in vitro* and *in vivo* effects, including inhibitory effects on endothelial cell growth, chemotaxis, polyamine synthesis, and various cytokine activities. In addition, it suppresses the generation of inflammatory mediators such as lipo-oxygenase products.[141]

Mechanism of resistance

Several biochemical mechanisms of resistance to MTX have been shown in cultured cells, including alteration in antifolate transport,[142] reduced capacity to polyglutamate MTX, and alterations in the target enzyme DHFR. Schimke[143] showed that amplification of the DHFR gene is one mechanism of resistance to antifolates. The amplified gene may be integrated into chromosomal DNA as homogenously staining regions, which is associated with stable resistance. Alternatively, amplified genes may exist in extra-chromosomal pieces of DNA known as double-minutes. These are unequally distributed during cell division, and cells eventually revert to a sensitive phenotype. An alternative mechanism is mutations that result in a DHFR protein with a reduced binding affinity to MTX. Decreased thymidylate synthase activity has also been reported as a mechanism of resistance. The clinical relevance of these mechanisms has not been fully elucidated.

To overcome resistance, high doses of MTX with leucovorin rescue may permit entry of MTX into cells with defective transport system and may give high intracellular concentrations to permit inhibition of elevated levels of DHFR.

Chemistry

Various heterocyclic substances with the 2,4-diamino structural configuration inhibit DHFR. They differ in their relative potency to block the enzyme from different species. Agents have been identified that have little effect on the human enzyme, but have strong activity against bacterial (trimethoprim) and parasitic (pyrimethamine) infections. MTX is a strong inhibitor of DHFR in all species.

Analytical methodology

Several methods have been developed to assay plasma MTX during high-dose therapy. Since the concentration is used to guide the dosing of the antidote leucovorin, all clinics giving high-dose therapy are supported by laboratory facilities to give a rapid response using commercially available antibody-based methods. In most treatment programmes, the plasma MTX concentration is followed until it falls below 0.2 μM. The current EMIT kit is not sufficiently sensitive at these levels. Some of the methods are more influenced by cross-reactivity of antibodies to 7-hydroxy-MTX and DAMPA.[144] Laboratories involved in MTX monitoring should have an HPLC method for verification if unexpected results are obtained, as sometimes occurs. One problem is the influence of sample haemolysis, giving elevated concentrations due to leakage of drug stored in erythrocytes.

We have devised a sensitive HPLC method for monitoring plasma MTX during low-dose therapy based on the fluorescence developed by MTX after photolytic cleavage.[145] Using this technique, it is possible to detect plasma MTX and 7-hydroxy-MTX during the entire dose interval after a dose of 15 mg/m² once weekly.

An alternative way of monitoring MTX therapy is to determine the intracellular MTX in red blood cells. Schmiegelow *et al.*[146] have shown that the simultaneous determination of thiopurine nucleotides and MTX in red blood cells from children on oral maintenance therapy for childhood leukaemia predict the outcome of the treatment.

Pharmacokinetics

MTX is readily absorbed from the gastrointestinal tract at the doses used in low-dose therapy. The absorption occurs via an active transport system utilized by dietary folate.[147] With optimal absorption, doses of 20 mg/m² produce peak plasma concentrations of about 1 μM 1–2 h after drug administration. At higher doses, the biovailability is reduced.

After intravenous administration, MTX disappears from the plasma in a triphasic pattern. The initial distribution phase is followed by a second phase with a half-life of 2–3 h, reflecting the renal clearance. The terminal phase reflects release of drug accumulated intracellularly as polyglutamates. Approximately 50% of MTX is bound to plasma proteins. 7-Hydroxy-MTX is the major metabolite, which unexpectedly is less soluble in water than the parent compound, especially at acid pH. Precipitation in the kidneys is potentially toxic if the urine has not been adequately alkalinized. Renal excretion of MTX occurs through a combination of glomerular filtration and tubular secretion. Weak organic acids like non-steroidal anti-inflammatory drugs can delay drug excretion.

Distribution of MTX into body spaces such as the pleural and peritoneal cavities occurs slowly. However, if such spaces are expanded (e.g. by ascites), they may act as storage pools and slowly release the drug, causing prolonged elevation of plasma concentrations.

Pharmacodynamics

The critical determinants of MTX cytotoxicity are drug concentration and duration of cell exposure. MTX can be transported into cells via a high-affinity carrier, referred to as the reduced folate carrier, with affinity constants in the nanomolar range.[148] The affinity of MTX for this carrier is much lower than the affinity of physiological reduced folates. There is also a second mechanism of uptake that operates at high MTX concentrations. This system transports MTX and reduced folates such as leucovorin with affinity constants in the micromolar range.[149] The relative importance of these two mechanisms is unclear.

The major physiological reduced folate in human plasma, 5-methyltetrahydrofolate, circulates with concentrations around 10 nM, which is inadequate to rescue cells. Administration of leucovorin (5-formyltetrahydrofolate) after high-dose MTX can prevent toxicity to the bone marrow and the gastrointestinal epithelium. The competitive nature of this rescue suggests that leucovorin does more than simply restore the intracellular pool of reduced folates. The administration of exogenous thymidine can also decrease MTX toxicity, but it is less effective than leucovorin since it will not restore purine nucleotides. Carboxypeptidase, an enzyme hydrolysing MTX to inactive metabolites, is currently undergoing clinical testing as an alternative form of rescue after high-dose MTX therapy.

Under experimental conditions, there is evidence of a clear concentration–response relationship. The plasma concentrations following high-dose administration in children have been associated with clinical outcome.[150]

Clinical toxicity

The primary toxicities of MTX affect the bone marrow and intestinal epithelium, with risks of bleeding, infections, and severe mucositis. The occurrence of these effects depends on the dose, schedule, and route of administration. Mucositis usually appears within a week after MTX administration and precedes the decrease in blood counts. Mucositis and myelosuppression are usually reversed within 2 weeks.

During high-dose MTX therapy, rapid renal excretion results in high urinary concentration which may cause intratubular precipitation and acute renal failure. This complication can be avoided by vigorous hydration and urinary alkalinization to increase drug solubility. Paradoxically, the 7-hydroxymetabolite is less soluble than the parent compound.

High-dose therapy is commonly associated with acute elevations in serum transaminases and bilirubin, but these usually return to normal within 10 days. Chronic administration of daily oral MTX, as has been used in psoriasis, is associated with hepatic fibrosis in as many as 25% of patients.[151] Cirrhosis of the liver has been described in this group. Weekly MTX, as used in patients with rheumatoid arthritis, is associated with lower incidence of hepatotoxicity.

MTX may cause pneumonitis characterized by fever, cough, and interstitial pulmonary infiltrates. A hypersensitivity reaction has been proposed as an explanation. Rechallenge with MTX does not uniformly result in return of symptoms. No specific therapy for MTX pneumonitis is recommended other than cessation of MTX during the acute episode.

The risk of second malignancy is low, judging from the vast experience of adjuvant therapy in breast cancer. However, there are reports of lymphomas in patients treated with MTX for rheumatoid arthritis. This might indicate that long-term therapy with low doses may lead to a greater risk than short-term intermittent therapy.

Intra tecal administration of MTX may lead to a chemical arachnoiditis characterized by severe headache, nuchal stiffness, vomiting, fever, and infiltration of inflammatory cells in the CSF. Other CNS symptoms may also occur. There is no evidence to support the use of leucovorin in patients developing neurotoxic symptoms.

A reversible defect in spermatogenesis occurs in men treated with high-dose MTX. There are no reports of defective reproductive function in women treated with MTX. MTX does not seem to cause second malignancies.

Novel antifolates

Several new antifolates have been developed in an attempt to overcome some of the mechanisms of resistance to MTX and to target folate-dependent enzymes other than DHFR.

Trimetrexate is more lipid soluble, its cellular uptake is not dependent on the reduced folate carrier system, and it is not polyglutamated. Therefore its intracellular half-life is much shorter than of MTX. It has a clinical role in the treatment of *Pneumocystis carinii*, but does not yet have any defined clinical role in the treatment of malignancies.

Raltitrexed (Tomudex®) is another antifolate which is a potent and specific inhibitor of thymidylate synthase. Like MTX, its cellular uptake is dependent on the reduced folate carrier system and it is highly polyglutamated. The inhibition of thymidylate leads to depletion of dTTP needed for synthesis and repair of DNA. It has shown interesting activity in patients with colorectal cancer.

References

1. Christensen LF, Broom AD, Robins MJ, *et al.* (1972) Synthesis and biochemical activity selected 2,6-disubstituted-(2-deoxy-α- and β-D-erythro-pentofuranosyl) purines. *J Med Chem*, **15**, 735–9.
2. Beutler E (1992) Cladribine. *Lancet*, **340**, 952–6.
3. Carson DA, Wasson DB, Beutler E (1984) Antileukemic and immunosuppressive activity of 2-chloro-2′-deoxyadenosine. *Proc Natl Acad Sci USA*, **81**, 2232–6.
4. Carson DA, Wasson DB, Kaye J, *et al.* (1980) Deoxycytidine kinase-mediated toxicity of deoxyadenosine analogs towards malignant human lymphoblasts *in vitro* and towards murine L1210 leukemia *in vivo*. *Proc Natl Acad Sci USA*, **77**, 6865–9.

5. Bryson H, Sorkin E (1993) Cladribine. A review of its pharmacodynamics, pharmacokinetics and therapeutic potential in the treatment of haematological malignancies. *Drugs*, **46**, 872–94.

6. Santana V, Mirro J, Cherrie H, *et al.* (1991) Phase I clinical trial of 2-chlorodeoxyadenosine in pediatric patients with acute leukemia. *J Clin Oncol*, **9**, 416–22.

7. Montgomery JA, Hewson K (1969) Nucleosides of 2-fluoroadenine. *J Med Chem*, **12**, 498–504.

8. Juliusson G, Heldal D, Hippe E, *et al.* (1995) Subcutaneous injection of 2-chlorodeoxyadenosine for symptomatic hairy cell leukemia. *J Clin Oncol*, **13**, 989–95.

9. Piro LD, Elison DJ, Saven A (1994) The Scripps Clinic experience with 2-chlorodeoxyadenosine in the treatment of hairy cell leukemia. *Leuk Lymphoma*, **14** (Suppl 1), 121–5.

10. Juliusson G, Christiansen I, Mørk-Hansen M, *et al.* (1996) Oral cladribine as primary therapy for patients with B-cell chronic lymphocytic leukemia. *J Clin Oncol*, **14**, 2160–6.

11. Juliusson G, Liliemark J (1996) Long-term survival following cladribine (2-chlorodeoxyadenosine) therapy in previously treated patients with chronic lymphocytic leukemia. *Ann Oncol*, **7**, 373–9.

12. Saven A, Carrera CJ, Carson D, *et al.* (1991) Chlorodeoxyadenosine treatment of refractory chronic lymphocytic leukemia. *Leuk Lymphoma*, **5** (Suppl), 133–8.

13. Saven A, Emanuele S, Kasty M, *et al.* (1995) 2-Chlorodeoxyadenosine activity in patients with untreated, indolent non-Hodgkin's lymphoma. *Blood*, **86**, 1710–16.

14. Kay A, Saven A, Carrera C, *et al.* (1992) 2-Chlorodeoxyadenosine treatment of low-grade lymphomas. *J Clin Oncol*, **10**, 371–7.

15. Liliemark J, Hagberg H, Cavallin-Ståhl E, *et al.* (1994) Cladribine (2-CdA) for early low grade non-Hodgkin's lymphoma (LG-NHL) *Blood*, **84** (Suppl l), 168a.

16. Liliemark J, Porwit A, Juliusson G (1997) Intermittent infusion of cladribine in previously treated patients with low-grade non-Hodgkin's lymphoma. *Leuk Lymphoma*, **25**, 313–8.

17. Piro LD, Petroni G, Barcos M, *et al.* (1995) Bolus infusion 2-chlorodeoxyadenosine (2CdA) as first line therapy of low-grade non-Hodgkin's lymphoma (NHL) *Blood*, **86** (Suppl 1), 274a.

18. Rummel MJ, Chow KU, Hoelzer D, *et al.* (1998) 2-CdA (2-chlorodeoxyadenosine) plus mitoxantrone in the treatment of low-grade non-Hodgkin's lymphomas—preliminary results of a phase-II study. *Blood*, **92** (Suppl 1), 413a.

19. Fidias P, Chabner BA, Grossbard ML (1996) Purine analogs for the treatment of low-grade lymphoproliferative disorders. *Oncologist*, **1**, 125–39.

20. Santana V, Mirro J, Kearns C, *et al.* (1992) 2-Chlorodeoxyadenosine produces a high rate of complete hematologic remissions in relapsed acute myeloid leukemia. *J Clin Oncol*, **10**, 364–70.

21. Eibschutz B, Baird SM, H, W.M., *et al.* (1995) Oral 2-chlorodeoxyadenosine in psoriatic arthritis. A preliminary report. *Arthritis Rheum*, **38**, 1604–9.

22. Beutler E, Sipe JC, Romine JS, *et al.* (1996) The treatment of chronic progressive multiple sclerosis with cladribine. *Proc Natl Acad Sci USA*, **93**, 1716–20.

23. Sipe JC, Romine JS, Koziol JA, *et al.* (1994) Cladribine in treatment of chronic progressive multiple sclerosis. *Lancet*, **334**, 9–13.

24. Langtry HD, Lamb HM (1998) Cladribine: A review of its use in multiple sclerosis. *BioDrugs*, **9**, 419–33.

25. Oberhuber G, Schmid T, Thaler W, *et al.* (1994) 2-Chlorodeoxyadenosine in combination with cyclosporine prevents rejection after allogeneic small bowel transplantation. *Transplantation*, **58**, 743–5.

26. Schmid T, Hechenleitner P, Mark W, *et al.* (1998) 2-Chlorodeoxyadenosine (cladribine) in combination with low-dose cyclosporin prevents rejection after allogeneic heart and liver transplantation in the rat. *Eur Surg Res*, **30**, 61–8.

27. Spriggs DR, Stopa E, Mayer RJ, *et al.* (1986) Fludarabine phosphate (NSC 312878) infusions for the treatment of acute leukemia: phase I and neuropathological study. *Cancer Res*, **46**, 5953–8.

28. Warrel RP, Jr, Berman E (1986) Phase I and II study of fludarabine phosphate in leukemia: therapeutic efficacy with delayed central nervous system toxicity. *J Clin Oncol*, **4**, 774–9.

29. Grever MR, Kopecky KJ, Coltman CA, *et al.* (1988) Fludarabine monophosphate: a potentially useful agent in chronic lymphocytic leukemia. *Nouv Rev Fr Hematol*, **30**, 457–9.

30. Keating MJ, Kantarjian H, Talpaz M, *et al.* (1989) Fludarabine: a new agent with major activity against chronic lymphocytic leukemia. *Blood*, **74**, 19–25.

31. Keating MJ, O'Brien S, Lerner S, *et al.* (1998) Long-term follow-up of patients with chronic lymphocytic leukemia (CLL) receiving fludarabine regimens as initial therapy. *Blood*, **94**, 1165–71.

32. Johnson S, Smith AG, Loffler H, *et al.* (1996) Multicentre prospective randomised trial of fludarabine versus cyclophosphamide, doxorubicin, and prednisone (CAP) for treatment of advanced-stage chronic lymphocytic leukaemia. *Lancet*, **347**, 1432–8.

33. McLaughlin P, Hagemeister FB, Romaguera JE, *et al.* (1996) Fludarabine, mitoxantrone, and dexamethasone: an effective new regimen for indolent lymphoma. *J Clin Oncol*, **14**, 1262–8.

34. Cheson CD (1992) The purine analogs—a therapeutic beauty contest. *J Clin Oncol*, **10**, 352–5.

35. Arner ES, Eriksson S (1995) Mammalian deoxyribonucleoside kinases. *Pharmacol Ther*, **67**, 155–86.

36. Wang L, Karlsson A, Arnér ES, *et al.* (1993) Substrate specificity of mitochondrial 2'-deoxyguanosine kinase. Efficient phosphorylation of 2-chlorodeoxyadenosine. *J Biol Chem*, **268**, 22847–52.

37. Saven A, Kawasaki H, Carrera CJ, *et al.* (1993) 2-Chlorodeoxyadenosine dose escalation in nonhematological malignancies. *J Clin Oncol*, **11**, 671–8.

38. Johansson M, Brismar S, Karlsson A (1997) Human deoxycytidine kinase is located in the cell nucleus. *Proc Natl Acad Sci USA*, **94**, 11941–5.

39. Albertioni F, Juliusson G, Eriksson S, *et al.* (1996) Intracellular pharmacokinetics of cladribine 5'-mono- and triphosphate following oral cladribine in patients with chronic lymphocytic leukemia. *Clin Cancer Res*.

40. Carson DA, Wasson DB, Teatle R, *et al.* (1983) Specific toxicity of 2-chlorodeoxyadenosine towards resting and proliferating human lymphocytes. *Blood*, **62**, 737–43.

41. Giblett ER, Anderson JE, Cohen F, *et al.* (1972) Adenosine-deaminase deficiency in two patients with severe impaired cellular immunity. *Lancet*, **2**, 1067–8.

42. Seto S, Carrera CJ, Kubota M, *et al.* (1985) Mechanism of deoxyadenosine and 2-chlorodeoxyadenosine toxicity to non-dividing human lymphocytes. *J Clin Invest*, **75**, 377–83.

43. Parker WB, Babat AR, Shen J-X, *et al.* (1988) Interaction of 2-halogenated dATP analogs (F, Cl, and Br) with human DNA polymerase, DNA primase, and ribonucleotide reductase. *Mol Pharmacol*, **34**, 485–91.

44. Lechleitner M, Auer B, Zilian U, *et al.* (1994) The immunosuppressive substance 2-chloro-2-deoxyadenosine modulates lipoprotein metabolism in a murine macrophage cell line (P388 cells). *Lipids*, **29**, 627–33.

45. Callasi J, Hentosh P (1997) Mitochondrial effects of 2-chlorodeoxyadenosine. *Proc Am Assoc Cancer Res*, **38**, A4050.

46. Huang P, Chubb S, Plunkett W (1990) Termination of DNA synthesis by 9-β-D-arabinofuranocyl-2-fluoroadenine: a mechanism of cytotoxicity. *J Biol Chem*, **265**, 16617–25.

47. Kamiya K, Huang P, Plunkett W (1996) Inhibition of 3′-5′ exonuclease of human DNA polymerase-epsilon by fludarabine-terminated DNA. *J Biol Chem*, **271**, 19428–35.

48. Albertioni F, Spasokoutskaja T, Pettersson B, *et al.* (1997) Mechanisms of 2-chloro-2′-arabinofluoro-2′deoxyadenosine resistance in a human lymphoid, CCRF-CEM cell line. *Proc Am Soc Cancer Res*, **37**.

49. Lofti K, Liliemark J, Pettersson B, *et al.* (1997) Cross resistance between purine analogs in human lymphoid cell lines, CCRF-CEM cells selected to cladribine and 2-chloro-2′-arabino-fluoro-2′-deoxyadenosine. *Proc Am Soc Cancer Res*, **38**, A686.

50. Leegwater PA, DeAbreau RA, Albertioni F (1998) Analysis of DNA methylation of the 5′ region of the deoxycytidine kinase gene in CCRF-CEM-sensitive and cladribine (CdA)- and 2-chloro-2′-arabino-fluoro-2′-deoxyadenosine (CAFdA)-resistant cells. *Cancer Lett*, **130**, 169–73.

51. Juliusson G, Elmhorn-Rosenborg A, Liliemark J (1992) Complete response to 2-chloro-deoxyadenosine (CdA) in B-cell chronic lymphocytic leukemia resistant to fludarabine. *N Engl J Med*, **327**, 1056–61.

52. Kawasaki H, Carrera CJ, Piro LD, *et al.* (1993) Relationship of deoxycytidine kinase and cytoplasmic 5′-nucleotidase to the chemotherapeutic efficacy of 2-chlorodeoxyadenosine. *Blood*, **81**, 597–601.

53. Schirmer M, Stegmann AP, Geisen F, *et al.* (1998) Lack of cross-resistance with gemcitabine and cytarabine in cladribine-resistant HL60 cells with elevated 5′-nucleotidase activity. *Exp Hematol*, **26**, 1223–8.

54. Robertson LE, Chubb S, Meyn RE, *et al.* (1993) Induction of apoptotic cell death in chronic lymphocytic leukemia by 2-chloro-2′-deoxyadenosine and 9-β-D-arabinosyl-2-fluoroadenine. *Blood*, **81**, 143–50.

55. Thomas A, Reed JC, Kobayashi H, *et al.* (1995) Fludarabine–camptothecin induced apoptosis in B-CLL: relationship of p53 gene mutation, bcl-2 and bax expression in drug resistance. *Proc Am Assoc Cancer Res*, **35**, 22.

56. Kazimierczuk Z, Vilpo J, Seela F (1992) Base-modified nucleosides related to 2-chloro-2′-deoxyadenosine. *Helv Chem Acta*, **75**, 2289–97.

57. Reichelova V, Albertioni F, Liliemark J (1994) Hydrophobicity parameters of 2-chloro-2′-deoxyadenosine and some related analogs and retention in reversed-phase liquid chromatography. *J Chromatogr*, **667**, 37–45.

58. Kazimierczuk Z, Cottam HB, Ravankar GR, *et al.* (1984) Synthesis of 2′-deoxytubercidin, 2′-deoxyadenosin and related 2′-deoxynucleosides via a novel direct stereospecific serum salt glycosylation procedure. *J Am Chem Soc*, **106**, 6379–82.

59. Malspeis L, Grever MR, Staubus AE, *et al.* (1990) Pharmacokinetics of 2-F-ara-A (9-β-D-arabinofuranosyl-2-fluoroadenine) in cancer patients during phase I clinical investigation of fludarabine phosphate. *Semin Oncol*, **17** (Suppl 8), 18–32.

60. Albertioni F, Pettersson B, Reichelovà V, *et al.* (1995) Analysis of 2-chloro-2′-deoxyadenosine in human blood samples and urine by high-performance liquid chromatography using solid-phase extraction. *Ther Drug Monit*, **16**, 413–8.

61. Liliemark J, Pettersson B, Juliusson G (1991) Determination of 2-chloro-2′-deoxyadenosine in human plasma. *Biomed Chromatogr*, **5**, 262–4.

62. Beutler E, Piro LD, Saven A, *et al.* (1991) 2-chlorodeoxyadenosine (2-CdA): a potent chemotherapeutic and immunosuppressive nucleoside. *Leuk Lymphoma*, **5**, 1–8.

63. Saven A, Cheung WK, Smith I, *et al.* (1996) Pharmacokinetic study of oral and bolus intravenous 2-chlorodeoxyadenosine in patients with malignancy. *J Clin Oncol*, **14**, 978–83.

64. Drug Master File for 2-Chloro-2′-deoxyadenosine. Foundation for the Development of Diagnostics and Therapy, Warsaw, 1992.

65. Hersh MR, Kuhn JG, Phillips JL, *et al.* (1986) Pharmacokinetic study of fludarabine phosphate (NSC 312887). *Cancer Chemother Pharmacol*, **17**, 277–280.

66. Danhauser L, Plunkett W, Keating M, *et al.* (1986) 9-β-D-arabinofuranosyl-2-fluoroadenine-5′-monophosphate pharmacokinetics in plasma and tumor cells of patients with relapsed leukemia and lymphoma. *Cancer Chemother Pharmacol*, **18**, 145–52.

67. Kemena A, Keating MJ, Plunkett W (1991) Plasma and cellular bioavailability of oral fludarabine. *Blood*, **78** (Suppl 1), 52a.

68. Albertioni F, Juliusson G, Liliemark J (1993) On the bioavailability of 2-chloro-2′-deoxyadenosine (CdA): the influence of food and omeprazole. *Eur J Clin Pharmacol*, **44**, 579–82.

69. Liliemark J, Albertioni F, Hassan M, *et al.* (1992) On the bioavailability of oral and subcutaneous 2-chloro-2′-deoxyadenosine in humans; alternative routes of administration. *J Clin Oncol*, **10**, 1514–18.

70. Liliemark J, Juliusson G (1995) Cellular pharmacokinetics of 2-chloro-2′-deoxyadenosine nucleotides: Comparison of intermittent and continuous intravenous

infusion and subcutaneous and oral administration in leukemia patients. *Clin Cancer Res*, 1, 385–90.

71. Liliemark J, Pettersson B, Engberg B, *et al.* (1990) On the paradoxically concentration dependant metabolism of 6-mercaptopurine by leukemic cells. *Cancer Res*, 50, 108–12.

72. Plunkett W, Liliemark JO, Adams TM, *et al.* (1987) Saturation of 1-β-D-arabinofuranosylcytosine 5'-triphosphate accumulation in leukemia cells during high-dose 1-β-D -arabinofuranosylcytosine therapy. *Cancer Res*, 47, 3005–11.

73. Eriksson S, Kierdaszuk B, Munch-Petersen B, *et al.* (1991) Comparison of the substrate specificities of human thymidine kinase 1 and 2 and deoxycytidine kinase towards antiviral and cytostatic nucleoside analogs. *Biochem Biophys Res Commun*, 176, 586–92.

74. Juliusson G, Johnson SAN, Christiansen J, *et al.* (1993) Oral 2-chlorodeoxyadenosine (CdA) as primary treatment for symptomatic chronic lymphocytic leukemia (CLL). *Blood* 10 (Suppl 1), 141a.

75. Karlsson K, Strömberg M, Johnson SAN, *et al.* (1996) Three-day three-weekly oral cladribine (2-CdA) for chronic lymphocytic leukemia. A preliminary report from a European phase II multicenter study. *Ann Oncol*, 7 (Suppl 3), 68.

76. Kato Y, Matsushita T, Uchida H, *et al.* (1992) Rectal bioavailability of 6-mercaptopurine in children with acute lymphoblastic leukemia: avoidance of "first pass" metabolism. *Eur J Clin Pharmacol*, 42, 619–22.

77. Liliemark J, Albertioni F, Edlund C, *et al.* (1995) Bioavailability and bacterial degradation of rectally administered 2-chloro-2'-deoxyadenosine. *J Pharm Biomed Anal*, 13, 661–5.

78. Albertioni F, Herngren L, Juliusson G, *et al.* (1994) On the protein binding of 2-chloro-2'-deoxyadenosine (CdA) in patients with leukemia: influence of pH, temperature and concentration. *Eur J Clin Pharmacol*, 46, 563–64.

79. Freireich E, Gehan E, Rall D, *et al.* (1996) Quantitative comparison of toxicity of anticancer agents in mouse, rat, hamster, dog, monkey, and man. *Cancer Chemother Rep*, 50, 219–44.

80. Liliemark J, Juliusson G (1991) On the pharmacokinetics of 2-chloro-2'-deoxyadenosine in humans. *Cancer Res*, 51, 5570–2.

81. Marks RS, Richardson RL, Reid JM, *et al.* (1994) A phase I and pharmacologic study of 2-chlorodeoxyadenosine in patients with chronic myelomonocytic and chronic granulocytic leukemias. *Proc Am Soc Clin Oncol*, 13, 415a.

82. Marks RS, Richardson RL, Reid JM, *et al.* (1994) A phase I and pharmacologic study of 2-chlorodeoxyadenosine in patients with advanced solid tumors. *Proc Am Soc Clin Oncol*, 13, 416a.

83. Avramis V, Champagne J, Sato J, *et al.* (1990) Pharmacology of fludarabine phosphate after a phase I/II trial by a loading bolus and continuous infusion in pediatric patients. *Cancer Res*, 50, 7226–31.

84. Kemena A, Fernandez M, Bauman J, *et al.* (1991) A sensitive fluorescence assay for quantitation of fludarabine and metabololites in biological fluids. *Clin Chim Acta*, 200, 95–106.

85. Malspeis L, Staubus AE, Lyon ME, *et al.* (1989) Oral bioavailability of 2-F-ara-A from fludarabine phosphate capsules in dogs. *Proc Am Assoc Cancer Res*, 30, 534.

86. Kearns CM, Blakley RL, Santana VM, *et al.* (1994) Pharmacokinetics of cladribine (2-chlorodeoxyadenosine) in children with acute leukemia. *Cancer Res*, 54, 1235–9.

87. Liliemark J, Juliusson G (1992) On the pharmacokinetics of 2-chloro-2'-deoxyadenosine (CdA) in cerebrospinal fluid (CSF). *Blood*, 80 (Suppl 1), 471a.

88. Richards AI (1995) Response of meningeal Waldenström's macroglobulinemia to 2-chlorodeoxyadenosine. *J Clin Oncol*, 13, 2476.

89. Santana VM, Hurwitz CA, Blakley RL, *et al.* (1994) Complete hematologic remissions induced by 2-chlorodeoxyadenosine in children with newly diagnosed acute myeloid leukemia. *Blood*, 84, 1237–42.

90. Albertioni F, Hassan M, Silberring J, *et al.* (1995) Kinetics and metabolism of 2-chloro-2'-deoxyadenosine and 2-chloro-2'-arabino-fluoro-2'-deoxyadenosine in the isolated rat liver. *Eur J Drug Metab Pharmacokinet*, 20, 225–32.

91. Gandhi V, Estey E, Keating MJ, *et al.* (1996) Chlorodeoxyadenosine and arabinocylcytosie in patients with acute myelogenous leukemia: pharmacokinetic, pharmacodynamic, and molecular interactions. *Blood*, 87, 256–64.

92. Juliusson G, Liliemark J (1994) 2-Chlorodeoxyadenosine therapy in chronic lymphocytic leukemia. *N Engl J Med*, 330, 1828–9.

93. Gandhi V, Kemena A, Keating MJ, *et al.* (1993) Cellular pharmacology of fludarabine triphosphate in lymphocytic leukemia cells during fludarabine therapy. *Leuk Lymphoma*, 10, 49–56.

94. Maerevoet M, Delannoy A, Ferrant A, *et al.* (1995) 2-Chlorodeoxyadenosine (CDA) therapy in chronic lymphocytic leukemia (CLL) and Waldenström's macroglobuliemia (WD): an update on 77 patients. *Blood*, 86(Suppl 1), 838a.

95. Mulligan SP, Eliadis P, Dale B, *et al.* (1995) 2-Chlorodeoxyadenosine (2-CDA) in previously untreated chronic lymphocytic leukemia (CLL)—preliminary analysis from the Australian leukemia study group trial. *Blood*, 86 (Suppl 1), 349a.

96. von Rohr A, Bacchi M, Fey MF, *et al.* (1995) 2-Chlorodeoxyadenosine (CDA) by subcutaneous bolus injection: a phase II study in hairy cell leukemia (HCL). *Blood*, 86 (Suppl 1), 350a.

97. Gandhi V, Estey E, Keating MJ, *et al.* (1993) Fludarabine potentiates metabolism of cytarabine in patients with acute myelogenous leukemia during therapy. *J Clin Oncol*, 11, 116–24.

98. Puccio CA, Mittelman A, Lichtman SM, *et al.* (1991) A loading dose/continuous infusion schedule of fludarabine phosphate in chronic lymphocytic leukemia. *J Clin Oncol*, 9, 1562–9.

99. Liliemark J, Arnér E, Juliusson G (1994) On the relationship between cladribine (CdA) plasma concentrations, intracellular CdA-nucleotide (CdAN) concentration, deoxycytidine kinase (dCK) and anti-leukemic response

in patients with chronic lymphocytic leukemia. *Proc Am Soc Clin Oncol*, **12**, 308.

100. Liliemark JO, Plunkett W, Dixon DO (1985) Relationship between 1-β-D -arabinofuranosylcytosine in plasma to 1-β-D-arabinofuranocylcytosine 5'-triphosphate levels in leukemic cells during treatment with high-dose 1-β-D-arabinofuranosylcytosine. *Cancer Res*, **45**, 5952–7.

101. Petzer AL, Bilgeri R, Zilian U, *et al.* (1991) Inhibitory effect of 2-chlorodeoxyadenosine on granulocytic, erythroid, and T-lymphocytic colony growth. *Blood*, **78**, 2583–7.

102. Avery TL, Regh JE, Lumm WC, *et al.* (1989) Biochemical pharmacology of 2-chlorodeoxyadenosine in malignant human hematopoietic cell lines and therapeutc effect of 2-bromodeoxyadenosine in drug combinations in mice. *Cancer Res*, **49**, 4972–8.

103. Arnér E, Spasokoutskaja T, Juliusson G, *et al.* (1994) Phosphorylation of 2-chlorodeoxyadenosine (CdA) in extracts of peripheral blood mononuclear cells of leukemic patients. *Br J Haematol*, **87**, 715–18.

104. Robertson LE, Hall R, Keating MJ, *et al.* (1993) High-dose cytosine arabinoside in chronic lymphocytic leukemia: a clinical and pharmacologic analysis. *Leuk Lymphoma*, **10**, 43–8.

105. Plunkett W, Iaconi S, Estey E, *et al.* (1985) Pharmacologically directed ara-C therapy. *Semin Oncol*, **12** (Suppl 1), 20–30.

106. Elion GB (1967) Biochemistry and pharmacology of purine analogs. *Fed. Proc.*, **26**, 898–903.

107. Burchenal JH, Murphy WL, Ellison RR (1953) Clinical evaluation of a new antimetabolite 6-mercaptopurine in the treatment of leukemia and allied diseases. *Blood*, **8**, 965–99.

108. Murray JE, Merrill JP, Harrison JH, *et al.* (1963) Prolonged survival of human kidney homographts by immunosuppressive drug therapy. *N Engl J Med*, **268**, 1315.

109. Janka-Schaub GE, Harms D, Erb N, *et al.* (1996) Randomized comparison of 6-mercaptopurine (MP) versus 6-thgioguanine (TG) in childhood ALL: pharmacology, hematological toxicity, and preliminary clinical results (abstract). *Med Pediatr Oncol*, **27**, 213.

110. Tidd DM, Paterson APP (1974) A biochemical mechanism for the delayed cytotoxic reaction of 6-mercaptopurine. *Cancer Res*, **34**, 738–46.

111. VanDiggelen OP, Donahue TF, Shin SI (1979) Basis for differential sensitivity to 8-azaguanine and 6-thioguanine. *J Cell Physiol*, **98**, 59.

112. Pettersson B, Söderhäll S, Almer S, *et al.* (1999) Role of thiopurine methyltransferase (TPMT) for the cytotoxicity of thiopurines. *Proc AACR*, **40**, abstr 2591.

113. Lennard L, Maddocks J (1983) Assay of 6-thioguanine nucleotide, a major metabolite of azathioprine, 6-mercaptopurine, and thioguanine, in human red blood cells. *J Pharm Pharmacol*, **35**, 15–18.

114. Weinshilboum RM, Sladek SK (1980) Mercaptopurine pharmacogenetics: monogenic inheritance of erythrocyte thiopurine methyltransferaseactivity. *Am J Hum Genet*, **32**, 651–25.

115. Zimm S, Collins JM, Riccardi R (1983) Variable bioavailability of oral mercaptopurine. *N Engl J Med*, **308**, 1005–9.

116. Lafolie P, Hayder S, Björk O, *et al.* (1991) Intraindividual variation in 6-mercaptopurine pharmacokinetics during oral maintenance therapy of children with acute lymphoblastic leukemia. *Eur J Clin Pharmacol*, **40**, 599–601.

117. Riccardi R, Balis F, Ferrasa P, *et al.* (1986) Influence of food intake on bioavailability of oral 6-mercaptopurine in children with acute lymphoblastic leukemia. *Pediatr Hematol Oncol*, **3**, 319–24.

118. Lafolie P, Björk O, Hayder S (1989) Variability of 6-mercaptopurine pharmacokinetics during oral maintenance therapy of children with acute leukemia. *Med Oncol Tumor Pharmacother*, **6**, 259–65.

119. Lancaster DL, Lennard L, Rowland K, *et al.* (1998) Thioguanine versus mercaptopurine for therapy of childhood lymphoblastic leukaemia: a comparison of haematological toxicity and drug metabolite concentrations. *Br J Haematol*, **102**, 439–43.

120. Erb N, Harms DO, Janka-Schaub G (1998) Pharmacokinetics and metabolism of thiopurines in children with acute lymphoblastic leukemia receiving 6-thioguanine versus 6-mercaptopurine. *Cancer Chemother Pharmacol*, **42**, 266–72.

121. Weinshilboum RM (1989) Methyltransferase pharmacogenetics. *Pharmacol Ther*, **43**, 77.

122. Jones CD, Smart C, Titus T, *et al.* (1993) Thiopurine methyltransferase activity in a sample of black subjects in Florida. *Clin Pharmacol Ther*, **53**, 348–53.

123. Klemetsdal B, Tollefsen E, Loennechen T, *et al.* (1992) Interethnic difference in thiopurine methyltransferase activity. *Clin Pharmacol Ther*, **51**, 24–31.

124. Park-Hah JO, Klemetsdal B, Lysaa R, *et al.* (1996) Thiopurine methyltransferase activity in a Korean population sample of children. *Clin Pharmacol Ther*, **60**, 68–74.

125. Szumlanski CL, Honchel R, Scott MC, *et al.* (1992) Human liver thiopurine methyltransferase pharmacogenetics: biochemical properties, liver–erythrocyte correlation and presence of isoenzymes. *Pharmacogenetics*, **2**, 148–59.

126. Hayder S, Lafolie P, Björk O, *et al.* (1989) 6-Mercaptopurine plasma levels in children with acute lymphoblastic leukemia: relationship to relapse risk and myelotoxicity. *Ther Drug Monit*, **11**, 617–22.

127. Koren G, Ferrazini G, Sulh H, *et al.* (1990) Systemic exposure to mercaptopurine as a prognostic factor in acute lymphoblastic leukemia. *N Engl J Med*, **323**, 17.

128. Hayder S, Lafolie P, Björk O, *et al.* (1988) 6-Mercaptopurine in cerebrospinal fluid during oral maintenance therapy of children with acute lymphoblastic leukemia. *Med Oncol Tumor Pharmacother*, **5**, 187–9.

129. Lennard L, Lilleyman JS, Loon JAV, *et al.* (1991) Genetic variation in response to 6-mercaptopurine for childhood acute lymphoblastic leukemia. *Lancet*, **336**, 225.

130. Bostrom B, Erdman G (1991) Cellular pharmacology of 6-mercaptopurine in acute lymphocytic leukemia. *Am J Pediatr Hematol Oncol*, **15**, 80.

131. Evans WE, Horner M, Chu YQ, *et al.* (1991) Altered mercaptopurine metabolism, toxic effects, and dosage requirement in a thiopurine methyltransferase-deficient child with acute lymphoblastic leukemia. *J Pediatr*, **119**, 985–9.

132. Farber S, Diamond LK, Mercer RD, *et al.* (1948) Temporary remissions in acute leukemia in children produced by folic antagonist 4-amethopteroylglutamic acid (aminopterin). *N Engl J Med*, **238**, 787–93.

133. Hertz R (1963) Folic acid antagonists: effects on the cell and the patient. Clinical staff conference at N.I.H. *Ann Intern Med*, **59**, 931–56.

134. Chabner BA, Allegra CJ, Curt GA, *et al.* (1985) Polyglutamation of methotrexate. Is methotrexate a prodrug? *J Clin Invest*, **76**, 907–12.

135. Borsi JD, Moe PJ (1987) A comparative study on the pharmacokinetics of methotrexate in a dose range of 0.5 to 33.6 g/m^2 in children with acute lymphoblastic leukemia. *Cancer*, **60**, 5–13.

136. Gustafsson G, Kreuger A, Clausen N, *et al.* (1998) Intensified treatment of acute childhood lymphoblastic leukemia has improved prognosis, especially in non-high-risk patients: the Nordic experience of 2648 patients diagnosed between 1981 and 1996. Nordic Society of Paediatric Haematology and Oncology. *Acta Paediatr*, **87**, 1151–61.

137. Chu E, Drake JC, Boarman D, *et al.* (1980) Mechanism of thymidylate synthase inhibition by methotrexate in human neoplastic cell lines and normal human myeloid progenitor cells. *J Biol Chem*, **265**, 8470–8.

138. Winick NJ, Kamen BA, Balis FM, *et al.* (1987) Folate and methotrexate polyglutamate tissue levels in rhesus monkeys following chronic low-dose methotrexate. *Cancer Drug Deliv*, **4.**, 25–31.

139. Poser RG, Sirotnak FM, Chello PL (1981) Differential synthesis of methotrexate polyglutamates in normal proliferative and neoplastic mouse tissues *in vivo*. *Cancer Res*, **41**, 441–6.

140. Jackson RC (1987) Unresolved issues in the biochemical pharmacology of antifolates. *NCI Monogr*, **5**, 9–15.

141. Kremer JM (1994) The mechanism of action of methotrexate in rheumatoid arthritis. The search continues. *J Rheumatol*, **21**, 1–5.

142. Assaref YG, Schimke RT (1987) Identification of methotrexate transport deficiency in mammalian cells using fluoresceinated methotrexate and flow cytometry. *Proc Natl Acad Sci USA*, **84**, 7154–8.

143. Schimke RT (1984) Gene amplification, drug resistance and cancer. *Cancer Res*, **44**, 1735–42.

144. Albertioni F, Rask C, Eksborg S, *et al.* (1996) Evaluation of clinical assays for measuring high-dose methotrexate in plasma. *Clin Chem*, **42**, 39–44.

145. Albertioni F, Pettersson B, Beck O, *et al.* (1995) Simultaneous quantitation of methotrexate and its two main metabolites in biological fluids by a novel solid-phase extraction procedure using high-performance liquid chromatography. *J Chromatogr B Biomed Appl*, **665**, 163–70.

146. Schmiegelow K, Schroder H, Gustafsson G, *et al.* (1995) Risk of relapse in childhood acute lymphoblastic leukemia is related to RBC methotrexate and mercaptopurine metabolites during maintenance chemotherapy. Nordic Society of Paediatric Haematology and Oncology. *J Clin Oncol*, **13**, 345–51.

147. Chungi VS, Bourne DWA, Dittert LW (1978) Drug absorption. VIII. Kinetics of gastrointestinal absorption of methotrexate. *J Pharm Sci*, **67**, 560–1.

148. Elwood PC (1989) Molecular cloning and characterization of the human folate binding protein cDNA from placenta and malignant tissue culture (KB) cells. *J Biol Chem*, **264**, 14893–901.

149. Allegra CJ (1996) In Chabner BA, Longo, DL (eds) *Cancer Chemotherapy and Biotherapy: Principles and Practice*. Philadelphia, PA: Lippincott–Raven, 109.

150. Evans WE, Relling MV, Rodman JH, *et al.* (1998) Conventional compared with individualized chemotherapy for childhood acute lymphoblastic leukemia. *N Engl J Med*, **338**, 499–505.

151. Zachariae H, Kragballe K, Sogaard H (1980) Methotrexate-induced cirrhosis. *Br J Dermatol*, **102**, 407.

7 | *Alkylating agents*

Alan V. Boddy

Introduction

Alkylating agents were among the first drugs to be used to treat malignant disease and form a major component of many regimens employed against both haematological and solid tumours. Their common mechanism of action is the formation of covalent adducts with the nucleotides of DNA. Subsequent processing or repair of these lesions leads to single- or double-strand breaks in the DNA and subsequently to cell death. The phar-

Summary

	Cyclophosphamide	Ifosfamide	Melphalan	Nitrosoureas
Brand names	Cytoxan, Endoxan	Holoxan, Mitoxana	Alkeran	CCNU, BiCnu
Other names	Cytoxan, NSC-26271	Isophosphamide, NSC-109724	NSC-8806, CB-3025, PAM	Lomustine (CCNU, NSC79037), Carmustine (BCNU, NSC-409962)
Molecular weight (Da)	261.1	261.1	305.2	233.7, 214
Mechanism of action	Alkylation and cross-linking of DNA	Alkylation and cross-linking of DNA	Alkylation and cross-linking of DNA	Alkylation of DNA
Cell-cycle specificity	None	None	None	None
Route of administration	IV and oral	IV and oral (but associated with higher toxicity)	Oral, sometimes IV	Oral (CCNU) or IV (BCNU)
Protein binding (%)	20	20	≥50	Unknown
Metabolism	Activating and inactivating pathways, involve CYP3A4 and CYP2B6; autoinduction	Activating and inactivating pathways, involve CYP3A4; Autoinduction	Spontaneous hydrolysis	Rapid; possible active metabolites
Elimination	Renal, minor route	Renal, minor route	Renal, ~10%	Mostly as metabolites
Terminal half-life	2–4 h	4–8 h	40–120 min	0.4–4.3 h (BCNU)
Toxicities	Haematological, cardiac, mucositis	Nephrotoxicity and encephalopathy	Haematological	Haematological, pulmonary fibrosis
Unique features	Prodrug, requires activation	Prodrug, requires activation	Analogue of phenyl alanine, substrate for specific amino acid uptake	Cumulative toxicity, crosses BBB

	Busulphan	Chlorambucil	Thiotepa	Temozolomide
Brand names	Myleran, Myelosan	Leukeran		Temodal
Other names	NSC-750, WR-19508	NSC-3088	NSC-6396, WR-45312	CCRG81045, M&B-39831, NSC-363856, SCH-52365
Molecular weight (Da)	246.3	304.2	189.2	194.2
Mechanism of action	Alkylation and cross-linking of DNA	Alkylation and cross-linking of DNA	Alkylation and cross-linking of DNA	Mono-alkylation of DNA
Cell-cycle specificity	None	None	None	None
Route of administration	Oral	Oral	IV or intravesicular instillation	Oral
Protein binding (%)	Unknown	98%	10%	Unknown
Metabolism	Rapid, autoinduction	Rapid to active phenyl-acetic acid mustard (PAA)	Rapid to possible active metabolite TEPA	Spontaneous breakdown to active MTIC
Elimination	Mostly as metabolites	<1% in urine	Mostly as metabolites	Renal?
Terminal half-life	2–3 h	1 – 1.5 h (PAA, 2–2.5 h)	2 h (10 h for TEPA)	1.8 h
Toxicities	Haematological; pulmonary fibrosis; hepatic veno-occlusive disease; neurological	Progressive and irreversible haemato-logical toxicity; also gastrointestinal and neurotoxicity	Haematological	Haematological
Unique features		Irreversible toxicity	Toxicity specific to bone marrow	Monofunctional

macologies of the various alkylating agents are relatively complex in that many require some chemical modification *in vivo* to form reactive species. The mechanisms underlying these modifications, the nature of the nucleotide binding, and the consequent mechanisms of cell death differ widely amongst these agents, as will be described in this chapter.

Recent interest in chemotherapy with alkylating agents has focused on two areas: high-dose chemotherapy (HDC) and overcoming resistance. Alkylating agents are good candidates for HDC in that they have a steep dose–response curve and relatively little non-haematological toxicity. The rapid elimination of most alkylating agents also makes them suitable for use prior to bone marrow or stem cell transplant. However, large doses of any chemotherapeutic agent, particularly those with complex metabolic pathways, pose new pharmacological questions. The field of resistance modification has centred mainly on inhibition of cellular inactivation and inhibition of DNA repair for the monofunctional alkylating agents.

Given the disparate nature of the alkylating chemotherapeutic agents, the pharmacology of each class of agent can be considered separately.

Cyclophosphamide and ifosfamide

Introduction

The oxazaphosphorines cyclophosphamide (CP) and ifosfamide (IFO) were among the first alkylating agents to be used therapeutically. Originally designed to exploit a postulated abundance of phosphoramidase enzymes in tumours compared with normal tissue, CP was thought to deliver nitrogen mustard selectively to malignant cells.[1] Although oxazaphosphorines do act as prodrugs, the exact pharmacological route to DNA alkylation is more complex and there is still some controversy as to the exact sequence of events.

Although CP and IFO have a spectrum of toxicities,[2] with interesting differences between the two agents, they continue to be widely used, with recent interest focusing on the use of high-dose CP followed by autologous haematological support.

Other oxazaphosphorines have been investigated, but the clinical use of these agents is as yet limited. These include trophosphamide, mafosfamide, and the activated 4-hydroperoxy form of CP.

Clinical use

The clinical use of the oxazaphosphorines includes both adult and paediatric tumours, and both haematological and non-haematological disease. CP is a component of regimens used for the treatment of breast and ovarian cancer, sarcomas, and lymphomas. One of the most common clinical applications of CP has been in the CMF adjuvant regimen for the treatment of breast cancer,[3] where it has been shown to be a key component. Ifosfamide has a similar spectrum of use, but in adult tumours is less common in first-line treatment. In paediatric malignancy, both CP and IFO are used in multicycle regimens, usually in conjunction with other agents. Combination regimens including CP or IFO usually also comprise a topo-isomerase inhibitor, vinca alkaloid, or other agent.

CP is employed in high-dose regimens for two purposes:[4] first, as a mobilizer of peripheral blood progenitor cells and, secondly, at higher doses as a bone marrow ablative.

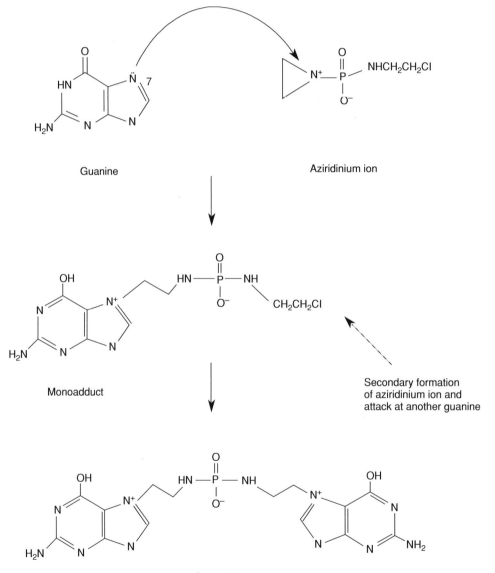

Figure 7.1. Mechanism of alkylation guanine by isophosphoramide mustard, the active metabolite of ifosfamide.

In antineoplastic therapy, both CP and IFO are usually administered intravenously dissolved in either dextrose 5% or NaCl 0.9%. A short infusion or bolus is often used and there is little clinical evidence for any benefit from more prolonged administration. Both drugs have been administered orally and both have high bioavailability.[5,6] However, oral administration of IFO is associated with a higher incidence of neurotoxicity, possibly due to first-pass metabolism.[7] Oral dosing of CP is mostly confined to its use as an immunosuppressive agent and some adjuvant breast cancer regimens.

IFO, and CP at high doses, must be given with the uroprotective agent *Mesna*. This prevents haemorrhagic cystitis, thought to be due to the toxic metabolites acrolein and chloroacetaldehyde. Mesna is usually given intravenously, but an oral formulation is also available.

Mechanism of action

Both CP and IFO form bifunctional *DNA adducts* through the action of their mustard metabolites (see below). Reaction occurs predominantly at the N-7 of guanine via formation of a reactive aziridinium intermediate (Fig. 7.1). The reaction of the second arm of the mustard leads to cross-links, with the differing configurations of the two mustards resulting in slightly different ranges of cross-linking. Subsequent processing or repair of these lesions is thought to result in cytotoxicity, although the exact mechanism is not known.

Mechanisms of resistance

Because of the need for metabolic activation, and the potential for metabolic inactivation, oxazaphosphorines have a number of possible mechanisms for resistance.[8] While these have been described in preclinical models, relatively little evidence exists for their clinical relevance.

As reactive alkylating species, oxazaphosphorines are able to form conjugates with other nucleophilic species such as glutathione. A number of cell lines have been described which have elevated glutathione or glutathione-*S*-transferase (GST) activity and are resistant to oxazaphosphorines.[9] However, the relevance of these observations for clinical resistance is unclear.

The inactivation of activated oxazaphosphorine intermediates by aldehyde dehydrogenase (ALDH) enzymes has been described[10] and may be a mechanism of clinical resistance.[11] The expression of ALDH isoforms in erythrocytes and in tumours may lead to either systemic or intratumoral inactivation.

Analytical methodology

Because oxazaphosphorines are prodrugs, analytical methods for the determination of parent drug do not provide information on the active species. Gas chromatography is probably the easiest and most sensitive method for the measurement of parent drug and of dechloroethylated and keto metabolites,[12] although high-pressure liquid chromatography (HPLC) may also be employed for parent drug at clinically relevant concentrations.[13]

Assay methods for the more relevant active metabolites have been described, but these species are unstable and so often require complex derivatization.[14] The relevance of systemic concentrations of the active metabolites is questionable.

Pharmacokinetics

When administered intravenously CP and IFO have half-lives of 4–6 h,[14,15] with clearance values reported to be 5.4 l/h for CP[15] and a lower value of 2.5–4 l/h for IFO.[15] The volume of distribution is hard to estimate due to the complex pharmacokinetics of these drugs, but is generally around 0.6 l/kg.[14,15] The majority of elimination is by metabolism, with less than 20% of a dose eliminated unchanged in the urine. There is no difference in pharmacokinetics between paediatric and adult patients. While hepatic disease might be expected to reduce the activation of oxazaphosphorines, there are few clinical data available to confirm this.[16]

Absorption

Both CP and IFO are absorbed well following oral administration, but bioavailability measures based on parent drug may mask qualitative and quantitative effects owing to metabolism in the gastrointestinal tract or first-pass metabolism.[7] Comparison of intravenous and oral data for CP, including data on metabolites, indicate almost complete bioequivalence of the two routes of administration.[6] However, the pharmacology of IFO is different following oral administration, with an unacceptably high incidence of encephalopathic episodes.[17]

Distribution

The oxazaphosphorines distribute throughout the body, with a low degree of protein binding in plasma.[14,15]

There is some evidence that distribution is increased in obese patients, resulting in a longer half-life for the parent drug.[18] Distribution of parent drug and metabolites has been determined in the cerebrospinal fluid

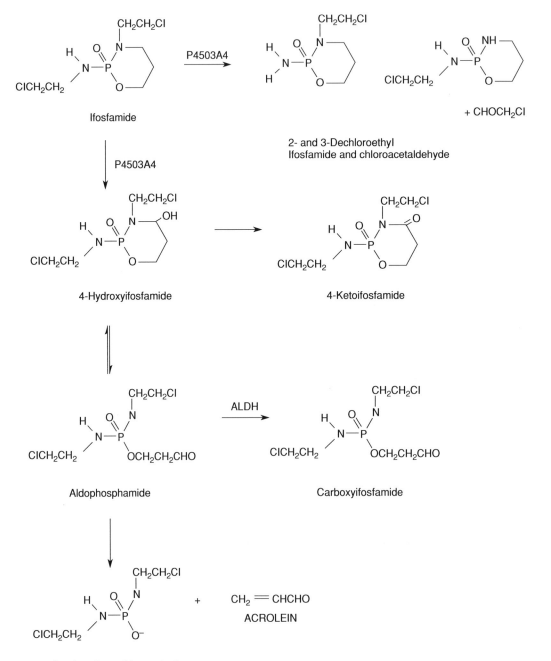

Figure 7.2. Metabolism of ifosfamide showing activating and inactivating pathways of metabolism. The structure of cyclophosphamide is similar to that of ifosfamide, but with both chloroethyl groups on the exocyclic nitrogen. The metabolism of cyclophosphamide is analogous, but with less dechloroethylation.

(CSF), with concentrations comparable to those seen in plasma.[19]

Metabolism and excretion

Oxazaphosphorines are prodrugs and require metabolic activation to form the DNA-reactive mustard species PM and IPM.[8] As well as the activation pathway, via 4-hydroxy and aldehyde intermediates, CP and IFO may form inactive dechloroethylated, carboxy, and keto metabolites (Fig. 7.2).[20,21] A further level of complexity is provided by the chiral nature of the phosphorus atom in the molecules, although the contribution of stereoselective metabolism or pharmacological effect appears to be of relatively minor significance.[22]

These complex metabolic pathways have led to much investigation, and speculation as to the role of different metabolites in the activity and toxicities observed. Of particular relevance is the question of the relative contributions of systemic and intratumoral activation, especially given the polarity and consequent poor cell penetration of the mustard species.

Investigations of the activation pathway for CP and IFO have indicated that the cytochrome P450 enzymes CYP3A4, CYP3A5, CYP2B6, and CYP2C9 are able to catalyse the formation of the 4-hydroxy metabolites.[23,24] Although these enzymes are expressed in hepatic and other host tissues, recent investigations have indicated that they may also be expressed in tumours,[25–27] leading to speculation that intratumoral activation may contribute significantly to activity.

Dechloroethylation is also mediated by CYP3A isoforms.[23] This inactivating reaction is much more significant for IFO, accounting for up to 50% of a dose[20] compared with less than 10% for CP.[28] The formation of chloroacetaldehyde in this reaction and the different spectrum of toxicities observed with the two drugs suggest some causative role for chloroacetaldehyde in IFO nephro- or neurotoxicity.[29]

Both CP and IFO induce their own metabolism following repeated or continuous administration.[30–32] This results in an increase in clearance, a decrease in half-life, and increased formation of both activated and inactivated metabolites. Autoinduction of metabolism occurs within 12–24 h of drug administration, but is reversed within 3 weeks.[33]

At high doses saturation of metabolism may also occur, with proportionately less metabolism of parent drug as the dose increases.[34] This is particularly relevant for CP when used in high-dose chemotherapy.[35]

The combination of autoinduction and non-linear metabolism of CP results in further complexity when given in high-dose fractionated regimens.

Pharmacokinetic drug interactions

As oxazaphosphorines are dependent on metabolism for activity, drug interactions resulting in modification of metabolism are particularly important. Drugs which may inhibit activation of CP and IFO include antifungal agents (ketoconazole and fluconazole), allopurinol, and chlorpromazine.[36,37] Thiotepa may inhibit CP metabolism in high-dose chemotherapy.[38] Conversely, other agents are inducers of hepatic metabolizing enzymes,[39] and increased metabolism of CP or IFO has been reported following prolonged administration of *steroids and anticonvulsants* (phenobarbitone and carbamazepine).[31,40] Since these agents are also substrates for the same metabolizing enzymes, a complex mixture of competition and induction exists when they are co-administered.

Since administration of CP or IFO induces drug-metabolizing enzymes, their administration may increase the rate of elimination of other substrates. There are few reports of any clinically significant interactions of this type.

Pharmacokinetic models

One or two-compartment models have been sufficient to describe the pharmacokinetics of either drug following a short intravenous infusion at conventional doses. However, more complex models involving time- and/or concentration-dependent pharmacokinetics have been proposed for prolonged or high-dose administration.[31,34] While these more complex models apply specifically to concentrations of parent drug in the plasma, they also have implications for the systemic formation of inactive and active metabolites.

Pharmacodynamics

Because of the prodrug nature of CP and IFO, pharmacodynamic models are difficult to formulate in terms of the parent drug. Also, in multi-agent chemotherapy regimens, it is difficult to identify the contribution of any one agent to therapeutic or toxic events. Perhaps the most significant observation relating to the pharmacodynamics of oxazaphosphorines is that an inverse relationship exists between the area under the plasma concentration–time curve (AUC) for parent CP and the likelihood of both response and cardiotoxicity.[41] This implies that the less metabolism (presumably activating) occurs, the less pharmacologically active the drug is. Conversely, attempts to determine a relationship between pharmacological effect and systemic concentrations of activated metabolites have been unsuccessful.

Melphalan

Introduction

Melphalan is a nitrogen mustard attached to a phenylalanine moiety (Fig. 7.3), which was synthesized in an attempt to exploit specific uptake of this amino acid by melanoma cells. Subsequently, melphalan has been shown to be active in breast and ovarian cancer and in multiple myeloma. As with other alkylating agents, melphalan is now being employed in high-dose regimens with haematological support.

Clinical use

Oral and intravenous preparations of melphalan may be used, but the intravenous route is used more commonly. Melphalan has activity in a number of malignancies, including multiple myeloma and ovarian cancer, but one of the major current uses is as myeloablative therapy in haematological malignancies prior to bone marrow or PBSC transplant. Doses of up to 220 mg/m² have been used, with the major non-haematological toxicity being mucositis.[42] Prolonged thrombocytopaenia is also a problem.

Mechanism of action

Melphalan is a mustard, forming mono and bifunctional adducts with DNA. Uptake into cells may be facilitated by amino acid transport systems,[43] but no tumour selectivity is gained by this mechanism.

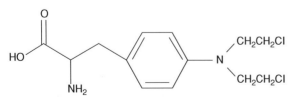

Figure 7.3.   Structure of melphalan.

Mechanisms of resistance

Like many alkylating agents, resistance to melphalan has been associated with glutathione and its associated transferase enzymes.[44] Clinical studies using buthionine sulfoximine, which depletes GSH, have been performed but have failed to show any advantage over melphalan alone.[45]

Chemistry

The half-life of melphalan in plasma *in vitro* is 2.2 ± 0.5 h.[46]

Analytical methodology

Melphalan concentrations in plasma can be determined by HPLC with UV detection.[47] Stability in aqueous solution is poor, but in plasma melphalan is stabilized by binding to albumin[48] and samples may be stored frozen prior to analysis.

Pharmacokinetics

Absorption

Oral dosing of melphalan results in a high degree of both inter- and intra-patient variability in plasma concentrations.[49] Appearance of the drug in the plasma may be delayed for 1–4 h,[50] with a half-life for absorption of 2–62 min.[51] Food also reduces the extent and rate of absorption,[51,52] with bioavailability reduced from 85% to 58%.[53,54] Bioavailability may be as low as 28%,[46] or as high as 100%,[51] as absorption may be dependent on active energy-dependent processes.

Protein binding

Binding of melphalan to plasma protein is modest, with 17–45% unbound fraction in plasma.

Central nervous system penetration

Only very low concentrations of melphalan are detectable in cerebrospinal fluid (CSF).[55]

Distribution

A volume of distribution of 20 ± 4 l/m² or 0.5 ± 0.2 l/kg has been reported after intravenous administration.[56,57]

Elimination

Melphalan is relatively stable due to the aromatic ring that deactivates the mustard group. Most of the drug is eliminated via hydrolysis of the chloroethyl side chains to mono- and dihydroxy forms,[46,56] with relatively little elimination in urine.[54] Elimination of melphalan after oral administration correlates with renal function [glomerular filtration rate (GFR)],[58] but this is not observed consistently.[59] Renal impairment does not result in a decreased rate of elimination, although patients with poor renal function may experience higher toxicity.

Half-life after oral dosing is 0.9 ± 0.5 h,[50] but may range up to 552 min.[46] After intravenous administration of low doses (10–20 mg/m^2) the half-life is 13–40 min,[60] whereas after higher doses it is biphasic with values of 8 ± 3 min and 108 ± 21.[56]

Pharmacokinetic drug interactions

Cimetidine produces a 30% reduction in melphalan absorption and a similar decrease in the half-life of melphalan administered orally.[61] The mechanism for this interaction of cimetidine is unclear, but it may be related to inhibition of active transport processes involved in intestinal absorption and renal tubular reabsorption.

Alterations with disease or age

The elimination of melphalan is largely independent of renal and hepatic function. Dose reductions are often recommended in renally impaired patients, based on an inverse correlation of AUC with GFR[62] and an increase in toxicity associated with renal insufficiency. However, studies of patients with creatinine clearance <40 ml/min show no difference in the pharmacokinetics of high-dose melphalan compared with patients with more normal renal function.[63] The pharmacokinetics of melphalan in children receiving 140 or 220 mg/m^2 intravenously were comparable to those in adults.[64]

Pharmacokinetic models

Although the elimination of melphalan is rapid, careful sampling shows a biphasic elimination with half-lives of 8 min and 46 min, respectively, in children and adults.[55] A longer terminal half-life of up to 6.5 h has also been reported.[42] Clearance ranges from 170 to 570 ml/min/m^2.

Pharmacodynamics

There are no pharmacodynamic data on melphalan in clinical studies.

Nitrosoureas

Introduction

This group of agents includes BCNU (carmustine), CCNU (lomustine), and fotemustine (Fig. 7.4). These agents form carbamoyl adducts with proteins, but their primary mechanism of action is alkylation of DNA. Although active in a number of tumour types, relatively little is known about the clinical pharmacology of the nitrosoureas owing to their instability in aqueous media and their complex metabolism *in vivo*.

Clinical use

The major clinical use of nitrosoureas is in brain tumours, myelomas, and Hodgkin's lymphoma.

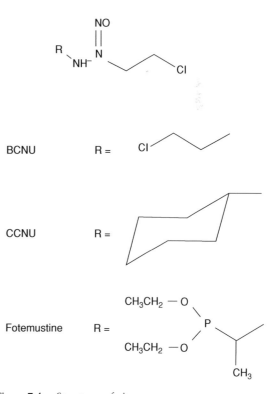

Figure 7.4.   Structures of nitrosoureas.

Mechanism of action

Nitrosoureas act by alkylation of DNA, and possibly by carbamoylation of protein.[65,66]

Mechanisms of resistance

There is some indication that glutathione may play a role in tumour resistance to nitrosoureas,[67] although the clinical relevance of this is unknown.

Chemistry and analytical methodology

The nitrosoureas are relatively unstable in aqueous solution. The reactive unstable intermediates formed hamper the analysis of drugs in plasma, and these problems have been overcome only recently.

Pharmacokinetics

Absorption

Absorption of BCNU is almost complete, with less than 1% of a radiolabelled oral dose recovered in the faeces.[68] However, first-pass metabolism may limit the systemic availability of other nitrosoureas such as CCNU.[69]

Distribution and central nervous system penetration

These compounds are lipid soluble and bind to lipids and lipoproteins,[70] and so distribute rapidly and extensively throughout the body. Volumes of distribution of 3–5 l/kg have been reported for BCNU,[71,72] although that of fotemustine is lower at 31 litres.[73]

Penetration of the brain by nitrosoureas is extensive, with CSF concentrations around 30% of those in plasma.[68,74] More sophisticated analysis using [11C]BCNU indicated a higher retention of drug in tumour than in normal brain[75] and an advantage of intra-arterial over intravenous administration for delivery of the drug to gliomas.[76]

Metabolism

The spontaneous decomposition of nitrosoureas results in reactive alkylating species such as the chloroethyl carbonium ion, analogous to that of the mustards.[77] Isocyanate may also be formed as part of the breakdown and carbamoylation pathways.[78] Metabolism, by

either dechlorination of fotemustine[79] or hydroxylation of CCNU, is mainly an inactivation mechanism.[80]

Elimination

The investigation of nitrosourea elimination from plasma is complicated by the spontaneous breakdown and rapid metabolism of these compounds. Early studies with radiolabelled BCNU indicated a half-life of up to 67 h,[68] but values of only 22 min were obtained with more specific assay methods.[71,72] The pharmacokinetics of BCNU may be dose dependent, with a longer half-life (up to 4.3 h) after higher doses.[81] CCNU is rapidly eliminated from the plasma, especially after oral administration,[69] possibly due to hepatic hydroxylation mediated by CYP450 enzymes.[80] First-pass metabolism has also been reported for fotemustine.[82] The clearance of this drug is very high (70–100 l/h) with a very short half-life (13–64 min)[73,83] For this reason, hepatic arterial administration of fotemustine has been advocated, as it should result in high concentrations in hepatic tumours but lower concentrations systemically.[84] Similarly, intracarotid infusion has been used for selective delivery to gliomas.[85]

Other properties

Owing to the instability of the nitrosoureas, relatively little is known about their pharmacokinetic or pharmacodynamic relationships, interactions, or variations with age and disease.

Busulphan

Introduction

The primary uses of busulphan (Fig. 7.5) are in the treatment of chronic myelogenous leukaemia or in myeloablative treatment prior to autologous or orthologous bone marrow transplant or other haematological support. The dosing of busulphan in this context is crucial, given the need to achieve adequate treatment and the narrow therapeutic window. Myeloablative treatment with busulphan is associated with haematological toxicity, but more significantly with hepatic veno-occlusive disease and pulmonary toxicities. Overall, the incidence of transplant-related mortality is relatively high and pharmacological knowledge has thus

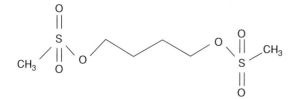

Figure 7.5. Structure of busulphan.

been developed to optimize busulphan dosage to overcome this.[86,87]

Clinical use

Busulphan is administered orally as intact tablets or crushed tablets, or as a suspension of the latter via a nasogastric tube. The dose is usually administered four times a day over four consecutive days and may be accompanied by other chemotherapy, such as cyclophosphamide. Anticonvulsants are frequently used prophylactically prior to busulphan administration, but may result in drug interactions.[40] Immunosuppressive treatment may also be given in the context of orthologous bone marrow transplant, to guard against graft versus host disease.

Mechanism of action

Busulphan is a bifunctional alkylating agent.

Mechanisms of resistance

Mechanisms of resistance are the same as with nitrosoureas and other alkylating agents.

Chemistry and analytical methodology

Busulphan is stable in plasma frozen at –20°C for up to 3 months.[88] Analytical methods include gas chromatography (GC), following derivatization with sodium iodide to form 1,4-diiodobutane[89] and HPLC following reaction with diethyldithiocarbamate. A gas chromatography–mass spectrometry (GC–MS) method has also been described.[90]

Pharmacokinetics

The pharmacokinetics of busulphan are highly variable and depend on age, circadian variation,[91] and disease type.[92] Since there is a large body of data relating both

therapeutic and toxic outcome to pharmacokinetics, dose adjustment based initially on body size (weight or surface area) and subsequently on plasma concentration (trough or AUC) has been advocated.[86] Although the data suggesting a link between low plasma concentrations of busulphan and rejection of graft in bone marrow transplant is relatively weak,[93] that between high concentrations and toxicity, particularly venoocclusive disease, is very strong.[86]

Absorption

Given that busulphan is usually administered orally, it is surprising that reliable data on bioavailability are lacking. Estimates range from 20% to 120%, and this variability probably underlies much of the reported variability in pharmacokinetics. Absorption is usually rapid, with maximum concentrations achieved in 30–120 min. Recent efforts towards formulating an intravenous preparation of busulphan may allow more precise dose individualization as well as providing more reliable estimates of bioavailability. In terms of dose absorbed, crushed tablets are equivalent to the intact dosage form.[89]

Central nervous system penetration and distribution

Busulphan enters the CNS easily, with CSF-to-plasma concentration ratios of 0.5–1.4.[94] Volume of distribution is estimated to be 27 ± 11 l/m² following oral administration in children.[94]

Elimination

The elimination of busulphan is rapid, with a half-life of less than 2 h for children with inherited diseases and 3 h for children with leukaemia.[94] Elimination is approximately twice as fast in children as in adults.[95]

Pharmacokinetic drug interactions

Pretreatment with anticonvulsants (phenytoin and phenobarbitone) may increase the rate of elimination of busulphan by about 20%,[96] although this interaction is confounded by possible time-dependent pharmacokinetics. Similarly, concurrent treatment with cyclophosphamide may increase busulphan clearance.[93]

Alterations with disease or age

Busulphan clearance is faster in paediatric patients (200 ml/min/m^2) than in adults (95 ml/min/m^2),[88,95] and within the paediatric group is fastest in patients aged less than 5 years.[91] Also, volume of distribution in children is higher than that in adults.[95]

Some, but not all, of the age dependence for elimination is removed by normalizing doses to surface area rather than weight[87,89] and results in higher doses (mg/kg) in young children than in older patients. This may be associated with a higher incidence of neurotoxicity.[97]

Leukaemic patients may eliminate the drug less rapidly than patients with non-neoplastic diseases. Although liver involvement is a common feature of non-malignant syndromes treated with busulphan, there is no relation between the degree of pre-existing hepatic dysfunction and busulphan pharmacokinetics.

Pharmacokinetic models

Busulphan pharmacokinetics is normally characterized by first-order absorption, with a single-compartment model for disposition.[98] Limited sampling models for the estimation of AUC by regression analysis have been proposed,[99] but the relative merits of these are disputed.

Pharmacodynamics

The influence of plasma concentrations of busulphan on toxicity has been demonstrated in numerous studies.[98] A threshold AUC for the occurrence of veno-occlusive disease has been identified at 1500 μM min, and dose adjustment to attain AUC values below this threshold advocated.[86] The effect of plasma concentrations on therapeutic outcome in terms of ensuring adequate treatment is unresolved; however, an association between high busulphan plasma concentrations and an increased risk of transplant-related mortality has been reported.[100]

Chlorambucil

Introduction

The attachment of an aromatic ring to a mustard group results in a more stable alkylating agent. Chlorambucil is an example of these aromatic mustards (Fig. 7.6),

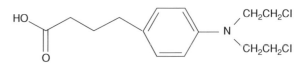

Figure 7.6.   Structure of chlorambucil.

and is used primarily in the treatment of chronic lymphocytic leukaemia and lymphomas.

Mechanisms of resistance

As with other alkylating agents, a role for glutathione in resistance to chlorambucil has been suggested[101] and disputed.[102] Recently, a role for mutant p53[103] and multidrug-resistance-associated protein[104] have also been proposed.

Analytical methodology

GC–MS is the method of choice for the analysis of chlorambucil and its metabolite,[105] although HPLC assays have also been described.[106,107]

Pharmacokinetics

Absorption

The preferred route of administration for chlorambucil is oral, with rapid absorption resulting in a maximum plasma concentration after 15–30 min.[108,109] Absorption may be delayed and reduced by the concomitant ingestion of food,[110] although this is not a consistent observation.[111]

Protein binding

About 98% of the drug in plasma is bound to protein.[109]

Central nervous system penetration

Only a small amount of drug is able to penetrate the blood–brain barrier, with low concentrations observed in the CSF.

Metabolism

Chlorambucil is metabolized to phenylacetic acid. The metabolite has a longer half-life (~150 min) and so has an AUC greater than or equal to that of the parent.[107,112,113] Phenylacetic acid has antitumour activity,[114] but may be more toxic to host tissues than is chlorambucil[115] and may be associated with chlorambucil-induced neurotoxicity.[109] Like other mustards, chlorambucil may undergo oxidative *N*-dechloroethylation, which again may be linked to neurotoxicity.[116]

Elimination

Less than 1% of the dose is excreted in the urine, either as chlorambucil or as phenylacetic acid.[117]

Pharmacokinetic models

Both chlorambucil and its metabolite phenylacetic acid mustard are eliminated in a mono-exponential fashion, with half-lives of 1.0 h and 1.9 h, respectively.[113]

Other properties

No specific information is available on pharmacokinetic drug interactions, alterations with disease or age, or on pharmacodynamics.

Thiotepa

Introduction

Thiotepa is a trisaziridino compound and thus potentially has three alkylating moieties (Fig. 7.7). In practice, only two of these react, forming mono- or bifunctional DNA adducts. Its metabolite, TEPA, retains some alkylating and cytotoxic activity.

Clinical use

Thiotepa may be used as single doses or cycles of 2–3 weeks. Recent studies have used higher doses with haematological support,[118–120] and some protocols have advocated the use of continuous infusion. In high-dose regimens for the treatment of breast cancer[121] or paediatric malignancies,[122] thiotepa is commonly used in conjunction with carboplatin or cyclophosphamide with doses of up to 500 mg/m^2/day divided over 3–4 days.

Mechanism of action

Studies with thiotepa and TEPA, in the presence or absence of a hepatic microsomal metabolizing system, reveal that high concentrations of thiotepa are necessary to form DNA inter-strand cross-links. In contrast, TEPA produces alkali labile DNA lesions, which are also seen when thiotepa is metabolized.[123]

Mechanisms of resistance

As for most alkylating agents, a role for GSH and GSTs in resistance to thiotepa has been suggested.[124] However, the clinical relevance of this remains unproven.

Chemistry

Thiotepa is unstable in aqueous solution, but is more stable at neutral than at acid pH. Stability is enhanced at lower temperatures. At 37°C, only 10% of thiotepa is lost at pH 6 or pH 7.[125] Thiotepa and TEPA also undergo hydrolytic cleavage to release aziridine, which may act directly to alkylate DNA.[126] Although TEPA is hydrolysed more quickly, it has less cytotoxic activity *in vitro*, which may indicate that thiotepa acts as a relatively stable carrier of aziridine to its target in cells.[127]

Analytical methodology

Determination of thiotepa and the metabolite TEPA is best achieved by solid phase extraction with GC and a nitrogen detector,[128,129] although HPLC with fluorescence derivatization has been described.[130]

Pharmacokinetics

Absorption

Thiotepa is rapidly absorbed after intra-peritoneal administration, with significant systemic concentrations of both parent drug and TEPA.[131,132]

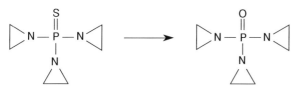

Figure 7.7. Structures of thiotepa and TEPA.

Protein binding

Thiotepa is only insignificantly (10%) bound to plasma protein.[133]

Central nervous system penetration

After intravenous injection, thiotepa and TEPA can be found in the CSF at concentrations equivalent to those in plasma.[134,135]

Distribution

As thiotepa is a small lipophilic molecule, its distribution is close to total body water, with volumes of distribution of 0.7 ± 0.1 l/kg.[136]

Metabolism

The conversion of thiotepa to TEPA can occur spontaneously in solution, but a role for active metabolism to an activated form, either TEPA or some other unidentified metabolite, has been reported.[137-139] The metabolism of thiotepa by CYP2B enzymes seems to result in inactivation of the enzyme.[138]

Elimination

Thiotepa is eliminated with a half-life of less than 2 h after an intravenous dose. In contrast, elimination of TEPA is slower, with a half-life of up to 10 h. Thus concentrations of TEPA exceed those of the parent drug soon after administration.[140] Excretion of drug in the urine is minimal (<6% combined metabolites).[136-140] The pharmacokinetics of thiotepa are dose dependent,[141] with less TEPA formed at higher doses of thiotepa (>55 mg/m²).

Pharmacokinetic drug interactions

In an attempt to reverse drug resistance based on inactivation by glutathione, clinical studies of the combination of thiotepa with GST inhibitors such as ethacrynic acid have been performed. Co-administration of ethacrynic acid results in a twofold increase in thiotepa AUC, with a reduction in the AUC of TEPA.[142]

Pharmacodynamics

Despite suggestions that TEPA is the active metabolite, haematological toxicity correlates most closely with the AUC of thiotepa.[141,143]

Temozolomide

Introduction

Temozolomide has been introduced relatively recently and has shown promising activity in glioma, astrocytoma, and melanoma. Because it has a relatively 'clean' mechanism of action as a monofunctional alkylator of DNA, it is favoured in combination regimens with inhibitors of DNA repair. The oral mode of administration also makes it an attractive drug for continued studies. The history of the synthesis and early studies with this agent have been reviewed recently.[144] The major advantage temozolomide offers over its predecessor *dacarbazine* is that it spontaneously releases the cytotoxic species 3-methyl-(triazen-1-yl)imidazole-4-carboxamide (MTIC) (Fig. 7.8), whereas the latter drug requires metabolic activation mediated by microsomal enzymes.[145]

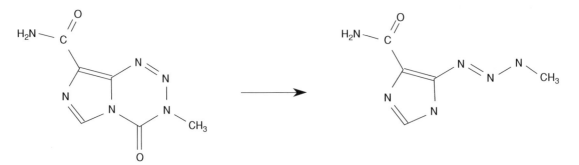

Figure 7.8.   Structure of temozolomide and its active metabolite MTIC.

Clinical use

Temozolomide follows a related series of compounds (dacarbazine and mitozolomide). The former requires metabolic activation, while the latter resulted in severe and unpredictable myelosuppression in early clinical trials.[144] Phase I trials of a 5 day schedule of temozolomide, identified as optimal from preclinical studies, established a phase II dose of 200 mg/m² each day for 5 days in the absence of myelosuppression. Dose-limiting toxicities were thrombocytopenia and leukopenia. Some patients may be particularly sensitive to the myelosuppressive effects of temozolomide.

A high response rate was reported in high-grade astrocytomas,[144] but subsequent studies have failed to repeat this, with little or no impact on overall survival. Nevertheless, an overall improvement in clinical status was observed in the majority of patients.[146] Similar results have been seen in glioma.[147,148] There has also been evidence of activity in melanoma, with a 21% overall response rate, with three complete responders, in 49 previously untreated patients.[149] Toxicity, mainly haematological, is mostly manageable and predictable.

In paediatric patients, activity has been observed in patients with high-grade astrocytoma and brain-stem glioma, at doses similar to those employed in adults.[150]

Chemistry and mechanism of action

Temozolomide breaks down spontaneously to form the methyl triazene MTIC, which can transfer its methyl group to a nucleophile such as DNA.[144] The residual chemical species 5-aminoimidazole-4-carboxamide (AIC) is a natural constituent of urine. The half-life of temozolomide at pH 7.4 and 37°C is 1.2 h.[151] It is stable under acid conditions, which assists oral absorption.

MTIC degrades rapidly at acid pH, but is sufficiently stable to act as an alkylating agent under physiological conditions. The major lesion is methylation of the N-7 of guanine (70% of total).[144] However, methylation also occurs at N-3 of adenine (9%) and O-6 of guanine (5%). Cytotoxicity correlates most closely with the formation of O-6-methylguanine adducts. This has been associated with the activity of the DNA mismatch repair pathway,[152] which recognizes the mismatched pairing of guanine with thymine, which is then repaired, mismatched again as replication continues, and repaired once more. This futile cycle of repair and mismatching is thought to trigger apoptotic cell death.

Mechanisms of resistance

The O-6-methyl adduct of guanine may be repaired by the DNA repair protein O-6-alkylguanine-DNA alkyltransferase (AGT, or MGMT, or Atase). This enzyme contains a cysteine residue which acts as an acceptor of the methyl group, irreversibly inactivating the enzyme. Other mechanisms of resistance have been suggested from *in vitro* experiments.[153]

Resistance may also result from mutations or inactivity of the DNA mismatch repair pathway.[152]

Analytical methodology

Determination of temozolomide and its metabolites in plasma requires stabilization under acid conditions. Following solid phase extraction from plasma, temozolomide can be assayed by HPLC.[154] An analytical method has also been described for the active metabolite MTIC.[155]

Pharmacokinetics

Absorption

After oral administration, the drug is rapidly absorbed, with a peak concentration being achieved in less than 1 h (range 20–240 min).[144,156]

Distribution and central nervous system penetration

The CNS penetration of temozolomide is high in preclinical models,[144] which accounts for the high activity of this agent against CNS tumours.

Patient studies using positron-emitting isotope labelling of temozolomide have demonstrated uniform distribution in extracranial tissues, but a selective distribution to tumour over normal brain tissue.[144]

Metabolism

The breakdown of temozolomide to MTIC occurs spontaneously. Other metabolites detectable in plasma are AIC and trace quantities of AM.[156] The active metabolite appears within 1 h of oral administration of temozolomide and parallels the concentrations and decline of the parent drug, but with an AUC of around 2.5% of that of the parent.[157]

Elimination

Elimination is first order with a half-life of 1.8 h, most of the drug being converted to MTIC.[144,156] While the majority of the drug is excreted in the urine, this may be in the form of a number of metabolites.[158]

Pharmacokinetic drug interactions

Administration of temozolomide with inhibitors of AGT result in both pharmacokinetic and pharmaco-dynamic interactions, as inhibition of AGT causes reduced elimination of the drug and reduces inactiva-tion.[144] As an inactivator of AGT, temozolomide itself can modulate its own activity and the optimal schedule is several days of repeated administration.

Toxicity of temozolomide is enhanced in patients with prior exposure to nitrosoureas, with recommended phase II doses being 125 mg/m^2 and 225 mg/m^2 for patients with and without prior exposure, respectively.[156]

Other properties

For this relatively new alkylating agent, little is yet known about alterations with disease or age or about pharmacodynamics.

Acknowledgements

This work was supported by the Cancer Research UK. The figures used in this chapter were prepared by Dr Elaine Johnstone.

References

1. Brock N (1989) Oxazaphosphorine cytostatics: past–present–future. *Cancer Res*, **49**, 1–7
2. Colvin M (1982) The comparative pharmacology of CP and ifosfamide. *Semin Oncol*, **9**, 2–7.
3. Bonadonna G, Valagussa P, Moliterni A, Zambetti M, Brambilla C (1995) Adjuvant cyclophosphamide, methotrexate and fluorouracil in node-positive breast cancer. *N Engl J Med*, **332**, 901–6.
4. Savarese DMF, Hsieh C, Stewart MF (1997) Clinical impact of chemotherapy dose escalation in patients with hematologic malignancies and solid tumors. *J Clin Oncol*, **15**, 2981–95.
5. Aeschlimann C, Kupfer A, Schefer H, Cerny T (1998) Comparative pharamcokinetics of oral and intravenous ifosfamide/mesna/methylene blue therapy. *Drug Metab Dispos*, **26**, 883–90.
6. Struck RF, Alberts DS, Horne K, Phillips HG, Peng Y-M, Roe DJ (1987) Plasma pharmacokinetics of cyclophos-phamide and its cytotoxic metabolites after intravenous versus oral administration in a randomized, crossover trial. *Cancer Res*, **47**, 2732–6.
7. Lind MJ, Roberts HL, Thatcher N, Idle JR (1990) The effect of route of administration and fractionation of dose on the metabolism of ifosfamide. *Cancer Chemother Pharmacol*, **26**, 105–11.
8. Sladek N (1988) Metabolism of oxazaphosphorines. *Pharmacol Ther*, **37**, 301–55.
9. Dirven HAAM, van Ommen B, van Bladeren PJ (1994) Involvement of human glutathione-*S*-transferase isoen-zymes in the conjugation of cyclophosphamide metabo-lites with glutathione. *Cancer Res*, **54**, 6215–20.
10. Dockham PA, Lee M-O, Sladek NE (1992) Identi-fication of human liver aldehyde dehydrogenases that catalyze the oxidation of aldophosphamide and retin-aldehyde. *Biochem Pharmacol*, **43**, 2453–69.
11. Sreerama L, Sladek NE (1994) Identification of the class-3 aldehyde dehydrogenases present in human MCF-7/0 breast adenocarcinoma cells and normal human breast tissue. *Biochem Pharmacol*, **48**, 617–20.
12. Juma FD, Rogers HJ, Trounce JR, Bradbrook ID (1978) Pharmacokinetics of intravenous cyclophosphamide in man, estimated by gas-liquid chromatography. *Cancer Chemother Pharmacol*, **1**, 229–31.
13. Burton LC, James CA (1988) Rapid method for the determination of ifosfamide and cyclophosphamide in plasma by high-performance liquid chromatography with solid-phase extraction. *J Chromatogr*, **431**, 450–4.
14. Kaijser GP, Beijnen JH, Bult A, Underberg WJM (1994) Ifosfamide metabolism and pharmacokinetics [review]. *Anticancer Res*, **14**, 517–32.
15. Moore MJ (1991) Clinical pharmacokinetics of cyclophosphamide. *Clin Pharmacokinet*, **20**, 194–208.
16. Juma FD (1984) Effect of liver failure on the pharmaco-kinetics of cyclophosphamide. *Eur J Clin Pharmacol*, **26**, 591–3.
17. Cerny T, Küpfer A (1992) The enigma of ifosfamide encephalopathy. *Ann Oncol*, **3**, 679–81.
18. Lind MJ, Margison JM, Cerny T, Thatcher N, Wilkinson PM (1989) Prolongation of ifosfamide elim-ination half-life in obese patients due to altered drug distribution. *Cancer Chemother Pharmacol*, **25**, 139–42.
19. Yule SM, Price L, Pearson ADJ, Boddy AV (1997) Cyclophosphamide and ifosfamide metabolites in the cerebrospinal fluid of children. *Clin Cancer Res*, **3**, 1985–92.
20. Boddy AV, Proctor M, Simmonds D, Lind MJ, Idle JR (1995) Pharmacokinetics, metabolism and clinical effect of ifosfamide in breast cancer patients. *Eur J Cancer*, **31A**, 69–76.
21. Hartley JM, Hansen L, Harland SJ, Nicholson PW, Pasini F, Souhami RL (1994) Metabolism of ifosfamide during a 3 day infusion. *Br J Cancer*, **69**, 931–6.
22. Masurel D, Houghton PJ, Young CL, Wainer IW (1990) Efficacy, toxicity, pharmacokinetics and *in vitro* metabolism of the enantiomers of ifosfamide in mice. *Cancer Res*, **50**, 252–5.

23. Walker D, Flinois J-P, Monkman SC, *et al.* (1994) Identification of the major human hepatic cytochrome P450 involved in activation and *N*-dechloroethylation of ifosfamide. *Biochem Pharmacol*, **47**, 1157–63.

24. Chang TKH, Weber GF, Crespi CL, Waxman DJ (1993) Differential activation of cyclophosphamide and ifosphamide by cytochromes P-450 2B and 3A in human liver microsomes. *Cancer Res*, **53**, 5629–37.

25. Murray GI, Weaver RJ, Paterson PJ, Ewen SWB, Melvin WT, Burke MD (1993) Expression of xenobiotic metabolizing enzymes in breast cancer. *J Pathol*, **169**, 347–53.

26. Murray GI, McKay JA, Weaver RJ, Ewen SWB, Melvin WT, Burke MD (1993) Cytochrome P450 expression is a common molecular event in soft tissue sarcomas. *J Pathol*, **171**, 49–52.

27. Janot F, Massaad L, Ribrag V, *et al.* (1993) Principal xenobiotic-metabolizing enzyme systems in human head and neck squamous cell carcinoma. *Carcinogenesis*, **14**, 1279–83.

28. Yule SM, Boddy AV, Cole M, *et al.* (1995) Cyclophosphamide metabolism in children. *Cancer Res*, **55**, 803–9.

29. Goren MP, Wright RK, Pratt CB, Pell FE (1986) Dechloroethylation of ifosfamide and neurotoxicity. *Lancet*, **ii**, 1219–20.

30. Kurowski V, Wagner T (1993) Comparative pharmacokinetics of ifosfamide, 4-hydroxyifosfamide, chloroacetaldehyde and 2- and 3-dechloroethylifosfamide in patients on fractionated intravenous ifosfamide therapy. *Cancer Chemother Pharmacol*, **33**, 36–42.

31. Boddy AV, Cole M, Pearson ADJ, Idle JR (1995) The kinetics of the auto-induction of ifosfamide metabolism during continuous infusion. *Cancer Chemother Pharmacol*, **36**, 53–60.

32. D'Incalci M, Bolis G, Facchinetti T, *et al.* (1979) Decreased half life of cyclophosphamide in patients under continual treatment. *Eur J Cancer*, **13**, 7–10.

33. Lewis LD (1996) A study of 5 day fractionated ifosfamide pharmacokinetics in consecutive treatment cycles. *Br J Clin Pharmacol*, **42**, 179–86.

34. Chen T-L, Passos-Coelho J, Noe D, *et al.* (1995) Nonlinear pharmacokinetics of cyclophosphamide in patients with metastatic breast cancer receiving high-dose chemotherapy followed by autologous bone marrow transplantation. *Cancer Res*, **55**, 810–16.

35. Busse D, Busch FW, Bohnenstengel F, *et al.* (1997) Dose escalation of cyclophosphamide in patients with breast cancer: consequences for pharmacokinetics and metabolism. *J Clin Oncol*, **15**, 1885–96.

36. Yule SM, Walker D, Pearson ADJ (1994) Potential inhibition of alkylating agent metabolism by fluconazole. *Eur J Clin Microbiol Infect Dis*, **13**, 1086–7.

37. Yule SM, Boddy AV, Cole M, *et al.* (1996) Cyclophosphamide pharmacokinetics in children. *Br J Clin Pharmacol*, **41**, 13–19.

38. Anderson L, Chen T-L, Colvin OM, *et al.* (1996) Cyclophosphamide and 4-hydroxycyclophosphamide/aldophosphamide kinetics in patients receiving high-dose cyclophosphamide chemotherapy. *Clin Cancer Res*, **2**, 1481–7.

39. Chang TKH, Yu L, Maurel P, Waxman DJ (1997) Enhanced cyclophosphamide and ifosfamide activation in primary human hepatocyte cultures: response to cytochrome P-450 inducers and autoinduction by oxazaphosphorines. *Cancer Res*, **57**, 1946–54.

40. Slattery JT, Kalhorn TF, McDonald GB, *et al.* (1996) Conditioning regimen-dependent disposition of cyclophosphamide and hydroxycyclophosphamide in human marrow transplantation patients. *J Clin Oncol*, **14**, 1484–94.

41. Ayash LJ, Wright JE, Tretyakov O, *et al.* (1992) Cyclophosphamide pharmacokinetics: correlation with cardiac toxicity and tumor response. *J Clin Oncol*, **10**, 995–1000.

42. Moreau P, Kergueris M-F, Milpied N, *et al.* (1996) A pilot study of 220 mg/m² melphalan followed by autologous stem cell transplantation in patients with advanced haematological malignancies: pharmacokinetics and toxicity. *Br J Haematol*, **95**, 527–30.

43. Vistica DT, Toal JN, Rabinovitz M (1978) Amino acid-conferred protection against melphalan- characterization of melphalan transport and corrleation of uptake with cytotoxicity in cultured L1210 murine leukemia cells. *Biochem Pharmacol*, **27**, 2865–70.

44. Alaoui-Jamali MA, Panasci L, Centurioni GM, Schecter R, Lehnert S, Batist G (1992) Nitrogen mustard-DNA interaction in melphalan-resistant mammary carcinoma cells with elevated intracellular glutathione and glutathione-S-transferase activity. *Cancer Chemother Pharmacol*, **30**, 341–7.

45. O'Dwyer PJ, Hamilton TC, Lacreta FP, *et al.* (1996) Phase-I trial of buthionine sulfoximine in combination with melphalan in patients with cancer. *J Clin Oncol*, **14**, 249–56.

46. Alberts DS, Chang SY, Chen H-SG, Evans TL, Moon TE (1979) Oral melphalan kinetics. *Clin Pharmacol Ther*, **26**, 737–45.

47. Chang SY, Alberts DS, Melnick LR, Walson PD, Salmon SE (1978) High-pressure liquid chromatographic analysis of melphalan in plasma. *J Pharm Sci*, **67**, 679.

48. Chang SY, Alberts DS, Farquhar D, Melnick LR, Walson TD, Salmon SE (1978) Hydrolysis and protein binding of melphalan. *J Pharm Sci* **67**, 682–4.

49. Choi KE, Ratain MJ, Williams SF, *et al.* (1989) Plasma pharmacokinetics of high dose oral melphalan in patients treated with triaklylator chemotherapy and autologous bone marrow reinfusion. *Cancer Res*, **49**, 1318–21.

50. Taha IA-K, Ahman RA, Gray H, Roberts CI, Rogers HJ (1982) Plasma melphalan and prednisolone concentrations during oral therapy for multiple myeloma. *Cancer Chemother Pharmacol*, **9**, 57–60.

51. Bosanquet AG, Gilby ED (1982) Pharmacokinetics of oral and intravenous melphalan during routine treatment of multiple myeloma. *Eur J Cancer Clin Oncol*, **18**, 355–62.

52. Bosanquet AG, Gilby D (1984) Comparison of the fed and fasting states on the absorption of melphalan in multiple myeloma. *Cancer Chemother Pharmacol*, **12**, 183–6.

53. Reece PA, Kotasek D, Morris RG, Dale BM, Sage RE (1986) The effect of food on oral melphalan absorption. *Cancer Chemother Pharmacol*, **16**, 194–7.

54. Reece PA, Hill HS, Green RM, *et al.* (1988) Renal clearance and protein binding of melphalan in patients with cancer. *Cancer Chemother Pharmacol*, **22**, 348–52.

55. Gouyette A, Hartmann O, Pico J (1986) Pharmacokinetics of high-dose melphalan in children and adults. *Cancer Chemother Pharmacol*, **16**, 184–9.

56. Alberts DS, Chang SY, Chen H-SG, *et al.* (1979) Kinetics of intravenous melphalan. *Clin Pharmacol Ther*, **26**, 73–80.

57. Zucchetti M, D'Incalci M, Willems Y, Cavalli F, Sessa C (1988) Lack of effect of cisplatin on i.v. L-PAM plasma pharmacokinetics in ovarian cancer patients. *Cancer Chemother Pharmacol*, **22**, 87–9.

58. Adair C, Bridges J, Desai Z (1986) Renal function in the elimination of oral melphalan in patients with multiple myeloma. *Cancer Chemother Pharmacol*, **17**, 185–8.

59. Kergueris M, Milpied N, Moreau P, Harousseau J, Larousse C (1994) Pharmacokinetics of high-dose melphalan in adults: influence of renal function. *Anticancer Res*, **14**, 2379–82.

60. Brox L, Birkett L, Belch A (1979) Pharmacology of intravenous melphalan in patients with multiple myeloma. *Cancer Treat Rev*, **6** (Suppl), 27–32.

61. Sviland L, Robinson A, Proctor SJ, Bateman DN (1987) Interaction of cimetidine with oral melphalan: a pharmacokinetic study. *Cancer Chemother Pharmacol*, **20**, 173–5.

62. Osterborg A, Ehrsson H, Eksborg S, Wallin I, Mellstedt H (1989) Pharmacokinetics of oral melphalan in relation to renal function in multiple myeloma patients. *Eur J Cancer Clin Oncol*, **25**, 899–903.

63. Tricot G, Alberts DS, Johnson C, *et al.* (1996) Safety of autotransplants with high-dose melphalan in renal failure. A pharmacokinetic and toxicity study. *Clin Cancer Res*, **2**, 947–52.

64. Taha IA-K, Ahmad RA, Rogers DW, Pritchard J, Rogers HJ (1983) Pharmacokinetics of melphalan in children following high-dose intravenous injection. *Cancer Chemother Pharmacol*, **10**, 212–16.

65. Reed DJ (1987) 2-Chloroethylnitrosoureas. In Powis G, Prough RA (eds) *Metabolism and Actions of Anticancer Drugs*. London: Taylor and Francis.

66. Lemoine A, Lucas C, Ings RMJ (1991) Metabolism of chloroethylnitrosoureas. *Xenobiotica*, **21**, 775–91.

67. Smith MT, Evans CG, Doane-Setzer P, Castro VM, Tahir MK, Mannervik B (1989) Denitrosation of 1,3-bis(2-chloroethyl)-1-nitrosourea by class mu glutathione transferases. *Cancer Res*, **49**, 2621–5.

68. DeVita VT, Denham C, Davidson JD, Oliverio VT (1967) The physiological disposition of the carcinostatic 1,3-bis(2-chloroethyl)-1-nitrosourea(BCNU) in man and animals. *Clin Pharmacol Ther*, **8**, 566–77.

69. Lee FYF, Workman P, Roberts JJ, Bleehen NM (1985) Clinical pharmacokinetics of oral CCNU (lomustine) *Cancer Chemother Pharmacol*, **14**, 125–31.

70. Weikam RJ, Finn A, Levin VA, Kane JP (1980) Lipophilic drugs and lipoproteins: partitioning effects on chloroethylnitrosourea reaction rates in serum. *J Pharmacol Exp Ther*, **214**, 318–23.

71. Levin VA, Hoffman W, Weinkam RJ (1978) Pharmacokinetics of BCNU in man: preliminary study of 20 patients. *Cancer Treat Rep*, **62**, 1305–12.

72. Henner WD, Peters WP, Eder JP, Antman K, Schnipper L, Frei E (1986) Pharmacokinetics and immediate effects of high-dose carmustine in man. *Cancer Treat Rep*, **70**, 877–80.

73. Tranchand B, Lucas C, Biron P, *et al.* (1993) Phase I pharmacokinetics study of high-dose fotemustine and its metabolite 2-chloroethanol in patients with high-grade gliomas. *Cancer Chemother Pharmacol*, **32**, 46–52.

74. Sponzo RW, DeVita VT, Oliviero VT (1973) Physiologic disposition of 1-(2-chloroethyl)-3-cyclohexyl-1-nitrosourea (CCNU) and 1-(2-chloroethyl(-3-(4-methyl cyclohexyl)-1-nitrosourea (MeCCNU) in man. *Cancer*, **31**, 1154–9.

75. Diksic M, Sako K, Feindel W, *et al.* (1984) Pharmacokinetics of position labelled 1,3-bis(2-chloroethyl)-nitrosourea (BCNU) in human brain tumors using positron emission tomography. *Cancer Res*, **44**, 3120–4.

76. Tyler JL, Yamamoto YL, Diksik M, *et al.* (1986) Pharmacokinetics of superselective intra-arterial and intra-venous [^{11}C]BCNU evaluated by PET. *J Nucl Med*, **27**, 775–80.

77. Colvin M, Brundrett B, Cowens W, Jardine I, Ludlum B (1976) A chemical basis of the antitumor activity of chloroethylnitrosoureas. *Biochem Pharmacol*, **25**, 695–9.

78. Wheeler GP, Bowdon BJ, Grimsley J, Lloyd HH (1974) Interrelationships of some chemical physiocochemical and biological activities of several 1-(2-haloethyl)-1-nitrosoureas. *Cancer Res*, **34**, 194–200.

79. Ings RMJ, Gray AJ, Taylor AR, *et al.* (1990) Disposition, pharmacokinetics and metabolism of ^{14}C-fotemustine in cancer patients. *Eur J Cancer*, **26**, 838–42.

80. Lee FYF, Workman P (1985) Misonidazole protects mouse-tumor and normal-tissues from the toxicity of oral CCNU. *Br J Cancer*, **51**, 85–91.

81. Mbidde EK, Selby PJ, Perren TJ, *et al.* (1988) High dose BCNU chemotherapy with autologous bone marrow transplantation and full dose radiotherapy for grade IV astrocytoma. *Br J Cancer*, **58**, 779–82.

82. Fety R, Lucas C, Solere P, Cour V, Vignoud J (1992) Hepatic intra-arterial infusion of fotemustine: pharmacokinetics. *Cancer Chemother Pharmacol*, **31**, 118–22.

83. Iliadis A, Launayiliadis MC, Lucas C, *et al.* (1996) Pharmacokinetics and pharmacodynamics of nitrosourea fotemustine—a French Cancer Center multicentric study. *Eur J Cancer*, **32A**, 455–60.

84. Hartmann JT, Schmoll E, Bokemeyer C, *et al.* (1998) Phase I pharmacological study of intra-arterially infused fotemustine for colorectal liver metastases. *Eur J Cancer*, **34**, 87–91.

85. Bobo H, Kapp JP, Vance R (1992) Effect of intra-arterial cisplatin and 1,3-bis(2-chloroethyl)-1-nitrosourea (BCNU) dosage on radiographic response and regional toxicity in malignant glioma patients: proposal of a new method of intra-arterial dosage calculation. *J Neurooncol*, **13**, 291–9.

86. Grochow LB (1993) Busulphan disposition: the role of therapeutic drug monitoring in bone marrow transplantation induction regimens. *Semin Oncol*, **20** (Suppl 4), 18–25.

87. Yeager AM, Wagner JE, Graham ML, Jones RJ, Santos GW, Grochow LB (1992) Optimization of busulfan dosage in children undergoig bone marrow transplantation: a pharmacokinetic study of dose escalation. *Blood*, **80**, 2425–8.

88. Pawlowska AB, Blazar BR, Angelucci E, Baronciani D, Shu XO, Bostrom B (1997) Relationship of plasma pharmacokinetics of high-dose oral busulfan to the outcome of allogeneic bone marrow transplantation in children with thalassemia. *Bone Marrow Transplant*, **20**, 915–20.

89. Shaw P, Scharping C, Brian R, Earl J (1994) Busulfan pharmacokinetics using a single daily high-dose regimen in children with acute leukemia. *Blood*, **84**, 2357–62.

90. Vassal G, Re M, Gouyette A (1988) Gas chromatographic-mass spectrometry assay for busulfan in biological fluids using a deuterated internal standard. *J Chromatogr*, **428**, 357–61.

91. Hassan M, Oberg G, Bekassy AN, et al. (1991) Pharmacokinetics of high dose busulphan in relation to age and chronopharmacology. *Cancer Chemother Pharmacol*, **28**, 130–4.

92. Vassal G, Fischer A, Challine D, et al. (1993) Busulfan disposition below the age of three: alteration in children with lysosomal storage disease. *Blood*, **82**, 1030–4.

93. Slattery JT, Sanders JE, Buckner CD, et al. (1995) Graft rejection and toxicity following bone marrow transplantation in relation to busulfan pharmacokinetics. *Bone Marrow Transplant*, **16**, 31–42.

94. Vassal G, Gouyette A, Hartmann O, Pico JL, Lemerle J (1989) Pharmacokinetics of high-dose busulfan in children. *Cancer Chemother Pharmacol*, **24**, 386–90.

95. Grochow LB, Krivit W, Whitley CB, Blazar B (1990) Busulfan disposition in children. *Blood*, **75**, 1723–7.

96. Hassan M, Oberg G, Bjorkholm M, Wallin I, Lindgren M (1993) Influence of prophylactic anticonvulsant therapy on high-dose busulphan kinetics. *Cancer Chemother Pharmacol*, **33**, 181–6.

97. Vassal G, Deroussent A, Hartmann O, et al. (1990) Dose-dependent neurotoxicity of high-dose busulfan in children: a clinical and pharmacological study. *Cancer Res*, **50**, 6203–7.

98. Grochow LB, Jones RJ, Brundrett RB, et al. (1989) Pharmacokinetics of busulfan: correlation with venoocclusive disease in patients undergoing bone marrow transplantation. *Cancer Chemother Pharmacol*, **25**, 55–61.

99. Chattergoon DS, Saunders EF, Klein J, et al. (1997) An improved limited sampling method for individualised busulphan dosing in bone marrow transplantation in children. *Bone Marrow Transplant*, **20**, 347–54.

100. Ljungman P, Hassan M, Bekassy AN, Ringden O, Oberg G (1997) High busulfan concentrations are associated with increased transplant-related mortality in allogeneic bone marrow transplant patients. *Bone Marrow Transplant*, **20**, 909–13.

101. Yang WZ, Begleiter A, Johnston JB, Israels LG, Mowat MRA (1992) Role of glutathione and glutathione-S-transferase in chlorambucil resistance. *Mol Pharmacol*, **41**, 625–30.

102. Bramson J, McQuillan A, Aubin R, et al. (1995) Nitrogen-mustard drug-resistant B-cell chronic lymphocytic-leukemia as an *in vivo* model for cross-linking agent resistance. *Mutat Res*, **336**, 269–78.

103. Morabito F, Filangeri M, Callea I, et al. (1997) Bcl-2 protein expression and p53 gene mutation in chronic lymphocytic leukemia: correlation with *in vitro* sensitivity to chlorambucil and purine analogs. *Haematologica*, **82**, 16–20.

104. Barnouin K, Leier I, Jedlitschky G, et al. (1998) Multidrug resistance protein-mediated transport of chlorambucil and melphalan conjugated to glutathione. *Br J Cancer*, **77**, 201–9.

105. Chang SY, Larcom BJ, Alberts DS, Larsen B, Walson PD, Sipes IG (1980) Mass spectrometry of chlorambucil, its degradation products and its metabolite in biological samples. *J Pharm Sci*, **69**, 80–4.

106. Leff P, Bardsley WG (1979) Pharmacokinetics of chlorambucil in ovarian carcinoma using a new HPLC assay. *Biochem Pharmacol*, **28**, 1289–92.

107. Oppitz MM, Musch E, Malek M, et al. (1989) Studies on the pharmacokinetics of chlorambucil and prednimustine in patients using a new high-performance liquid chromatography assay. *Cancer Chemother Pharmacol*, **23**, 208–12.

108. Alberts DS, Chang SY, Chen H-SG, Larcom BJ, Evans TL (1980) Comparative pharmacokinetics of chlorambucil and melphalan in man. *Recent Results Cancer Res*, **74**, 124–31.

109. Newell DR, Calvert AH, Harrap KR, McElwain TJ (1983) Studies on the pharmacokinetics of chlorambucil and prednimustine in man. *Br J Clin Pharmacol*, **15**, 253–8.

110. Adair CG, McElnay JC (1986) Studies on the mechanism of gastrointestinal absorption of melphalan and chlorambucil. *Cancer Chemother Pharmacol*, **17**, 95–8.

111. Ehrsson H, Wallin I, Simonsson B, Hartvig P, Oberg G (1984) Effect of food on pharmacokinetics of chlorambucil and its main metabolite, phenylacetic acid mustard. *Eur J Clin Pharmacol*, **27**, 111–14.

112. Bastholt L, Johansson CJ, Pfeiffer P, et al. (1991) A pharmacokinetic study of prednimustine as compared with prednisolone plus chlorambucil in cancer-patients. *Cancer Chemother Pharmacol*, **28**, 205–10.

113. Hartvig P, Simonsson B, Oberg G, Wallin I, Ehrsson H (1988) Inter- and intraindividual differences in oral chlorambucil pharmacokinetics. *Eur J Clin Pharmacol*, **35**, 551–4.

114. Godeneche D, Madelmont JC, Moreau MF, Plagne R, Meyniel G (1980) Comparative physico-chemical properties, biological effects, and disposition in mice of four nitrogen mustards. *Cancer Chemother Pharmacol*, **5**, 1–9.

115. McLean A, Newell D, Baker G, Connors T (1980) The metabolism of chlorambucil. *Biochem Pharmacol*, **29**, 2039–47.

116. Lee FYF, Coe P, Workman P (1986) Pharmacokinetic basis for the comparative antitumour activity and toxicity of chlorambucil, phyenylacetic acid mustard and b,b-difluorochlorambucil (CB7103) in mice. *Cancer Chemother Pharmacol*, **17**, 21–9.

117. Alberts DS, Chang SY, Chen H-SG, Larcom BJ, Jones SE (1979) Pharmacokinetics and metabolism of chlorambucil in man: a preliminary report. *Cancer Treat Rev*, **6** (Suppl), 9–17.

118. Lazarus HM, Reed MD, Spitzer TR, Rabba MS, Blumer JL (1987) High-dose IV thiotepa and cryopreserved autologous bone marrow transplantation for therapy of refractory cancer. *Cancer Treat Rep*, **71**, 689–95.

119. Hara J, Osugi Y, Ohta H, *et al.* (1998) Double-conditioning regimens consisting of thiotepa, melphalan and busulfan with stem cell rescue for the treatment of pediatric solid tumors. *Bone Marrow Transplant*, **22**, 7–12.

120. Henner WD, Shea TC, Furlong EA, *et al.* (1987) Pharmacokinetics of continuous-infusion high-dose thiotepa. *Cancer Treat Rep*, **71**, 1043–7.

121. Antman K, Ayash L, Elias A, *et al.* (1992) A phase II study of high-dose cyclophosphamide, thiotepa and carboplatin with autologous marrow support in women with measurable advanced breast cancer responding to standard-dose therapy. *J Clin Oncol*, **10**, 102–10.

122. Dunkel IJ, Boyett JM, Yates A, *et al.* (1998) High-dose carboplatin, thiotepa, and etoposide with autologous stem-cell rescue for patients with recurrent medulloblastoma. *J Clin Oncol*, **16**, 222–8.

123. Cohen NA, Egorin MJ, Snyder SW, *et al.* (1991) Interaction of N,N′,N″-triethylenethiophosphoramide and N,N′,N″-triethylenephosphoramide with cellular DNA. *Cancer Res*, **51**, 4360–6.

124. Dirven HAAM, Dictus ELJT, Broeders NLHL, van Ommen B, van Bladeren PJ (1995) The role of human glutathione-S-transferase isoenzymes in the formation of glutathione conjugates of the alkylating cytostatic drug thiotepa. *Cancer Res*, **55**, 1701–6.

125. Cohen BE, Egorin MJ, Balachandran Nayar MS, Gutierrez PL (1984) Effects of pH and temperature on the stability and decomposition of N,N′,N″-triethylenethiophosphoramide in urine and buffer. *Cancer Res*, **44**, 4312–16.

126. Musser SM, Pan S, Egorin MJ, Kyle DJ, Callery PS (1992) Alkylation of DNA with aziridine produced during the hydrolysis of N,N′,N-triethylenethiophosphoramide. *Chem Res Toxicol*, **5**, 95–9.

127. Teicher BA, Waxman DJ, Holden SA, *et al.* (1989) Evidence for enzymatic activation and oxygen involvement in cytotoxicity and antitumor activity of N,N′,N-triethylenethiophosphoramide. *Cancer Res*, **49**, 4996–5001.

128. McDermott BJ, Double JA, Bibby MC (1985) Gas chromatographic analysis of triethylenethiophosphoramide and triethylenephosphoramide in biological specimens. *J Chromatogr*, **338**, 335–45.

129. van Maanen RJ, vanOoijen RD, Beijnen JH (1997) Determination of N,N′,N-triethylenthiophosphoramide in biological samples using capillary gas chromatography. *J Chromatogr B*, **698**, 111–21.

130. Sano A, Matsutani S, Takitani S (1988) High-performance liquid chromatography of the antitumour agent triethylenethiophosphoramide and its metabolite triethylenephosphoramide with sodium sulphide, taurine, O-phthalaldehyde as pre-column fluorescent derivatization reagents. *J Chromatogr*, **458**, 295–301.

131. Lewis C, Lawson N, Rankin EM, *et al.* (1990) Phase I and pharmacokinetic study of intraperitoneal thioTEPA in patients with ovarian cancer. *Cancer Chemother Pharmacol*, **26**, 283–7.

132. Wadler S, Egorin MJ, Zuhowski EG, *et al.* (1989) Phase I clinical and pharmacokinetic study of thiotepa administered intraperitoneally in patients with advanced malignancies. *J Clin Oncol*, **7**, 132–9.

133. Hagen B, Nilsen OG (1987) The binding of thio-TEPA in human serum and to isolated serum protein fractions. *Cancer Chemother Pharmacol*, **20**, 319–23.

134. Strong JM, Collins JM, Lester C, Poplack DG (1986) Pharmacokinetics of intraventricular and intravenous N,N′,N-triethylenethiophosphoramide (thiotepa) in Rhesus monkeys and humans. *Cancer Res*, **46**, 6101–4.

135. Heideman RL, Cole DE, Balis F, *et al.* (1989) Phase I and pharmacokinetic evaluation of thiotepa in the cerebrospinal fluid and plasma of pediatric patients: evidence for dose-dependent plasma clearance of thiotepa. *Cancer Res* **49**, 736–41.

136. Cohen BE, Egorin MJ, Kohlhepp EA, Aisner J, Gutierrez PL (1986) Human plasma pharmacokinetics and urinary excretion of thiotepa and its metabolites. *Cancer Treat Rep*, **70**, 859–64.

137. Ng S-F, Waxman DJ (1993) Activation of thio-TEPA cytotoxicity toward human breast cancer cells by hepatic cytochrome P450. *Int J Oncol*, **2**, 731–8.

138. Ng S-F, Waxman DJ (1990) Biotransformation of N,N′,N -triethylenethiophosphoramide: oxidative desulfuration to yield N,N′,N -triethylenephosphoramide associated with suicide inhibition of a phenobarbital inducible hepatic P450 monooxygenase. *Cancer Res*, **50**, 466–71.

139. Ng S, Waxman D (1991) N,N′,N -triethylenethiophophoramide (thio-tepa) oxygenation by constitutive hepatic P450 enzymes and modulation of drug-metabolism and clearance *in vivo* by P450-inducing agents. *Cancer Res*, **51**, 9.

140. Hagen B, Neverdal G, Walstad RA, Nilsen OG (1990) Long-term pharmacokinetics of thio-TEPA, TEPA and total alkylating activity following i.v. bolus administration of thio-TEPA in ovarian cancer patinets. *Cancer Chemother Pharmacol*, **25**, 257–62.

141. O'Dwyer PJ, LaCreta F, Engstrom PF, *et al.* (1991) Phase I/pharmacokinetic re-evaluation of ThioTEPA. *Cancer Res*, **51**, 3171–6.

142. O'Dwyer PJ, LaCreta F, Nash S, *et al.* (1991) Phase I study of thiotepa in combination with the glutathione transferase inhibitor ethacrynic acid. *Cancer Res*, **51**, 6059–65.

143. Hagen B (1991) Pharmacokinetics of thio-TEPA and TEPA in the conventional dose-range and its correlation to myelosuppressive effects. *Cancer Chemother Pharmacol*, **27**, 373–8.

144. Newlands ES, Stevens MFG, Wedge SR, Wheelhouse RT, Brock C (1997) Temozolomide: a review of its discovery, chemical properties and clinical trials. *Cancer Treat Rev*, **23**, 35–61.

145. Tsang LLH, Quarterman CP, Gescher A, Slack JA (1991) Comparison of the cytotoxicity *in vitro* of temozolomide and dacarbazine, prodrugs of 3-methyl-(triazen-1yl)imidazole-4-carboxamide. *Cancer Chemother Pharmacol*, **27**, 342–6.

146. O'Reilly SM, Newlands WS, Glaser MG, *et al.* (1993) Temozolomide—A new oral acytotoxic chemotherapeutic agent with promising activity against primary brain-tumors. *Eur J Cancer*, **29A**, 940–2.

147. Newlands ES, O'Reilly SM, Glaser MG, *et al.* (1996) The Charing Cross Hospital experience with temozolomide in patients with gliomas. *Eur J Cancer*, **32A**, 2236–41.

148. Bower M, Newlands ES, Bleehen NM, *et al.* (1997) Multicentre CRC phase II trial of temozolomide in recurrent or progressive high-grade glioma. *Cancer Chemother Pharmacol*, **40**, 484–8.

149. Bleehen NM, Newlands ES, Lee SM, *et al.* (1995) Cancer Research Campaign phase II trial of temozolomide in metastatic melanoma. *J Clin Oncol*, **13**, 910–13.

150. Pearson ADJ, Estlin EJ, Lashford L, *et al.* Phase I study of temozolomide in pediatric patients with advanced cancer. *Proceedings of the American Society for Clinical Oncology, Philadelphia, PA,* 1996.

151. Stevens MFG, Hickman JA, Langdon SP, *et al.* (1987) Antitumor activity and pharmacokinetics of 8-carbamoyl-3-methylimidazo[5,1-d]-1,2,3,5-tetrazin-4(3H)-one (CCRG 81045:M&B 39831), a novel drug with potential as an alternative to dacarbazine. *Cancer Res*, **47**, 5846–52.

152. Liu LL, Markowitz S, Gerson SL (1996) Mismatch repair mutations override alkyltransferase in conferring resistance to temozolomide but not to 1,3-bis(2-chloroethyl)nitrosourea. *Cancer Res*, **56**, 5375–9.

153. Bobola MS, Tseng SH, Blank A, Berger MS, Silber JR (1996) Role of O-6-methylguanine-DNA methyltransferase in resistance of human brain-tumor cell-lines to the clinically relevant methylating agents temozolomide and streptozotocin. *Clin Cancer Res*, **2**, 735–41.

154. Shen F, Decosterd LA, Gander M, Leyvraz S, Biollaz J, Lejeune F (1995) Determination of temozolomide in human plasma and urine by high-performance liquid chromatography after solid-phase extraction. *J Chromatogr*, **667**, 291–300.

155. Kim HK, Lin CC, Parker D, Veals J, *et al.* (1997) High performance liquid chromatographic determination and stability of 5-(3-methyltriazen-1-yl)-imidazo-4-carboximide, the biologically active product of the antitumor agent temozolomide, in human plasma. *J Chromatogr*, **703**, 225–33.

156. Dhodapkar M, Rubin J, Reid JM, *et al.* (1997) Phase I trial of temozolomide (NSC 362856) in patients with advanced cancer. *Clin Cancer Res*, **3**, 1093–1100.

157. Reid JM, Stevens DC, Rubin J, Ames MM (1997) Pharmacokinetics of 3-methyl-(triazen-1-yl) imidazole-4-carboximide following administration of temozolomide to patients with advanced cancer. *Clin Cancer Res*, **3**, 2393–8.

158. Tsang LLH, Farmer PB, Gescher A, Slack JA (1990) Characterisation of urinary metabolites of temozolomide in humans and mice and evaluation of their cytotoxicity. *Cancer Chemother Pharmacol*, **26**, 429–36.

8 | Epipodophyllotoxins

Howard L. McLeod

Introduction

The podophyllotoxins have a long therapeutic history, with references as early as AD 900 to the use of the roots of wild chervil to treat cancer.[1] Sandoz Pharmaceuticals synthesized nearly 600 derivatives of podophyllin in the 1950s and 1960s and identified two active compounds, etoposide and teniposide (Fig. 8.1) with a unique mechanism of action.[1] Previous analogues had arrested cells in mitosis, but the new derivatives prevented proliferating cells from entering mitosis and reduced the mitotic index to zero. Subsequent studies identified topoisomerase II as a primary cellular target of epipodophyllotoxins.

Summary

	Etoposide	Teniposide
Brand name	Vepesid	Vumon
Previous names	VP-16, NSC 141540	VM-26, NSC 122819
Molecular weight (Da)	588.6	656.7
Mechanism of action	Topoisomerase II inhibitor	Same as etoposide
Cell-cycle specificity	G_2–M	Same as etoposide
Route of administration	Oral, intravenous, intraperitoneal	Intravenous
Protein binding (range) (%)	90 (51–95)	99 (98–99.7)
Metabolism	Yes, partially by P450 3A4	Yes, partially by P450 3A4
Elimination	Renal, biliary	Biliary
Terminal half-life (range) (h)	6 (2–20)	9 (3–30)
Toxicities	Neutropenia, muscositis	Same as etoposide
Unique features	Plasma concentration correlated with haematological toxicity	Plasma concentration correlated with haematological toxicity; infusion >100 mg/h associated with acute toxicity

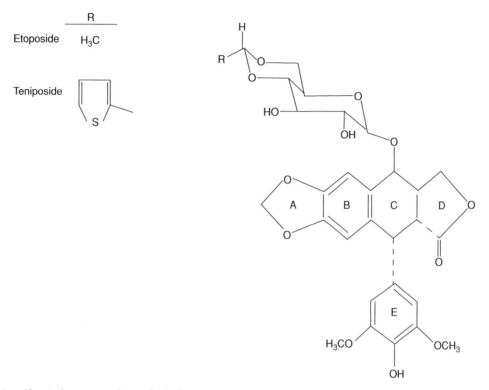

Figure 8.1. Chemical structure of epipodophyllotoxin compounds.

Clinical use

Teniposide and etoposide are widely used in the treatment of adult and paediatric malignancies.[2] Although both etoposide and teniposide have activity against adult malignancies, etoposide has been more broadly used in front-line therapy for small-cell lung cancer; germ-cell tumours, and Karposi's sarcoma, and as part of preparative regimens for bone marrow transplantation. Etoposide has also demonstrated activity against Hodgkin's disease, non-Hodgkin's lymphoma, ovarian carcinoma, and acute non-lymphoblastic leukaemias. Both etoposide and teniposide are used in front-line therapy for childhood cancers, including acute lymphoblastic leukaemia, neuroblastoma, rhabdomyosarcoma, and germ cell tumours.

Etoposide is commercially available as intravenous (20 mg/ml) and oral (10 and 50 mg gelatin capsules) formulations. Etoposide is poorly soluble in water and is formulated for intravenous use in polysorbate 80, polyethylene glycol 300, benzyl alcohol, citric acid, and ethanol. Preparations of etoposide for intravenous administration are stable in NaCl 0.9% or dextrose 5% at concentrations less than 0.5 mg/ml.

Etoposide capsules contain citric acid, glycerol, poylethylene glycol 400, and water. Teniposide is available only as an intravenous formulation (10 mg/ml). The intravenous formulation contains benzyl alcohol, ethanol, maleic acid, N_1N-dimethylacetamide, and polyoxyethylated castor oil (cremophor). Preparations of teniposide for intravenous administration are stable in NaCl 0.9% or dextrose 5% at 0.2 mg/ml for 4 h. Both etoposide and teniposide should be administered over at least 30–60 min to reduce acute toxicity. Teniposide has been associated with a greater frequency of hypersensitivity reactions than etoposide, presumably due to the presence of polyoxyethylated castor oil in the formulation. Detectable ethanol levels have been observed after intravenous administration of both etoposide and teniposide. Etoposide phosphate, a bioequivalent form of etoposide which is more water soluble, has recently completed early clinical evaluation, demonstrating antitumour activity with a decreased incidence of infusion-related toxicity compared with etoposide.

Mechanism of action

DNA topoisomerase II (topo II) is a key cellular target for both etoposide and teniposide. Topo II is a nuclear enzyme which alters DNA tertiary structure by creating transient double-stranded breakage of the DNA backbone, thus allowing subsequent passage of a second intact DNA duplex through the break (Fig. 8.2).[3] Etoposide seems to exert its action on topo II by inhibiting the ability of the enzyme to religate the cleaved DNA duplex. Etoposide can bind to *DNA in* the absence of topo II protein, but does so with relatively low affinity. Cleavage-site mapping suggests that etoposide is predisposed to induce topo-II-mediated DNA cleavage at sites that are immediately 3' to cytosine residues. Recent data show that etoposide–topo II (rather than drug–DNA) interactions mediate cleavage complex formation.[4] Through its role in assisting DNA passage, topo II generates transient double-stranded breaks in the nucleic acid backbone. Topo II then forms a bridge over the cleaved DNA (frequently referred to as the cleavable complex), which is normally a short-lived intermediate from the catalytic cycle of the enzyme. However, the presence of high levels of cleavable complex, due to poisoning of topo II by etoposide or teniposide, is potentially toxic, promoting mutation, permanent double-stranded DNA breaks, illegitimate recombination, and *apoptosis*.

There are two isoforms of topo II in mammalian cells, which are the products of different genes.[3] These isoforms are termed topo IIa (a 170 Da protein) and topo IIb (a 180 Da protein). Topo IIa is produced primarily in the late S phase and during the G_2–M phase of the cell cycle, whereas topo IIb is expressed throughout the cell cycle. In humans, the gene encoding topo IIa is mapped to chromosome 17q21–22 and topo IIb is mapped to chromosome 3p24. Several studies in human cancer cell lines have suggested that etoposide cytotoxicity is significantly correlated with topo IIb protein concentrations, but not significantly correlated with protein levels of topo IIa.[5] The relevance of this finding to the treatment of patients with etoposide or teniposide has not been fully evaluated.

A strong correlation between the cytotoxicity of etoposide and teniposide has been demonstrated, suggesting that there are no striking differences between the mechanisms of cytotoxicity for the two compounds. Teniposide is approximately 10 times more potent than etoposide on a molar basis, in terms of both *in vitro* cytotoxicity against human cell lines and ability to create DNA strand breaks.[1] The difference in antitumour activity is less apparent *in vivo*, where teniposide is only 1.5–3 times more potent.[1] The difference between *in vitro* and *in vivo* potency is probably due to the differences in lipophilicity, protein binding, hepatic metabolism, and related pharmacokinetic factors between the two compounds.

Mechanisms of resistance

A number of variables have been found to influence the cytotoxicity of etoposide and teniposide. Both epipodophyllotoxins are substrates for membrane efflux

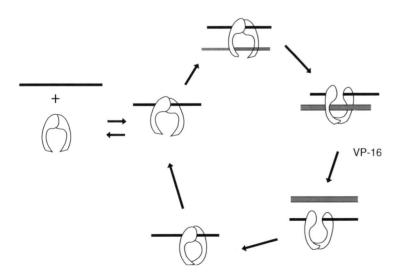

Figure 8.2. The topoisomerase II catalytic cycle. The enzyme is shown as a homodimer, the passing DNA strand is grey, and the cleaved DNA stand is black.

pumps, including p-glycoprotein 170. This pump results in the classical form of multidrug resistance, whereby a large number of structurally unrelated compounds display decreased activity in cell lines with high p-glycoprotein levels (see Chapter 1 for more details). Over-expression of p-glycoprotein is thought to enhance the ability of the cell to pump out the anticancer agents, thereby decreasing the drug concentration at intracellular target sites. Clinical studies combining etoposide with non-cytotoxic substrates for p-glycoprotein have been performed in attempts to circumvent this mechanism of drug resistance, with *PSC 833* being the most widely studied agent. Another form of resistance to epipodophyllotoxins is alteration in the level of topo II within the cell. Mutations in the topo II genes, altered topo II mRNA production, and decreased concentrations of topo II protein have all been described in cell lines with derived resistance to either etoposide or teniposide.

Chemistry

Teniposide and etoposide are 4-dimethyl-epipodophyllo-toxins with molecular weights of 656.7 Da and 588.6 Da, respectively. Teniposide only differs from etoposide in the substitution of a thenylidene ring in place of a methyl group (Fig. 8.1). Structure–activity studies have demonstrated that stereochemical restraints are needed on the C ring to maximize antitumour activity. Substitution at the 4-hydroxyl functional group on the E ring leads to decreased cytotoxic activity.

Analytical methodology

A number of analytical methods for quantitation of both etoposide and teniposide have been developed, with the majority using high-pressure liquid chromatography (HPLC).[2] Methods using UV spectroscopy, fluorescence, or electrochemical detection have been described Assay sensitivity in human plasma is approximately 400 nM for UV detection and 30 nM for electrochemical detection. Electrochemical detection methods are prone to poor linearity at high drug concentrations. An enzyme-linked immunosorbent assay (ELISA) method for etoposide has been described, with a sensitivity of 7.5 nM; however, specificity for parent drug is poor and the level of cross-reactivity with metabolites is not known.[2] Regardless of the approach used, simple, sensitive, reproducible, and automated assays are available for quantification of etoposide and teniposide in human biological fluids.

Pharmacokinetics and pharmacokinetic models

Absorption

The half-life for the absorption of etoposide following oral administration is 20–30 min, with peak concentrations occurring between 0.5 and 4 h. Delayed absorption patterns have been observed in patients receiving concurrent narcotics.[6] Oral bioavailability (%*F*) of the soft gelatin capsule formulation of etoposide in adult subjects is approximately 60%, with extensive variability (range 24–137%). Similar absorption (mean 48%) was observed in children receiving oral doses of the intravenous solution diluted in orange juice (range 35–88%). The P450 enzymes which metabolize etoposide and teniposide (e.g. P450 3A4) are known to be present in high abundance in gastrointestinal tissue. This may contribute to the reduced bioavailability of oral etoposide.

Etoposide oral absorption appears to be non-linear, with decreased bioavailability at doses above 200 mg (Fig. 8.3).[7] These findings suggest that, in attempts to increase therapy intensity, more frequent oral administration of lower doses of etoposide may be preferable to escalating oral doses above 200 mg/m[2] per dose. Etoposide phosphate has a mean bioavailability of 76% (range 37–144%), but again a trend toward decreasing %*F* at higher doses. There are no published reports of oral administration of teniposide.

Both disease risk factors (alcoholism, smoking) and treatment (surgery) of gastrointestinal tract malignancies can potentially effect the absorption of etoposide. Bioavailability was low (1–21%) in patients with advanced cancer of the head and neck, but altered absorption was not observed in patients with partial gastrectomy for gastric carcinoma.[8,9]

Protein binding

Etoposide and teniposide are extensively bound to plasma proteins, such that variability in plasma protein levels, and hence free (unbound) drug concentrations, may influence drug disposition and pharmacological effects. No evidence of saturation of protein binding has been observed *in vitro* for etoposide (1.7–425 μM)

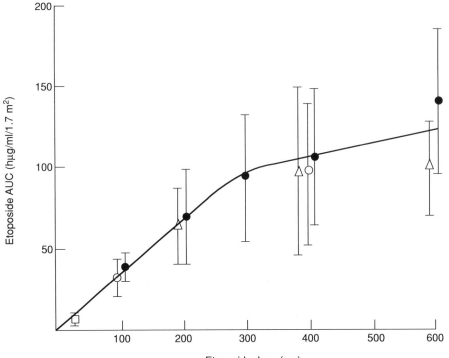

Figure 8.3. The influence of oral etoposide dose administered on measured AUC. Reproduced with permission from Hande *et al.* (1993) *J Clin Oncol*, **11**, 374–7.

or teniposide (15.2–304.6 μM). Etoposide is approximately 90% bound to plasma proteins in patients with normal serum albumin and bilirubin; however, wide inter-patient variability in the percentage of unbound drug (free fraction) has been reported in patients with cancer (range 5–49%).[10] *In vitro* studies have identified a single class of moderate affinity, and high-capacity binding sites in human plasma and etoposide protein binding were significantly correlated with albumin concentration. A model for predicting etoposide plasma protein binding in humans, based on serum albumin and total bilirubin concentrations, has been prospectively validated in cancer patients, with a slight bias towards overprediction of f_u in patients with normal bilirubin (< 1.5 mg/ml) or low albumin (< 3.3 g/dl) concentrations:[11]

% unbound = [1.4 × total bilirubin (mg/d1) − 6.8 × serum albumin (g/dl)] + 34.4.

Unbound etoposide systemic exposure (i.e. free AUC, free C_{ss}) is more precisely correlated with haematological toxicity than total etoposide systemic exposure, emphasizing the importance of measuring or estimating the concentration of compound that is available to exert a pharmacological effect.[12] Thus unbound (i.e. free) etoposide concentrations may be a better parameter to use for therapeutic drug monitoring, especially in patients where aberrant protein binding is anticipated (e.g. hypoalbuminaemia).

A higher degree of protein binding is observed with teniposide (> 98% bound to plasma proteins). The fraction of unbound teniposide is highly variable among patients (~10-fold) and is inversely linear related to serum albumin concentration. Teniposide free AUC correlated significantly with the percentage decrease in white blood cell count in children with acute lymphoblastic leukaemia, whereas the correlation for total teniposide AUC was not as strong.[13]

Central nervous system penetration

Penetration of etoposide into cerebrospinal fluid (CSF) is highly variable, ranging from undetectable to 2.5 μM 1–4 h after intravenous infusion or oral administration.[14,15] The concentration of etoposide in CSF varies between 0.09% and 4.2% of that measured simultaneously in plasma. No accumulation of eto-poside in CSF has been observed. Since the low level of protein in CSF results in less protein binding of etopo-side or teniposide, the amount of unbound (active) drug in CSF will be much greater at any given total drug concentration. For example, if etoposide protein binding is 95% in plasma versus 5% in CSF, a total CSF concentration of 0.2 μM would have an unbound (active) concentration comparable with a plasma con-centration of 3.8 μM (unbound, 0.19 μM for each).

Teniposide disposition in CSF has not been well defined. Teniposide CSF concentrations in a single patient reached 0.09 μM 2.5 h after a dose of 200 mg/m² intravenously.[16] The CSF-to-plasma ratio varied from 0.03% to 0.55%, and teniposide was detectable in the CSF 24 h after the first dose. These limited data for teniposide are consistent with those described for etoposide in CSF.

The disposition of etoposide after intrathecal admin-istration has been evaluated in a very small number of patients. The CSF-to-plasma ratio 1 h after a 0.01 mg/kg intrathecal etoposide injection was 1659:1.[17] Concentrations of etoposide in CSF 1–3 h after injec-tion were 1.9–8.8 μM, higher than that observed after intravenous injection. Concentrations above 0.3 μM were maintained in the CSF for at least 24 h after the single intrathecal injection.

Both etoposide and teniposide have been detected in brain tumour tissue after intravenous and oral drug administration, and concentrations in peritumoural tissue were lower than in tumour tissue.[18,19]

Peritoneal distribution

Teniposide distribution into malignant ascites after intravenous administration is highly variable, with

peak concentrations in ascitic fluid ranging from 2% to 21% of concentrations in serum.[20] Elimination of teni-poside from the peritoneal cavity is slow (median ter-minal half-life, 53 h), and intraperitoneal administration of teniposide yielded concentrations in ascitic fluid 8–20 times higher than those in plasma, although rapid distribution of teniposide into the systemic circulation was observed.[21] Very few studies of etoposide dis-position in the peritoneum have been performed. Concentrations of etoposide were 25–30 times higher in ascitic fluid than in plasma after continuous intraperitoneal infusion for 72 h.[22] The distribution of intravenous etoposide into malignant ascites has not been described.

Metabolism

Although the non-renal clearance of etoposide and teniposide is known to account for up to 70% and 90%, respectively, of elimination in humans, the meta-bolic fate of the drugs remains only partly elucidated. Several metabolites have been previously described in humans, including the hydroxyacid, glucuronide, and sulphate conjugates, and the *cis* or picro forms of the drugs. However, these metabolites have been recovered as only a minor percentage (<30%) of the administered dose and have limited or no *in vitro* cytotoxicity. In subjects with normal liver function, urinary excretion of etoposide glucuronide accounted for 3–29% of the administered dose. Although teniposide undergoes ex-tensive non-renal clearance, only trace quantities of teniposide metabolites have been found in humans. There is no evidence for saturation of *in vivo* etoposide or teniposide metabolism in children or adults.

In vitro studies have identified O-demethylation of the dimethoxyphenolic E ring of etoposide and tenipo-

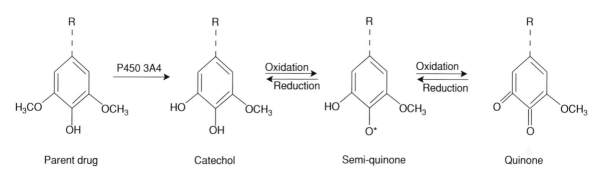

Figure 8.4. Pathway of P450-mediated O-demethylation of teniposide and etoposide to their catechol derivatives, with further oxidation to the semiquinone and quinone forms: R, remaining chemical structure for etoposide and teniposide (see Fig. 8.1).

side to their catechol and quinone forms (Fig. 8.4), with wide variability in maximum catechol formation rates.[23] The maximal formation rate is lower for teniposide catechol than fo etoposide catechol, and the rate of metabolism of both compounds is greater in normal than in diseased livers. Formation of both teniposide and etoposide catechol is catalysed by human P450 3A4. These reactions have important implications not only as routes of elimination but also, more importantly, because the reactive catechol metabolites can covalently bind to DNA and cellular proteins and have intrinsic cytotoxic activity.

Elimination

Etoposide is more rapidly eliminated than teniposide, with faster systemic clearance, greater renal clearance, and a shorter elimination half-life (Table 8.1). As the volume of distribution is similar for both drugs, the differences in disposition may be largely explained by differences in renal elimination, hepatic metabolism, and the more extensive binding of teniposide to plasma proteins. Approximately 30–70% of the excretion of an etoposide dose can be accounted for by renal and hepatic elimination, compared with 5–20% with teniposide. A linear relationship between etoposide systemic clearance and either measured or estimated creatinine clearance has been described for both adult and paediatric patients.[24,25] Renal clearance of etoposide is 10–50% of systemic clearance; however, the impact of this route of etoposide elimination appears to be influenced by the duration of intravenous administration. Renal clearance accounted for 30–50% of systemic clearance after etoposide infusion for 0.5–4 h, compared with 10–20% when the drug was administered as a 72 h infusion. Some authors have recommended a 30% decrease in etoposide dose for patients with serum creatinine > 120 μM (1.4 mg/dl) to

yield similar systemic exposure to patients with normal renal function.[26] In contrast, the renal clearance of teniposide is approximately 10% of systemic clearance in both adults and children. The biliary excretion of teniposide has not been well characterized; biliary clearance of parent drug or conjugated etoposide is a minor route of elimination (< 5%).

Pharmacokinetic drug interactions

Drug-induced alterations in etoposide and teniposide elimination have been described following co-administration of anticonvulsants, platinum complexes, and cyclosporines. As teniposide and etoposide rely on hepatic metabolism for a large degree of elimination, induction of hepatic enzymes by anticonvulsants (e.g. phenytoin, phenobarbital) or other agents may be of clinical importance. In a study of children receiving teniposide for acute lymphoblastic leukaemia (ALL), mean systemic clearance was 2.5 times faster in patients treated with *anticonvulsants* than in controls (Fig. 8.5).[27] In a single patient with multiple pharmacokinetic studies before and after the initiation of anticonvulsant therapy, teniposide clearance increased two- to threefold on anticonvulsants.[27] Alterations in etoposide clearance have also been observed in patients receiving prophylactic anticonvulsants during bone marrow transplantation.[28] Thus patients receiving anticonvulsant therapy will require higher doses of teniposide or etoposide to achieve a systemic exposure to parent drug that is comparable with that attained in the absence of interacting drug therapy.

The concurrent infusion of etoposide and *platinum* complexes does not appear to influence the pharmacokinetics of either drug. However, high cumulative doses of *cisplatin* have been associated with lower systemic clearance of etoposide in children. In addition, a 35–50%

Table 8.1　Epipodophyllotoxin disposition in patients with normal organ function

	Clearance (range) (ml/min/m^2)	Volume of distribution (range) (l/m^2)	Elimination half-life (range) (h)	Renal clearance (range) (ml/min/m^2)
Etoposide				
Adults i.v.	21 (9.5–44.8)	10 (2.1–22)	6 (2.1–41)	9 (4.4–24.6)
Children i.v.	20 (6.8–49)	7 (1.7–17.5)	5 (1.3–39)	8 (3–22)
Etoposide phosphate				
Adults i.v.	19 (8–30)	8 (3–18)	7 (3–20)	5.5 (2–11)
Teniposide				
Adults i.v.	15 (5.8–26.1)	11 (6–43.6)	8 (3–48.7)	NA
Children i.v.	13.5 (3.7–31.6)	8 (2.1–37.8)	9 (3.7–50.1)	NA

Pooled values (range) from multiple studies are presented. For more detailed evaluation see McLeod and Evans.[2]
NA, not available.

decrease in systemic clearance has been observed when etoposide was administered 24–48 h after either cisplatin or carboplatin.[28,29] These studies are consistent with an effect of platinum complexes on etoposide pharmacokinetics, through either altered renal elimination or decreased metabolism, or both.

Altered etoposide disposition has been observed when cyclosporin or its analogue *PSC 833* is co-administered in an attempt to modulate multi-drug resistance.[30] Systemic etoposide clearance (40–65% decease) and volume of distribution (40–50% increase) are both altered, resulting in a change in half-life. A decrease in both renal and non-renal clearance was noted, and these alterations suggest inhibition of P450 metabolism, perturbation of P-glycoprotein function, and/or modulation of other mechanisms of etoposide elimination.

Alterations with disease or age

Teniposide total systemic clearance in children with ALL was significantly lower at the time of disease relapse relative to patients in first remission.[13] Total systemic clearance then increased to values greater than in first-remission patients after a subsequent remission was achieved. The precise reasons for these changes are not clear, but they may involve altered protein binding secondary to hypoalbuminaemia resulting from the co-administration of 1-asparaginase.

Age-dependent changes in the disposition of etoposide and teniposide have not been observed in most pharmacokinetic studies to date. The systemic clearance of etoposide in children is similar to that observed in adults and infants (< 1 year), and teniposide systemic clearance (ml/min/m²) was similar to that observed in children (1–19 years).[31] However, clearance when normalized to body weight was lower in the children used.[31] These findings support the use of body surface area, rather than body weight, to achieve a similar degree of systemic exposure regardless of body size. Systemic clearance is lower in subjects aged over 70 years, which may reflect the decrease in glomerular filtration rate observed with increasing age.[32]

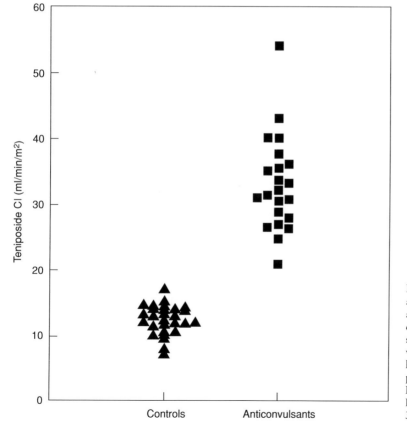

Figure 8.5. Teniposide systemic clearance values for all treatment courses administered to six children receiving concurrent anticonvulsant therapy and six control children. All clearance values for the control patients were lower than all clearance values for the patients treated with anticonvulsants. Reproduced with permission from Baker *et al.* (1992) *J Clin Oncol*, **10**, 311–15.

Pharmacokinetic models

The disposition of etoposide and teniposide has been described by both compartmental and non-compartmental pharmacokinetic models. Two- and three-compartment models have been most widely used, with the G phase usually only detectable after administration of high-dose therapy.

Limited sampling strategies for intravenous and oral etoposide have primarily used linear regression analysis to generate equations for the prediction of etoposide AUC from a small number of samples, while maintaining acceptable bias and precision.[2] All models have restricted analysis to sampling times post-infusion and have demonstrated good performance on a validation dataset. However, there are no published prospective validation studies for any model when used in a separate laboratory. The use of linear regression or multivariate analysis to generate predictive models for pharmacokinetic parameters has many statistical and practical problems. The stepwise regression approach assumes that the sampling time point of most influence in a single-sample model will continue to be important in models with a greater number of sample points. This is not always the case, as a single-sample model may select a mid-elimination time point while a two-sample model selects time points which reflect multiple elimination phases. This approach is also restrictive in the specific times at which samples must be taken. For example, in clinical practice the 4 h time point may actually be obtained 2–6 h after infusion. Also, if the drug is not given as a bolus, stepwise regression models may not compensate for differences in duration of admission. Linear mathematical equations do not have the flexibility to accomodate such deviations, thus restricting their application. Such difficulties have lead to Bayesian algorithms which can better manage data with imprecise sampling or variation in administration duration, and therefore are more amenable to adaptive control trials.

Somewhat more complex methodology has been applied to adaptive control trials of teniposide using Bayesian estimation strategies. The intersubject variability in teniposide clearance required a threefold range of doses to produce similar plasma AUC.[33] This approach has resulted in a 50% increase in exposure intensity over that previously possible with standard fixed doses, with no increase in acute non-haematological toxicity, by reducing the variability in teniposide AUC.

Pharmacodynamics

Etoposide

The influence of etoposide systemic exposure (AUC, C_{ss}, trough concentrations, etc) on haematological toxicity has been demonstrated in many clinical trials (reviewed by McLeod and Evans[2]). A linear relationship between leukocyte survival fraction (ratio of nadir count to pretreatment count) and C_{ss} has been observed in patients receiving etoposide as continuous infusions for 72 h to 14 days.[34–36] The etoposide C_{ss} associated with a 50% decrease in leukocyte count ranged from 0.7 to 1.9 μM with the 14 day infusions to 7.8 μM with the 72 h infusion. Similar correlations have been observed with etoposide AUC during and after 24 h continuous infusions, mean or trough concentration with hyperfractionated or once daily oral administration for 21 days, and systemic clearance with 1 h infusions on three consecutive days.[37,38] The addition of *cisplatin* to oral etoposide monotherapy altered the etoposide C_{mean} associated with a 50% decrease in leukocyte count (1.8 μM for etoposide alone versus 0.7 μM for etoposide plus cisplatin).[37]

A relationship between etoposide pharmacokinetic parameters and tumour response has been described in a small number of patients with solid tumours. Both etoposide plasma concentrations at steady-state and AUC, but not dose, correlated with response.[39] A stepwise relationship was observed in patients receiving a 14 day infusion of etoposide, where a partial response was observed in one of ten patients with $C_{ss} < 1.7$ μM, two of eight with $C_{ss} = 1.7–2.0$ μM, and five of 11 with $C_{ss} \geq 2.0$ μM.[36] There is evidence for schedule dependency for etoposide therapy.[40] The length of time that etoposide concentrations exceeded a threshold concentration is an additional variable which appears to have a significant influence on both the degree of haematological toxicity and the antitumour activity of the drug. An increase in the probability of severe haematological toxicity (>80% decrease in neutrophil count) was observed as a function of the time that etoposide concentrations exceeded 1.7 μM in children receiving oral etoposide therapy for 21 days.[6] The incidence of toxicity ranged from no to four patients with <2 h to three of five patients when plasma concentrations exceeded 1.7 μM for >6 h after the initial dose (Fig. 8.6).[6] The number of hours that the etoposide concentrations were above 1.7 μM has also been correlated with drug activity in patients with previously untreated extensive small-cell lung cancer.[40] A greater overall response rate was observed in a 5 day regimen than the same dose administered over 24 h (85% versus 10%).[41] This difference was associated with the number of hours thatetoposide concentrations were greater than 1.7 μM (94.5 h versus 46 h). Etoposide AUC was not different between the two groups. A follow-up comparison of etoposide 500 mg/m², as five daily 100 mg/m² infusions or eight daily 62.5 mg/m² infusions, found a similar overall response rate (81% versus 87%).[42] As with the initial trial, the time that etoposide concentrations exceeded 1 μg/ml was a significant predictor of response. The timethat concentrations exceeded 0.5 μg/ml was significantly greater in the 8-day arm, with no improvement in antitumour activity, suggesting that 0.5 μg/ml is below the critical threshold. The 8-day arm had a lower degree of haematological toxicity than the 5-day arm, which was best associated with the time that etoposide concentrations exceeded 2–3 μg/ml.[42] This suggests that there is a therapeutic index for infusional etoposide where maximal tumour activity can be achieved with minimal haematological toxicity. Prospective trials are under way to evaluate the feasibility and outcome of such an approach

The above data suggest that a threshold concentration is required for effective inhibition of the primary cellular target, topo II. Concentrations exceeding the threshold may not confer greater activity, but rather contribute to normal tissue toxicity. The sensitivity threshold will probably differ for specific tumour types, individual tumours, and possibly each tumour cell. As topo II isoforms show a degree of cell-cycle-dependent expression,[3] maintaining etoposide concentrations over a prolonged period may enhance drug action.

The introduction of etoposide therapy has had a direct bearing on survival rates in lymphoma, leukaemia, and some solid tumours. As more patients survive longer after treatment with epipodophyllotoxins, long-term toxicities appear. The most devastating of these long-term toxicities is secondary leukaemia. The occurrence of secondary leukaemia, specifically secondary acute myelogeneous leukaemia, has been associated with regimens which utilize frequent etoposide administration (weekly or alternating weeks) as opposed to intermittent treatment as used in high-dose therapy (bone marrow transplantation, some solid tumours).[43] These observations suggest that the frequent administration of teniposide or etoposide leads to transforming mutations in normal haematopoietic progenitor cells. By stabilizing the complex between DNA and topo II and inhibiting its repair, epipodo-

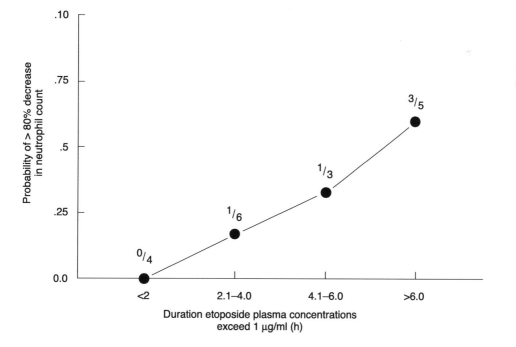

Figure 8.6. Relationship between the estimated duration that plasma etoposide concentrations exceed 1 mg/ml at steady state and the development of severe neutropenia (>80% decrease in the absolute neutrophil count from baseline). Reproduced with permission from Sonnichsen *et al.* (1995) *Clin Pharmacol Ther*, **58**, 99–107.

phyllotoxins induce single- and double-strand DNA breaks which have been related to cytotoxic effects. Recent *in vitro* studies suggest that etoposide causes illegitimate V(D)J recombination in human lymphoid leukaemic cells.[44] These recombination events occurred in a dose-dependent manner and increased to highest levels after prolonged exposure (6 days). Importantly, recombinogenesis was not inextricably linked to cytotoxicity.[45] Thus the ratio of cytotoxicity to genetic recombination increased with prolonged exposure, suggesting that long-term administration of epipodophyllotoxins decreases the risk of drug-induced acute leukaemia without compromising treatment efficacy. Clinical evaluation of this hypothesis is of great importance as it may help to define the future use of prolonged administration regimens (i.e. oral for 21 days).

Teniposide

The pharmacodynamics of teniposide has not been as extensively studied as etoposide. However, clinical pharmacokinetic studies of teniposide have also demonstrated correlations with toxicity and tumour response. In a study of children with relapsed leukaemia or lymphomas, C_{ss} was significantly higher in those patients who responded (median 24.4 versus 8.1 μM) owing to faster teniposide clearance in the non-responding group (Fig. 8.7).[46] While the incidence of both toxicity and response increased with increasing teniposide C_{ss}, a favourable therapeutic index was found at an AUC of 1200–1800 μM h when teniposide was given as a 72 h infusion, providing a high probability of response with an acceptable level of reversible toxicity. This has led to studies of adaptive control dosing of teniposide, where Bayesian analysis is used to individualize patient dose to achieve a target C_{ss} or AUC.[33,47] Escalation of teniposide by AUC led to a 50% increase in intensity of systemic exposure over that possible with standard fixed doses (mg/m^2).[33] A prospective clinical trial was then performed in children with ALL, where 188 patients were randomized to receive consolidation (post-acute remission) therapy with methotrexate, teniposide, and cytarabine at a conventional fixed dose (mg/m^2) or an individualized dose to achieve a target AUC.[47] The target AUC corresponded to the fiftieth to ninetieth percentile for children treated with conventional therapy (teniposide 200 mg/m^2 over 4 h, 360–525 μM h). Intra-patient variation in teniposide systemic clearance was lower (median CV, 17%) than inter-patient variability (median CV, 40%).[47] In the

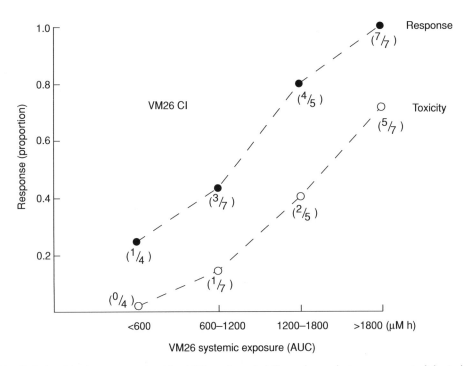

Figure 8.7. Relationship between teniposide AUC and probability of oncolytic response (solid circles) or grade 2–4 gastrointestinal toxicity (open circles) Reproduced with permission from Evans *et al.* (1998) *N Engl J Med*, **338**, 499–505.

individualized study arm, patients required a threefold range in teniposide dose to reach the target AUC (158–424 mg/m^2).[47] Analysis of outcome identified a significantly better relapse-free survival for children with B-cell ALL in the individualized chemotherapy arm with a twofold relative risk of relapse in the conventional therapy group. However, on more detailed analysis the greatest impact was observed with methotrexate systemic exposure, and the risk of relapse was not significantly related to teniposide AUC.[47]

References

1. Stähelin HF, von Wartburg A (1991) The chemical and biological route from podophyllotoxin glucoside to etoposide: Ninth Cain Memorial Award Lecture. *Cancer Res*, 51, 5–15.
2. McLeod HL, Evans WE (1998) Epipodophyllotoxins. In Grochow LB, Ames MM (eds) *A Clinician's Guide to Chemotherapy Pharmacokinetics and Pharmacodynamics*. Baltimore, MD: Williams & Wilkins, 259–87.
3. Watt PM, Hickson ID (1994) Structure and function of type II DNA topoisomerases. *Biochem J*, 303, 681–95.
4. Burden DA, Kingma PS, Froelich-Ammon SJ, Bjornsti MA, Patchan MW, Thompson RB (1996) Topoisomerase II etoposide interactions direct the formation of drug induced enzyme DNA cleavage complexes. *J Biol Chem*, 271, 29238–444.
5. Brown GA, McPherson JP, Lie G, Hedley DW, Toso R, Deuchars KL (1995) Relationship of DNA topoisomerase IIα and β expression of cytotoxicity of antineoplastic agents in human acute lymphoblastic leukemia cell lines. *Cancer Res*, 55, 78–82.
6. Sonnichsen DS, Ribeiro RC, Luo X, Mathew P, Relling MV (1995) Pharmacokinetics and pharmacodynamics of 21 day continuous oral etoposide in pediatric solid tumor patients. *Clin Pharmacol Ther*, 58, 99–107
7. Hande KR, Krozely MG, Greco FA, Hainsworth JD, Johnson DH (1993) Bioavailability of low-dose oral etoposide. *J Clin Oncol*, 11, 374–7.
8. Desoize B, Woirin V, Legros M, Coninx P (1992) Reduced oral etoposide bioavailability in patients with advanced cancer of the head and neck. *J Natl Cancer Inst*, 84, 348–50.
9. Taal BG, Beijnen JH, Teller FGM, Huinink WWT, Dubbelman R, Boot H (1994) Bioavailability of oral etoposide in gastric cancer. *Eur J Cancer*, 30A, 420–1.
10. Stewart CF, Arbuck SG, Pieper JA, Evans WE (1989) Altered protein binding of etoposide in patients with cancer. *Clin Pharmacol Ther*, 45, 49–55.
11. Stewart CF, Fleming RA, Arbuck SG, Evans WE (1990) Prospective evaluation of a model for predicting etoposide plasma protein binding in cancer patients. *Cancer Res*, 50, 6854–6.
12. Stewart CF, Arbuck SG, Fleming RA, Evans WE (1991) Relation of systemic exposure to unbound etoposide and hematologic toxicity. *Clin Pharmacol Ther*, 50, 385–93.
13. Evans WE, Rodman JH, Relling MV, Petros WP, Stewart CF, Pui CH (1992) Differences in teniposide disposition and pharmacodynamics in patients with newly diagnosed and relapsed acute lymphoblastic leukemia. *J Pharmacol Exp Ther*, 260, 71–7.
14. Postmus PE, Holthuis JJM, Haaxma-Reiche H, *et al.* (1984) Penetration of VP 16–213 into cerebrospinal fluid after high-dose intravenous administration. *J Clin Oncol*, 2, 215–20.
15. Relling MV, Mahmoud HH, Pui C-H, *et al.* (1996) Etoposide achieves potentially cytotoxic concentrations in CSF of children with acute lymphoblastic leukemia. *J Clin Oncol*, 14, 399–404.
16. Holthuis JJM, de Vries EGE, Postmus PE, *et al.* (1987) Pharmacokinetics of high-dose teniposide. *Cancer Treat Rep*, 71, 599–604.
17. van der Gaast A, Sonneveld P, Mans DRA, Splinter TAW (1992) Intrathecal administration of etoposide in the treatment of malignant meningitis: feasibility and pharmacokinetic data. *Cancer Chemother Pharmacol*, 29, 335–7.
18. Zuchetti M, Rossi C, Knerich R, *et al.* (1991) Concentrations of VP16 and VM26 in human brain tumors. *Ann Oncol*, 2, 63–6.
19. Kiya K, Uozumi T, Ogasawara H, *et al.* (1992) Penetration of etoposide into human malignant brain tumors after intravenous and oral administration. *Cancer Chemother Pharmacol*, 29, 339–42.
20. Canal P, Bugat R, Michel C, *et al.* (1985) Pharmacokinetics of teniposide (VM 26) after IV administration in serum and malignant ascites of patients with ovarian carcinoma. *Cancer Chemother Pharmacol*, 15, 149–52.
21. Chatelut E, de Forni M, Canal P, *et al.* (1991) Teniposide and cisplatin given by intraperitoneal administration: preclinical and phase I/pharmacokinetic studies. *Ann Oncol*, 2, 217–21.
22. Isonish S, Kirmani S, Kim S, *et al.* (1991) Phase I and pharmacokinetic trial of intraperitoneal etoposide in combination with the multidrug-resistance modulating agent dipyridamole. *J Natl Cancer Inst*, 83, 621–6.
23. Relling MV, Nemec J, Schuetz EG, *et al.* (1994) O-demethylation of epipodophyllotoxins is catalyzed by human cytochrome P450 3A4. *Mol Pharmacol*, 45, 352–8.
24. Stewart CF (1994) Use of etoposide in patients with organ dysfunction: pharmacokinetic and pharmacodynamic considerations. *Cancer Chemother Pharmacol*, 34, S76–83.
25. Lowis SP, Pearson ADJ, Newell DR, Cole M (1993) Etoposide pharmacokinetics in children: the development and prospective validation of a dosing equation. *Cancer Res*, 53, 4881–9.
26. Joel SP, Shah R, Slevin ML (1994) Etoposide dosage and pharmacodynamics. *Cancer Chemother Pharmacol*, 34, S69–75.
27. Baker DK, Relling MV, Pui C-H, Christenson ML, Evans WE, Rodman JH (1992) Increased teniposide clearance with concomitant anticonvulsant therapy. *J Clin Oncol*, 10, 311–15.
28. Rodman JH, Murry DJ, Madden T, Santana VM (1994) Altered etoposide pharmacokinetics and time to engraft-

ment in pediatric patients undergoing autologous bone marrow transplantation. *J Clin Oncol*, **12**, 2390–7.

29. Relling MV, McLeod HL, Bowman LC, Santana VM (1994) Etoposide pharmacokinetics and pharmaco-dynamics after acute and chronic exposure to cisplatin. *Clin Pharmacol Ther*, **56**, 503–11.

30. Lum BL, Kaubisch S, Yahanda AM, Adler KM, Jew L, Ehsan MN (1992) Alteration of etoposide pharmacokinetics and pharmacodynamics by cyclosporine in a phase I trial to modulate multidrug resistance. *J Clin Oncol*, **10**, 1635–42.

31. McLeod HL, Relling MV, Crom WR, Silverstein K, Groom S, Rodman JH (1992) Disposition of antineoplastic agents in the very young child. *Br J Cancer*, **66**, S23–9.

32. Pflüger K-H, Hahn M, Holz J-B, Schmidt L, Köhl P, Fritsch HW (1993) Pharmacokinetics of etoposide: correlation of pharmacokinetic parameters with clinical conditions. *Cancer Chemother Pharmacol*, **31**, 350–6.

33. Rodman JH, Furman WL, Sunderland M, Rivera G, Evans WE (1993) Escalating teniposide systemic exposure to increase dose intensity for pediatric cancer patients. *J Clin Oncol*, **11**, 287–93.

34. Ratain MJ, Mick R, Schilsky RL, Volgelzang NJ, Berezin F (1991) Pharmacologically based dosing of etoposide: a means of safely increasing dose intensity. *J Clin Oncol*, **9**, 1480–6.

35. Kunitoh H, Watanabe K (1994) Phase I/II and pharmacologic study of long-term continuous infusion etoposide combined with cisplatin in patients with advanced non-small-cell lung cancer. *J Clin Oncol*, **12**, 83–9.

36. Minami H, Shimokata K, Saka H, *et al.* (1993) Phase I clinical and pharmacokinetic study of a 14-day infusion of etoposide in patients with lung cancer. *J Clin Oncol*, **11**, 1602–8.

37. Minami H, Ando Y, Sakai S, Shimokata K (1995) Clinical and pharmacologic analysis of hyperfractionated daily oral etoposide. *J Clin Oncol*, **13**, 191–9.

38. Miller AA, Tolley EA, Niell HB, Griffin JP, Mauer AM (1993) Pharmacodynamics of prolonged oral etoposide in patients with advanced non-small-cell lung cancer. *J Clin Oncol*, **11**, 1179–88.

39. Desoize B, Marechal F, Cattan A (1990) Clinical pharmacokinetics of etoposide during 120 hours continuous infusions in solid tumours. *Br J Cancer*, **62**, 840–1.

40. Lowis SP, Newell DR (1996) Etoposide for the treatment of paediatric tumours. What is the best way to give it? *Eur J Cancer*, **32A**, 2291.

41. Slevin ML, Clark PI, Joel SP, *et al.* (1989) A randomized trial to evaluate the effect of schedule on the activity of etoposide in small-cell lung cancer. *J Clin Oncol*, **7**, 1333–40.

42. Clark PI, Slevin ML, Joel SP, *et al.* (1994) A randomized trial of two etoposide schedules in small-cell lung cancer: the influence of pharmacokinetics on efficacy and toxicity. *J Clin Oncol*, **12**, 1427–35.

43. Pui CH, Relling MV, Rivera GK, *et al.* (1995) Epipodophyllotoxin related acute myeloid leukemia—a study of 35 cases. *Leukemia*, **9**, 1990–5.

44. Chen C-L, Fuscoe JC, Liu O, Relling MV (1996) Etoposide causes illegitimate V(D)J recombination in human lymphoid leukemic cells. *Blood*, **88**, 2210–18.

45. Chen C-L, Fuscoe JC, Liu O, Pui CH, Mohmoud HH, Relling MV (1996) Relationship between cytotoxicity and site-specific DNA recombination after *in vitro* exposure of leukemia cells to etoposide. *J Natl Cancer Inst*, **88**, 1840–7.

46. Evans WE (1988) Clinical pharmacodynamics of anticancer drugs: a basis for extending the concept of dose-intensity. *Blut*, **56**, 241–8.

47. Evans WE, Relling MV, Rodman JH, Crom WR, Boyett JM, Pui CH (1998) Conventional compared with individualized chemotherapy for childhood acute lymphoblastic leukemia. *N Engl J Med*, **338**, 499–505.

9 | Anthracyclines

Jacques Robert

Introduction

Daunorubicin was the first anthracycline isolated, in France and Italy simultaneously in 1963, from the fermentation broth of an actinobacteria *Streptomyces peucetius*, and its antileukaemic properties in the clinic were rapidly acknowledged. While the French group at Rhône-Poulenc developed semisynthetic derivatives, the Italian group at Farmitalia focused on naturally occurring analogues and isolated doxorubicin (adriamycin, 14-hydroxy-daunorubicin) from the variant *S.peucetius caesius*, whose anticancer activity was rapidly shown to extend to solid tumours.[1]

The high potency of these drugs encouraged the pharmaceutical industry in Europe and Japan to isolate or synthesize a huge number of molecules, but only a

Summary

	Doxorubicin	Epirubicin	Daunorubicin	Idarubicin
Brand names	Adriblastin	Farmorubicin	Cerubidine	Zavedos
Other names	Adriamycin	4′-epi-adriamycin	Rubidomycin, daunomycin	4-Demethoxy-daunorubicin
Molecular weight (Da)	580	580	564	534
Cell-cycle specificity	No phase specificity	No phase specificity	No phase specificity	No phase specificity
Route of administration	Intravenous (also intraperitoneal and intra-arterial))	Intravenous	Intravenous	Intravenous, oral
Protein binding (%)	70	80	80	>80
Metabolism to 13-dihydro derivatives	Low	Low	High	High
Elimination	Mainly hepatic (renal, 10%)	Mainly hepatic (renal, 10%)	Mainly hepatic (renal, 10%)	Mainly hepatic (renal, 10%)
Terminal half-life (h)	20–30	18–24	15–18	12–16
Toxicities	Neutropenia, mucositis, alopecia, cardiomyopathy	Less toxic than doxorubicin	Same as doxorubicin	Same as doxorubicin

	Doxorubicin	Epirubicin	Daunorubicin	Idarubicin
Indications	Mainly used in solid tumours (breast and other adenocarcinomas, sarcomas, lymphomas)	Mainly used in solid tumours (breast and other adenocarcinomas, sarcomas, lymphomas)	Essentially used in haematology (acute leukaemias)	Essentially used in haematology (acute leukaemias)
Special features	Chronic cardiac toxicity related to cumulative dose	Chronic cardiac toxicity related to cumulative dose	Chronic cardiac toxicity related to cumulative dose	Chronic cardiac toxicity related to cumulative dose

few have been brought to clinical trial and even fewer have entered routine clinical use. We will only consider here the four anthracyclines that are presently marketed in most Western countries and Japan: doxorubicin, epirubicin, daunorubicin, and idarubicin. Two special formulations of anthracyclines in liposomes have also been marketed and will be discussed.

Doxorubicin remains the most widely used anthracycline and is the benchmark against which all new compounds in this series are compared. Although these compounds have closely related structures (Fig. 9.1), they are characterized by different metabolic pathways and pharmacokinetics. The mechanism of action of anthracyclines has been the matter of much debate; it is now generally accepted that their primary target for cytotoxicity is the nuclear enzyme DNA topoisomerase II (topo II), but the high number of cellular effects of

these drugs may still explain some features, especially at the level of their toxic effects.

Chemistry

Anthracyclines are constituted of a planar polyaromatic ring system (the chromophore) bearing a quinone moiety, which is linked by an O-glycosidic bond to an aminosugar. Several hundred structural analogues have been obtained by synthetic modification of daunorubicin or doxorubicin.[1] The key carbon atoms for modification are as follows: (i) on the chromophore, C-4 (methoxylated in daunorubicin and doxorubicin, no substituent in idarubicin); (ii) on the side chain, C-13 (reduced from ketone to hydroxyl to generate dihydro derivatives; or bearing various substituents in the series developed by Rhône-Poulenc); C-14, being either a methyl group (daunorubicin and idarubicin) or a hydroxymethyl group (doxorubicin, epirubicin and pirarubicin); (iii) on the sugar, C-4' (hydroxyl oriented downwards in doxorubicin, upwards in epirubicin, or bearing an O-tetrahydropyranyl group in pirarubicin); C-3', bearing the characteristic amino group, which can be substituted by a morpholinyl group in a series of special anthracyclines in development. It appears that only few atoms can be modified in the structure to generate molecule which is still active, and that these modifications can be very subtle (e.g. epimerization of a sugar) and give rise to a quite distinct molecule.

Anthracyclines present an intense orange-red colour and absorb light in both the UV (at 254 nm) and visible (~480 nm) regions of the spectrum. They are highly sensitive to light. The polyaromatic structure of the aglycone results in an intense fluorescence, allowing their detection and quantification by high-pressure liquid chromatography (HPLC) and several cellular techniques (flow cytometry, confocal laser imaging, etc.). Intercalation of anthracyclines in DNA produces a 98% quenching of this fluorescence, which has to be

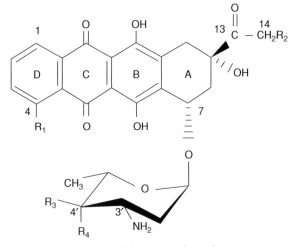

Figure 9.1.   Structure of the main anthracyclines.

R$_1$	R$_2$	R$_3$	R$_4$
Doxorubicin	OCH$_3$	OH	H	OH
Epirubicin	OCH$_3$	OH	OH	H
Daunorubicin	OCH$_3$	H	H	H
Idarubicin	H	H	H	OH

taken into account for subcellular distribution studies by fluorescence imaging.

All anthracyclines are currently used in the hydrochloric form, which allows good solubility in both water and polar organic solvents (methanol, acetonitrile). The pKa of the amino group of anthracyclines (daunorubicin, doxorubicin, idarubicin), which have an unsubstituted daunosamine, is approximately 8.2. It is lower for 4'-substituted molecules such as epirubicin (pKa = 7.7) or iododoxorubicin (pKa = 6.5). The lipophilicity of anthracyclines increases in the order doxorubicin < epirubicin < daunorubicin < idarubicin < pirarubicin, and this parameter governs cellular uptake of these drugs. The molecular weight of doxorubicin (hydrochloride) is 580 Da. The molecular extinction at 477 nm is 13 050, and this value should be used for calibration in quantitative studies. Anthracyclines have a tendency to form dimeric aggregates in solution, with an association constant of 10^4 M^{-1}. This can lead to erroneous spectrophotometric evaluations in concentrated solutions.

Mechanism of action

It was rapidly recognized that anthracyclines inhibit DNA and RNA syntheses.[1] It was shown that anthracyclines were able to interact directly with the DNA molecule; the planar ring system intercalates between DNA base pairs, and the amino sugar interacts in the major groove with the negatively charged phosphate moieties.[2,3] Anthracyclines have a very high affinity for DNA, with an association constant of about 10^6 M^{-1}. It was believed that intercalation itself caused anthracycline cytotoxicity by inhibiting DNA replication and transcription. Subsequently, the ability of anthracyclines to generate oxygen free radicals,[4] together with the discovery that they were responsible for DNA breaks, was believed to be the molecular mechanism of action of anthracyclines.[5] This hypothesis has now been clearly excluded.[6] Finally, it was shown in 1984 that the primary molecular target of anthracyclines was the nuclear enzyme DNA topo II,[7] and it is now universally agreed that this represents the molecular mechanism of action of this class of drugs.[8]

Topo II is a nuclear enzyme responsible for modifications of the tertiary structure of DNA, especially in regulating the level of supercoiling of the double helix, which is required for DNA replication and transcription. To achieve these topological alterations, topo II first recognizes a DNA sequence, then nicks the two strands of DNA, cleaving two phosphodiester bonds at a four-base interval, and finally religates the two breaks, restoring DNA continuity. In the meantime, another DNA chain can pass through the *break*, generating knotting and unknotting operations or creating positive or negative supercoils of DNA. In this situation, the continuity of the DNA molecule only exists through the covalent binding of the 5'-phosphate end of each break with a tyrosine of each subunit of topo

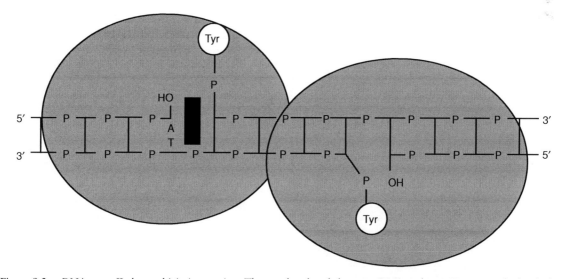

Figure 9.2.   DNA–topo II–doxorubicin interaction. The covalent bonds between DNA and topo II occur at the level of two tyrosines, which are both linked to a 5'-phosphate group of the cleaved DNA. The black rectangle schematizes the intercalation of doxorubicin between two base pairs at the level of one of the DNA breaks, with an adenine at position −1.[9,10]

II, and four groups of hydrogen bonds between DNA bases (Fig. 9.2). The 'cleavable complex' might be deleterious to the cell *in vivo* if the religation step is delayed. A number of drugs of different classes are able to stabilize the cleavable complex, thus transforming topo II into a cellular poison. Some of these drugs are intercalators (anthracyclines, mitoxantrone, dactinomycin, amsacrine); others are not (epipodophyllotoxins). It has been shown that the DNA sequences where topo II generates a cleavable complex are not the same for the class of drugs stabilizing the complex,[9] which might explain the specificity of antitumour activity of each drug family. It has also been shown that, among anthracyclines, there are differences in the degree of stabilization of the cleavable complex,[10] which may explain the different potency of each drug.

There are a number of arguments supporting the possibility that stabilization of the cleavable complex is only a signal generating a message for active cell death.[11] *Apoptosis* appears as a common final path for the cytotoxicity of most anticancer drugs, especially those acting through stabilization of cleavable complexes of DNA with topoisomerases. It is likely that anthracyclines do not escape this general rule, even though there is no definitive proof that anthracycline-induced cell death always satisfies all the criteria of programmed cell death.

Anthracyclines are able to generate oxygen free radicals by at least two distinct pathways,[4] but it is very doubtful if this contributes to cell death and antiproliferative effects. However, it is generally admitted that this could explain, at least partially, the cardiotoxicity of these molecules.[6] In the presence of NADH or NADPH, several flavoproteins can induce a one-electron reduction of anthracyclines, generating a reduced semi-quinone radical form (Fig. 9.3). One of the possible fates of this form is the restoration of the original anthracycline through reduction of molecular oxygen (redox cycling). The superoxide anion can be detoxified by successive actions of superoxide dismutase and catalase, but in the presence of iron (Fe^{3+}) it can generate the hydroxyl radical $OH^{\bullet}$, which is toxic for all the molecules present in its immediate vicinity, leading to DNA and protein breaks or lipid peroxidation. Flavoproteins able to perform the one-electron reduction of doxorubicin can be found in the endoplasmic reticulum (cytochrome P450 reductase) or in the mitochondria (NADH dehydrogenase). It does not seem possible that these free radicals, which have a very short lifetime, can reach the nucleus and nick DNA. In contrast, the high affinity of anthracyclines for the mitochondrial lipid cardiolipin, which is of the same order of magnitude as their affinity for DNA, might account for mitochondrial disruption, for instance at the level of the double bonds of unsaturated lipids. Some evidence has been presented in favour of this mechanism of anthracycline cardiotoxicity, which is clearly due to a mitochondrial injury. The abundance of mito-

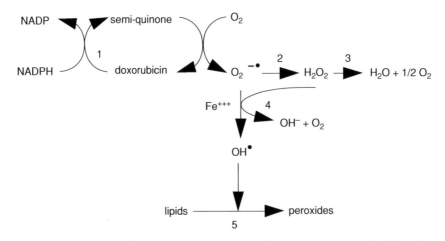

Figure 9.3. Anthracycline redox cycling. Doxorubicin can be converted into a semi-quinone radical form by a monoelectronic reaction involving NADPH and an oxidoreductase such as cytochrome P-450 reductase (1); in the presence of molecular oxygen, the semi-quinone reduces oxygen to a superoxide ion $O_2^{-\bullet}$ which can be detoxified by superoxide dismutase (2) and catalase (3) In the presence of ferric ions, the superoxide anion can generate, with hydrogen peroxide, the hydroxyl radical $OH^{\bullet}$ (Haber–Weiss reaction) (4), which is particularly aggressive for the molecules of its environment, generating in particular peroxides from lipid aliphatic chains (5).

chondria, together with the lack of antioxidant defence in the heart, might render this organ especially susceptible to anthracycline-induced lipid peroxidation.[6]

Mechanisms of resistance

The over-expression of P-glycoprotein constitutes a major mechanism of cellular resistance to anthracyclines.[12] This protein is responsible for the multidrug resistance (MDR) phenotype, characterized by cross-resistance between anthracyclines, vinca alkaloids, epipodophyllotoxins, taxanes, etc. It appears that most anthracyclines are equally subjected to P-glycoprotein action. However, the cross-resistance appears lower for the most lipophilic drugs of the series such as idarubicin; this is due to the faster uptake of these analogues rather than to their slower extrusion.[13] It is likely that MDR has clinical relevance, especially in haematological malignancies and childhood tumours.[14] A number of compounds, such as verapamil, quinine, or cyclosporine A, are able to reverse MDR and restore drug accumulation within the cell.[15] Such compounds are presently under clinical development.

Another membrane ATPase, called MDR-related protein (MRP), also causes resistance to anthracyclines and other drugs with a slightly different pattern of cross-resistance compared with P-glycoprotein.[16] MRP has been shown to extrude drugs and xenobiotics preferentially after their conjugation to glutathione. However, no glutathione conjugate of doxorubicin has ever been identified in any kind of cell. The question has been raised as to whether there is an intracellular redistribution of anthracyclines in cells overexpressing the MRP gene, since some MRP lines do not present any reduction of doxorubicin accumulation. This suggests that it may exist in intracellular sequestration compartments, preventing doxorubicin to reach its nuclear target.[17]

Alterations in DNA topo II also explain resistance to anthracyclines as well as to other topo-II-interfering drugs such as epipodophyllotoxins. These alterations may be quantitative (decrease of enzyme expression at its expected site of action) or qualitative (point mutations preventing either the enzyme to realize the cleavable complex or the drug to stabilize this complex).[18] A number of other alterations have been observed in cell lines rendered resistant to doxorubicin, but none of them has proved to be actually involved in resistance. In particular, they may concern non-specific defence mechanisms developed in response to any aggression.

The lowered level of free-radical formation and lipid peroxidation, which has been noticed in doxorubicin-resistant cell lines, does not contribute directly to doxorubicin resistance but may be part of this kind of general response.[19]

Clinical use

Doxorubicin is widely used in the treatment of adult solid tumours, with indications in breast cancer, small-cell lung cancer, bladder cancer, soft-tissue and osteogenous sarcoma, Hodgkin's disease and non-Hodgkin's lymphomas, ovarian and gastric carcinoma, etc. It is also active in adult and paediatric acute leukaemias and in childhood solid tumours. *Epirubicin* has roughly the same anticancer profile, but is generally used in adult solid tumours rather than in other malignancies. *Daunorubicin and idarubicin are* restricted to the treatment of adult and paediatric acute *leukaemias* (both myeloblastic and lymphoblastic), although they may also be of interest in the treatment of *lymphomas* or breast cancer. So far, liposomal daunorubicin and doxorubicin are only indicated for Kaposi's sarcoma.

Doxorubicin and epirubicin are both available as intravenous formulations of 10, 50, 150, or 200 mg of product. They are presented either as lyophilized powders, and should be reconstituted with sterile apyrogenic water to reach a concentration of 2 mg/ml, or as ready-to-use liquid formulations at the same concentration. Daunorubicin and idarubicin are available only as lyophilized powders containing 20 mg daunorubicin, or 5 or 10 mg idarubicin. In addition, oral formulations of idarubicin containing 1, 5, 10 or 20 mg of drug are available. *Liposomal daunorubicin and doxorubicin* are formulated as ready-to-use suspensions containing 50 mg daunorubicin or 10 mg doxorubicin (2 mg/ml). In all cases, further dilution of the concentrated drug solutions or suspensions in glucose 5% is recommended.

Doxorubicin is generally administered as a direct intravenous bolus at a dose of 35–70 mg/m^2 repeated every 3 weeks.[20] Other administration schedules have been developed but are less common, especially prolonged infusions over 2–5 days with a mean dose of 15 mg/m^2/day,[21] which significantly reduced the risk of congestive heart failure.[22] Intracavitary and intra-arterial routes, particularly through the hepatic artery, are feasible but have never entered routine use.

Epirubicin is generally administered like doxorubicin by bolus injections at 3-week intervals. The maximum tolerated dose per injection was initially estimated to be about 75 mg/m^2; this has recently been re-evaluated and is now estimated to be about 120 mg/m^2.

Daunorubicin and idarubicin doses are generally fractionated over 3–5 days at doses of 30–45 mg/m^2/day for daunorubicin and 8–15 mg/m^2/day for idarubicin. Weekly administration of daunorubicin is also routinely used in the treatment of childhood acute lymphoblastic leukaemias, and oral idarubicin is also proposed on a weekly schedule at a dose of 30–50 mg/m^2.

Analytical methodology

A number of analytical techniques have been developed for the determination of anthracyclines and their metabolites. Most of them can be used indifferently for any anthracycline with minor adaptations. Extraction of the drugs from biological fluids can be achieved with either organic solvents at alkaline pH[23] or C-18 cartridges.[24] Separation and quantitation is generally obtained by HPLC using reversed phase columns (C-18 or ODS) and a solvent made from a mixture of acetonitrile or methanol and aqueous buffer at pH 2–4.[25] With reversed phase silicagel columns, the order of elution ranges from the most polar to the least polar compound. Detection of anthracyclines in HPLC systems must be achieved by fluorometry, which combines the advantages of high sensitivity and high selectivity, and allows a lower limit of quantification of approximately 1 ng/ml.

Anthracycline accumulation in cells can be evaluated by flow cytometry or fluorescence microscopy, using various conditions of incubation, in leukaemia cells obtained from patients or grown in continuous lines.[26] Fluorescence quenching of anthracyclines in the nucleus has been profitably used for evaluating accumulation of anthracycline in living cells.[27] This consists in the continuous recording of the fluorescence emitted by a cell suspension placed in a nutrient medium in a 1 cm spectrofluorometer cuvette under continuous stirring. The addition of an anthracycline is followed by the occurrence of a fluorescence signal which progressively decreases upon uptake of the drug by the cells and its intercalation in DNA.

Metabolism

A common biotransformation for all anthracyclines is the reduction of the ketone on C-13, yielding 13-dihydro derivatives with a hydroxyl moiety. These compounds are usually named after the parent anthracycline with the suffix -ol (daunorubicinol, doxorubicinol, etc.). The enzyme responsible for this transformation is a ubiquitous aldoketoreductase located in the cytoplasm of all cells and tissues, especially erythrocytes, liver, and kidney,[28] but not in plasma. This enzyme has a higher affinity for daunorubicin and idarubicin than for doxorubicin and epirubicin; hence the plasma concentrations of the 13-dihydro derivatives are much higher than those of the unchanged compounds for the anthracyclines of the daunorubicin family. *In vitro*, the 13-dihydro derivatives are much less cytotoxic than the parent anthracyclines, except for idarubicinol which is as active as idarubicin.[29] However, they may be responsible for the largest part of anthracycline cardiotoxicity.[30]

Deglycosylation of anthracyclines, leading to inactive aglycones, has been shown to occur *in vitro* by the action of microsomal enzymes in anaerobic conditions.[31] This enzyme was originally characterized as a glycosidase. Whether this transformation occurs *in vivo* has been the subject of much debate. The 7-deoxyaglycones of anthracyclines and their 13-dihydro derivatives are often observed in plasma and urine of patients treated with anthracyclines, especially epirubicin, but their appearance is generally transient and unpredictable, and their concentrations always remain lower than those of the parent drug and its 13-dihydro derivative. The structure of the metabolites of doxorubicin is presented in Figure 9.4.

In addition to the formation of epirubicinol and aglycones, epirubicin undergoes conjugation to β-glucuronic acid to form β-*O*-glucuronide conjugates, which is a unique metabolic pathway specific to humans.[32] These metabolites are inactive, but are quantitatively important in plasma since the AUC ratio of metabolite to unchanged drug may reach 1.0.

Pharmacokinetics

Plasma pharmacokinetics

After bolus administration, doxorubicin disappears from plasma following a triexponential decay characterized by three successive half-lives close to 3–5 min, 1–2 h, and 24–36 h,[33–37] although a biexponential model sometimes gives a better description of the decay of drug concentrations in plasma.[38] A typical profile of doxorubicin decay from plasma after bolus administration of a standard dose is given in Figure 9.5. The total

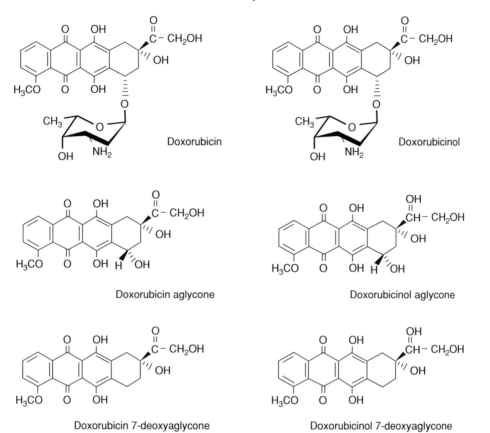

Figure 9.4. Structure of metabolites and/or degradation products of doxorubicin.

plasma clearance of doxorubicin is around 30 l/h/m² and its total volume of distribution at steady state is approximately 800 l/m² (Table 9.1). The plasma peak concentration after a bolus injection is very high and $AUC_{(0-20\ min)}$ contributes 30–40% to $AUC_{(0-\bullet)}$. Therefore the early phase may play a role in determining of the efficacy or toxicity of the treatment.[39] The kinetics of doxorubicin are linear, i.e. no significant change of drug clearance occurs with increasing dose.[40] During prolonged infusions lasting for 2–6 days at a dose of 9–25 mg/m²/day, the plasma clearance obtained is the same as after bolus injection,[41,42] which means that the kinetics of doxorubicin are not schedule dependent. In that case, the plateau concentration is obtained within 24 h of the infusion. Doxorubicinol is the only metabolite regularly found in the plasma of patients treated with doxorubicin. After a bolus injection, its plasma concentration rapidly increases and then decreases in parallel to that of doxorubicin; thereafter, this metabolite disappears from plasma with a half-life similar to or slightly longer than that of dox-

orubicin. The ratio of $AUC_{(0-\infty)}$ of doxorubicinol to $AUC_{(0-\infty)}$ of doxorubicin is generally in the range 0.3–0.5.

It is remarkable that the other anthracyclines of interest systematically have a faster clearance and a larger volume of distribution at steady state than doxorubicin. This is due to their higher tissue fixation, their higher lipophilicity, and their increased metabolism. The pharmacokinetic parameters that have been obtained in selected studies are summarized in Table 9.1. However, these parameters are subject to important individual variations.

Epirubicin has similar kinetics to doxorubicin, although plasma levels at equivalent doses are always lower than those of doxorubicin, even at steady state.[34,35,43,44] Epirubicin has a 50–100% faster plasma clearance than doxorubicin. As for doxorubicin, the plasma peak concentration of epirubicin after a bolus injection is very high and $AUC_{(0-20\ min)}$ contributes 30–40% to $AUC_{(0-\infty)}$. The pharmacokinetics are linear.[45–47] Epirubicinol has a similar pharmacokinetic behaviour

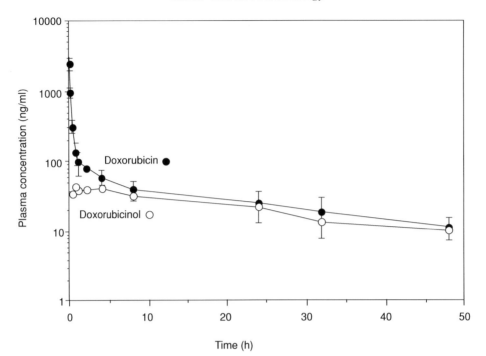

Figure 9.5. Plasma pharmacokinetics of doxorubicin. Evolution of plasma concentrations of doxorubicin and doxorubicinol obtained after bolus administration of 50 mg/m^2 in sarcoma patients.[33]

Table 9.1 Main pharmacokinetic parameters of some anthracyclines of clinical use

Author & Ref.	No of courses	Dose (mg/m^2)	$T_{1/2}$ (α) (mm)	$T_{1/2}$ (β) (h)	$T_{1/2}$ (γ) (h)	TPCl (l/h/m^2)	VD_{SS} (l/m^2)	$T_{1/2}$ (metab) (h)	AUC metab / AUC drug
Doxorubicin									
Robert *et al.* [33]	26	50–75	4.18	1.60	34.7	29.5	885	29.3	0.33
Mross *et al.* [34]	8	40–60	2.46	0.79	25.8	34.7	988	32.8	0.34
Camaggi *et al.* [35]	8	60	4.84	2.56	48.5	32.7	1371		0.66
Jacquet *et al.* [36]	18	25–72			28.5	25.7	1016	34.4	0.53
Twelves *et al.* [37]	5	75	4.80	2.4	33.0	44.1	2198		0.44
Christen *et al.* [38]	6	60	5		29.8	30.1	1287		0.52
Epirubicin									
Mross *et al.* [34]	8	40–60	1.80	0.49	15.3	50.1	592	31.5	0.20
Camaggi *et al.* [35]	8	60	2.92	1.08	31.4	43.1	1272		0.35
Jakobsen *et al.* [436]	16	60	3.92	1.94	24.3	47.8	776		0.42
Robert & Bui [44]	5	100	2.73	1.95	21.7	52.6	851	27.4	0.74
Daunorubicin									
Rahman *et al.* [48]	4	60	5.40	3.50	14.2	95.0	1334	23.4	3.97
Speth *et al.* [49]	4	45	20		18	50.0	1582		
Idarubicin									
Zanette *et al.* [50]	9	8–15			12.6	46.2		71.6	5.11
Stewart *et al.* [51]	13	15	5.40		15.5	56	1138	51.4	3.0
Camaggi *et al.* [52]	21	12	2.73	0.94	16.2	58.0	955	48.7	4.85

in plasma to that of doxorubicinol after an injection of doxorubicin. The glucuronides of epirubicin and epirubicinol reach a high C_{max} 1–2 h after epirubicin bolus administration, and disappear from plasma with a faster half-life than the parent drug (12–15 h). Their $AUC_{(0–48\ h)}$ values are of the same order of magnitude as those of the unconjugated compound.

The terminal half-life of unchanged daunorubicin is about 15–20 h.[48] The daunorubicin plasma peak concentration after bolus intravenous injection is much lower than that of doxorubicin or epirubicin, and the first phase of the kinetics represents only a small fraction of the total $AUC_{(0–\infty)}$. The pharmacokinetics of

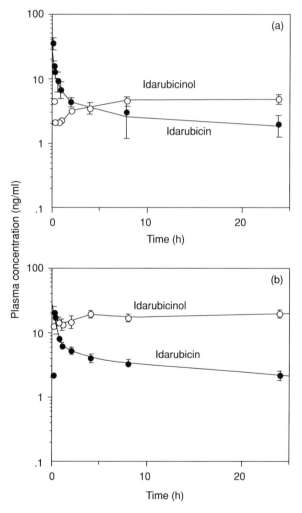

Figure 9.6. Plasma pharmacokinetics after iterative injections of idarubicin. Evolution of plasma concentrations of idarubicin and idarubicinol obtained after (a) the first and (b) the last bolus intravenous administration of a series of five daily doses of 8 mg/m² in leukaemia patients.[53]

daunorubicin did not appear to be schedule dependent in the 72-h infusions studied by Speth *et al.*[49] The circulating plasma levels of daunorubicinol in humans largely exceed those of daunorubicin and the AUC ratio of metabolite to unchanged drug is about 2–5. Daunorubicinol becomes the major circulating compound 1–2 h after an injection of daunorubicin and disappears from plasma with a terminal half-life of about 30 h. Repetitive daily administration of daunorubicin is not followed by a significant accumulation of the drug or metabolite in plasma.

The pharmacokinetics of idarubicin after intravenous administration is most often described by a biexponential model, with half-lives of 20 min and 15–20 h.[50–52] As for daunorubicin, the 13-dihydro derivative is a major metabolite, with an AUC ratio of metabolite to unchanged drug of 2–5 and an elimination half-life of 40–60 h. Owing to the rapid transformation to the 13-dihydro-derivative, the total plasma clearance of the idarubicin is very high, about 60 l/h/m². After oral administration, the terminal half-lives of idarubicin and idarubicinol are no different from those observed by intravenous administration, but idarubicinol has increased concentrations so that the AUC ratio of metabolite to unchanged drug is even higher than after intravenous injection. The bioavailability of idarubicin has been estimated to be 20–30%.[50–52] However, since idarubicinol is as active as idarubicin, the total bioavailability of the active species is about 40–50%. The repetitive daily administration of idarubicin is followed by a significant increase in idarubicinol plasma concentrations from day to day.[53] A typical profile of idarubicin and idarubicinol plasma concentrations after the first and last administrations of a series of five daily doses is shown in Figure 9.6.

Drug distribution and elimination

The plasma protein binding of doxorubicin has been estimated to be about 70%; that of the other anthracyclines, which all are more lipophilic than doxorubicin, appears to be substantially higher.[54] Anthracycline concentrations in tumours and normal tissues largely exceed those found in plasma.[55] The highest accumulation of drug is generally seen in the liver. Speth *et al.*[56] showed that white blood cells accumulated 100–200 times the plasma concentration of doxorubicin, independently of the schedule of administration. Disappearance of doxorubicin from white blood cells was estimated to proceed with a half-life of about 100 h, much longer than the half-life of the drug in the plasma compartment.

Epirubicin accumulation in white blood cells is systematically higher than that of doxorubicin evaluated under the same conditions, reflecting its higher lipophilicity. However, it is eliminated more rapidly from cells than doxorubicin, and its elimination half-life from white blood cells is about 50 h.[57] In the case of daunorubicin and idarubicin, cellular concentrations are 400–500 times higher than plasma concentrations, and the metabolite is proportionally much less concentrated than the parent drug in white blood cells. Daunorubicin and idarubicin disappeared from white blood cells with a half-life similar to that found for drug elimination from plasma.[48,58]

Anthracyclines do not cross the blood–brain barrier in significant quantities, and barely detectable concentrations are found in the cerebrospinal fluid (CSF) after intravenous injections (P. Cappelaere and J. Robert, unpublished results). It has been reported that idarubicinol was able to cross the blood–brain barrier in significant quantities, but this feature has never been reported for other anthracyclines.[59] In fact, the CSF levels of idarubicinol are extremely low (median value, 0.5 ng/ml). In the absence of clear clinical results showing activity of idarubicin against meningeal invasion by leukaemia cells, the use of idarubicin as a prophylactic treatment of such leukaemic extensions should not be recommended.

Elimination of anthracyclines mainly proceeds through the bile, and urinary excretion barely exceeds 10% of the dose injected.[60] The metabolites present in bile and urine are the same as those found in plasma, namely the 13-dihydro derivatives, aglycones, and eventually conjugates. Several observations tend to show that renal elimination of idarubicin is more important than the estimation obtained from fluorescent drug and metabolite, and that urinary non-fluorescent unidentified metabolites could well account for the excretion balance of idarubicin.

Alterations of pharmacokinetics in disease

Alterations of renal function have not been shown to modify the pharmacokinetics of most anthracyclines significantly. In contrast, liver dysfunction, whether or not due to neoplastic invasion, may profoundly alter the disposition of doxorubicin[61] and epirubicin.[62] This has led to empirical dosage reductions of doxorubicin or epirubicin according to total bilirubin plasma levels (50% when bilirubinaemia reaches 25 μM, and 100% when bilirubinaemia reaches 50 μM). Twelves et al.[63] have observed that serum aspartate aminotransferase is a better predictor of anthracycline clearance than bilirubinaemia; there is a strong inverse correlation between the logarithm of aspartate aminotransferase activity and epirubicin clearance, irrespective of bilirubin levels.

An additional reduction in the dosage of idarubicin should be recommended for treating patients with renal dysfunction (creatinine clearance <60 l/h) whatever the route of administration.[52]

Pharmacokinetic drug interactions

Only a few drug-induced alterations in anthracycline kinetics have been described. Concerning combinations with other cytostatics, Cummings et al.[64] have shown that etoposide co-administration could increase doxorubicin clearance up to twofold. *Paclitaxel* has been shown to be responsible for a non-linear disposition of doxorubicin and doxorubicinol, as evidenced from repetitive administrations of the combination in metastatic breast cancer patients.[65] This has been attributed, without clear evidence, to competition between the two drugs at the level of P-glycoprotein-mediated biliary excretion. The interaction between high-dose aracytine and daunorubicin or idarubicin pharmacokinetics has never been studied in detail.

The association of doxorubicin with MDR reverters has been studied in some detail. Cyclosporin A and its analogue PSC-833 are able to decrease doxorubicin clearance significantly (by ~50%).[66,67] Similar observations were made for *etoposide* or taxol. The alteration of doxorubicin pharmacokinetics by MDR reverters must lead to a modification of the strategy used for the development of these drugs: Sikic[68] has proposed that, instead of maintaining the usual dosage of the anticancer drug and increasing the reverter dose to the maximum tolerated dose of the combination, it would be wiser to use the reverter at its maximum tolerated dose and to increase the dose of the anticancer drug progressively to a predetermined level of myelosuppression.

The pharmacokinetics of the interactions of anthracyclines with antiemetics, antibiotics, or anti-inflammatories have not been described in the literature. The combination of doxorubicin or epirubicin with dexrazoxane (ICRF-187), a cardioprotector used in combination with doxorubicin, does not seem to modify their pharmacokinetics[69] and the usual doxorubicin clearance of 30–35 l/h/m^2 is maintained at dexrazoxane doses up to 600 mg.

Limited sampling strategies

Based upon the pharmacokinetic data, several authors have developed limited-sampling models in order to calculate the total plasma clearance of doxorubicin or epirubicin from two or three selected plasma samples. Such limited samplings allow the establishment of population kinetic data for individual dose monitoring. For doxorubicin, the best time points for sampling have been determined to be about 30 min and 24 h after injection,[70] and 2 h and 48 h after injection.[71] Bayesian approaches have also been developed[72] and have been proved of practical use for the study of pharmacokinetic drug interactions. For epirubicin, it has been shown that two samplings obtained 2 and 24 h after administration, or a single sample obtained 6 h after administration, could predict correctly for clearance.[73] A Bayesian approach has been developed by Wade *et al.*,[74] who have shown that age and gender are significant covariates for epirubicin clearance, which decreases with age and is slightly higher in males than in females.

Pharmacodynamics

Anthracyclines are very cytotoxic molecules that are part of a number of well-established protocols in many types of cancer. Owing to the dose dependence of their activity, which has been demonstrated for doxorubicin[75] and epirubicin[76] in particular, the administration of the highest tolerable doses is desired. However, owing to the considerable toxicity of these drugs, both immediate (myelosuppression and mucositis) and delayed (cardiac toxicity), there is a need for an individual

adaptation of doses and schedules. Unfortunately, this has never been done. Alternative important PIG and PD variability in toxicity warrants adaptive dosing.

Few studies have related doxorubicin efficacy in patients to its pharmacokinetics. A correlation between the peak plasma concentration and short-term response to the drug has been shown in a study of 12 patients with locally advanced breast cancer treated primarily with doxorubicin.[77] The doxorubicin plasma concentration obtained 3 h after administration was shown to be significantly correlated with the outcome of remission induction therapy in 45 patients treated for acute non-lymphocytic leukaemia.[78] In both studies, the distribution phase of the pharmacokinetics was an important determinant of drug efficacy.

Only two documented studies have shown a pharmacokinetic–pharmacodynamic relationship for doxorubicin toxicity. Ackland *et al.*[79] were able to show a correlation between doxorubicin plasma concentration at steady state (C_{ss}) of a prolonged infusion and the nadir of white blood cells. Piscitelli *et al.*[61] found that plasma AUC values after a bolus of 45–72 mg/m^2 doxorubicin correlated with the relative decrease in white blood cells (WBCs) according to the equation

WBC survival fraction = $0.219\exp(-0.00026 \times \text{AUC})$
($r = 0.57$, $p = 0.0025$).

This equation shows that 10% cell survival is obtained for AUC ≈ 3000 h ng/ml, and the corresponding graph is shown in Figure 9.7.

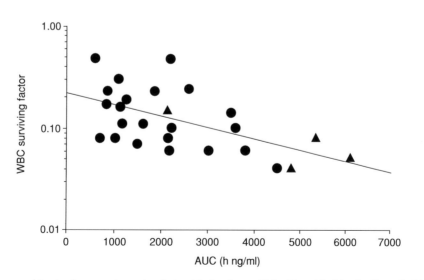

Figure 9.7. Pharmacokinetic-pharmacodynamic relationship for doxorubicin. The white blood cell survival fraction is plotted as a function of doxorubicin AUC in patients with (triangles) and without (circles) liver impairment.[61] The relationship is significant: $r = 0.57$, $p < 0.0025$.

For epirubicin, Jakobsen *et al.*[73] have shown a positive correlation between the plasma AUC value of epirubicin and its toxic effects on bone marrow, evaluated as the survival fraction of white blood cells at nadir, according to the equation

WBC survival fraction = 0.84exp(–0.00044 × AUC)
(r = 0.61, p = 0.0001).

Thus 10% cell survival is obtained for AUC ≈ 4800 h ng/ml. In both cases, the AUC can be calculated with an acceptable precision using the limited-sampling strategies that have been developed and validated by several authors.

Concerning daunorubicin and idarubicin, it appears more difficult for antileukaemic drugs to establish pharmacokinetic–pharmacodynamic relationships using absolute or relative drops in white blood cell counts, since the purpose of the remission induction treatment is precisely to reach leukaemic cell aplasia. Galettis *et al.*[80] tried to correlate daunorubicin disposition with the response of acute leukaemias to induction therapy. No correlation was found between daunorubicin plasma pharmacokinetic parameters and the occurrence of remissions. In contrast, daunorubicin and daunorubicinol accumulation in leukaemic cells was significantly correlated with response. Stewart *et al.*[51] observed a significant relationship between granulocyte nadirs and idarubicinol AUC value in whole blood, suggesting that the release of idarubicinol from erythrocyte pools could contribute to the cytotoxicity of the chemotherapy. In metastatic *breast* cancer patients treated with oral idarubicin, Elbaek *et al.*[81] observed that total idarubicin plus idarubicinol AUC value over 3 weeks of treatment correlated with the relative drop in leucocyte counts, but not with the absolute leucocyte counts at nadir.

Cardiac toxicity of anthracyclines remains a relatively rare event, especially because therapists are aware of the dramatic increase in the risk of congestive heart failure when the cumulative dose of doxorubicin reaches 550 mg/m². This dose has been established empirically by the study of several thousand chemotherapy courses which had generated a limited number of cardiac events.[82] It has been shown that this cumulative dose could still be increased by the use of continuous infusion therapy.[22] Pharmacokinetics has been of no help in establishing predictive indicators for cardiotoxicity either for new anthracyclines in general or for a given anthracycline in individual patients. The only published study is that of Cummings *et al.*[83], who noticed that patients who had early doxorubicin-induced cardiotoxicity had the highest plasma levels of 7-deoxyaglycones. This is consistent with the view that doxorubicin cardiotoxicity depends on free-radical formation in the doxorubicin redox cycle, which may lead to the formation of 7-deoxyaglycones. For monitoring individual patients, measuring left ventricular ejection fraction by isotopic ventriculography remains the best predictor of the risk of congestive heart failure when cumulative dosage approaches 550 mg/m² or when special risk factors exist.[84] The major problem with cardiac toxicity of anthracyclines concerns children who are cured of acute leukaemias and solid tumours with anthracycline-containing therapies and who may develop congestive heart failure 10–15 years after completion of the treatment.

Loco-regional administration of anthracyclines

A number of approaches have been used to increase intra-tumoral anthracycline concentrations, with the aim of increasing drug activity and reducing its systemic toxicity. Benefit from loco-regional delivery can be expected only for drugs with specific pharmacokinetic characteristics, especially a high total body clearance and a high extraction rate by the target organ. This is the case for doxorubicin, but other anthracyclines might be better candidates in this respect.

Intra-arterial administration of *doxorubicin and epirubicin* has been used in head and neck cancer, limb sarcoma, breast carcinoma, and bladder cancer without convincing improvement over systemic administration.[85] The theoretical advantage of infusion of doxorubicin in the *hepatic artery* is not very high, and the ratio of local to systemic plasma concentrations or AUC values may not exceed 2; however, it should be higher for other anthracyclines with a faster total plasma clearance, such as epirubicin.[86] In order to increase tumour selectivity and drug accumulation, the use of lipiodol suspensions of doxorubicin or epirubicin might overcome the problem of low drug extraction.[87] *Lipiodol* undergoes embolization in the tumour vasculature and this considerably reduces the flow rate, improving then the ratio of local to systemic drug concentrations.

Intraperitoneal administration of anthracyclines is feasible, especially for the treatment of peritoneal ovarian metastases. It allows high local concentrations of the drug to be achieved with a minimal systemic passage.[88] This is due to the low regional exchange rate between peritoneal fluid and plasma, typically of the order of 5–25 ml/min. Doxorubicin disappears from the peritoneal fluid with a half-life of about 2 h.[89] Intraperitoneal doxorubicin administration is not routine in clinical use because it is often associated with sterile peritonitis and peritoneal sclerosis.

Intravesical anthracycline instillations can be performed for the treatment of localized bladder cancer. Only negligible amounts of drug reach the systemic circulation,[90] and measurable concentrations of doxorubicin or epirubicin are found in the bladder wall associated with a good tolerance of the bladder mucosa.[91]

New and potent anthracyclines

Only a very few of the numerous molecules of the anthracycline family that have entered clinical trials in the past decade are still under consideration for further development and deserve special mention. Morpholinyl anthracyclines, especially methoxymorpholinyl-doxorubicin, present several original features:[92] they appear to be about 100 times more potent than classical anthracyclines, they are not cardiotoxic at therapeutic doses in animal models, they are active in MDR tumours, they have a novel mechanism of action, which is probably distinct from that of other anthracyclines, and they can be converted by cytochrome P-450 to more active species that produce DNA cross-linking and therefore behave as alkylating agents.

The existence of a cytochrome-P-450-mediated metabolic activation pathway raises new problems which had not been encountered in anthracycline research. It is well known that CYP 3A isoenzymes can be expressed at different levels in tumour tissues, exhibit a highly variable expression in the liver, and can be activated by a number of common drugs. These characteristics can profoundly affect the clinical use of the morpholinyl derivatives. Metabolic tests for activation should be done before administration in individual patients to predict potential activity, which may rather complicate the routine use of these drugs.

The pharmacokinetics of methoxymorpholinyl-doxorubicin has been determined in 18 patients during a phase I study.[93] The kinetics was linear in the range of tested doses (1–2.25 $\mu g/m^2$) and was characterized by a biexponential decay with a terminal half-life of 40 h, a mean plasma clearance of 39 l/h/m^2, and a volume of distribution at steady state of about 2000 l/m^2. A 13-dihydro metabolite was identified as the only fluorescent metabolite in plasma.

In addition to the morpholinyl anthracyclines, one can also cite the anthracycline disaccharides[94] which

present numerous interesting features compared with the classical anthracyclines, especially at the level of their interaction with topo II. These compounds are now entering clinical trials.

Anthracycline carriers and vehicles

In addition to the continuous development of hundreds of analogues, considerable efforts have been put into the development of anthracycline carriers in recent years. The general aim of this development is to increase drug selectivity, either by positive targeting of the drug to the tumour or by diverting the drug from highly sensitive targets such as the heart. Important modifications of the pharmacokinetics of anthracyclines occur, whether they are covalently bound or non-covalently entrapped in carriers.

Two anthracycline liposomal formulations have been marketed: *liposomal doxorubicin* prepared with Stealth liposomes (Caelyx® or Doxil®, Liposome Technology and Sequus) and *liposomal daunorubicin* (DaunoXome®, NeXstar). One of the major indications for liposomal anthracyclines can be found in the treatment of AIDS-related *Kaposi's sarcoma*, but other malignancies are probably sensitive to these formulations.

Using a classical liposomal formulation of doxorubicin, Gabizon *et al.*[95] observed pharmacokinetic behaviour which was roughly similar to that of free doxorubicin (elimination half-life between 11 and 110 h, total plasma clearance of 35.6 l/h/m^2, and volume of distribution at steady state of 845 l/m^2). This suggests that most of the drug had leaked out of the liposomes very rapidly. In studies with TLC D-99, which is also a 'classical' liposomal formulation of doxorubicin, the same characteristics were found: distribution and elimination half-lives were within the range of the values usually found for free doxorubicin, and total plasma clearance and volume of distribution at steady state were two to four times lower than expected for free doxorubicin.[96]

Studies with doxorubicin entrapped in Stealth liposomes gave very different results.[97] Doxil is eliminated from plasma with two successive half-lives of 2 h and 45 h (the usual elimination phase with a half-life of 5 min is completely missing), its total plasma clearance is about 0.1 l/h, and its volume of distribution at steady state is about 4 litres. These values are respectively 300 and 200 times lower than the values usually reported for free doxorubicin. DaunoXome is a preparation of daunorubicin entrapped in gel phase lipo-

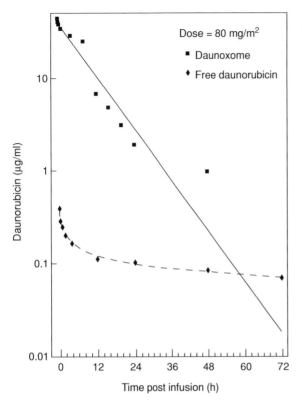

Figure 9.8. Plasma pharmacokinetics of liposome-encapsulated daunorubicin. Evolution of plasma concentrations of total daunorubicin after administration of 100 mg/m^2 in patients.[98]

somes. The pharmacokinetic behaviour of this formulation is quite unusual (Fig. 9.8); it has a relatively short terminal half-life (4–8 h), a total plasma clearance of 0.4–1 l/h/m^2 and a volume of distribution at steady state of 3–4 litres.[98]

Of the various anthracycline conjugates that have been proposed for clinical testing on the basis of preclinical activity, *doxorubicin*-N-(2-hydroxypropyl) methacrylamide *copolymers* of high molecular weight (~24 kDa), are worth mentioning. The drug is covalently bound to the polymer, at a rate of about 7% (w/w), via its aminosugar.[99] It has been suggested that the conjugate cannot diffuse through cellular membranes and is activated through proteolytic degradation in the tumour extracellular tissue rather than within the cells. In animal models, this polymer has shown a significant antitumour activity and reduced cardiac toxicity, which warrants further evaluation in humans. It also displays a lower volume of distribution, a lower peak plasma concentration, and a longer plasma half-life than free doxorubicin.[100] A clinical evaluation is ongoing but no results are available yet.

References

1. Arcamone F (1981) *Doxorubicin, Anticancer Antibiotics*. New York: Academic Press.
2. Zunino F, Gambetta R, Di Marco A (1975) The inhibition *in vitro* of DNA polymerase and RNA polymerase by daunomycin and adriamycin. *Biochem Pharmacol*, **24**, 309–17.
3. Aubel-Sadron G, Londos-Gagliardi D (1984) Daunorubicin and doxorubicin, anthracycline antibiotics: a physicochemical and biological review. *Biochimie*, **66**, 333–52.
4. Sinha BK (1989) Free radicals in anticancer drug pharmacology. *Chem Biol Interact*, **69**, 293–317.
5. Doroshow JH (1986) Role of oxygen peroxide and hydroxyl radical formation in the killing of Ehrlich tumor cells by anticancer quinones. *Proc Natl Acad Sci USA*, **83**, 4514–18.
6. Keizer HG, Pinedo HM, Schuurhuis GJ, Joenje H (1990) Doxorubicin (adriamycin): a critical review of free radical-dependent mechanisms of cytotoxicity. *Pharmacol Ther*, **47**, 219–31.
7. Tewey KM, Chen GL, Nelson EM, Liu LF (1984) Intercalative antitumor drugs interfere with the breakage-reunion reaction of mammalian DNA topoisomerase II. *J Biol Chem*, **259**, 9182–7.
8. Osheroff N, Corbett AH, Robinson MJ (1995) Mechanism of action of topoisomerase II-targeted antineoplastic drugs. *Adv Pharmacol*, **29B**, 105–26.
9. Pommier Y, Capranico G, Orr A, Kohn K (1991) Distribution of topoisomerase II cleavage sites in simian virus 40 DNA and the effects of drugs. *J Mol Biol*, **222**, 909–24.
10. Capranico G, Zunino F, Kohn K, Pommier Y (1990) Sequence-selective topoisomerase II inhibition by anthracycline derivatives in SV40 DNA: relationship with DNA affinity and cytotoxicity. *Biochemie*, **29**, 562–9
11. Ling YH, Priebe W, Perez-Soler R (1993) Apoptosis induced by anthracycline antibiotics in P388 parent and multidrug-resistant cells. *Cancer Res*, **53**, 1845–52.
12. Gottesman MM, Pastan I (1993) Biochemistry of multidrug resistance mediated by the multidrug transporter. *Annu Rev Biochem*, **62**, 385–427.
13. Mulder HS, Dekker H, Pinedo HM, Lankelma J (1995) The P-glycoprotein-mediated relative decrease in cytosolic free drug concentration is similar for several anthracyclines with varying lipophilicity. *Biochem Pharmacol*, **50**, 967–74.
14. Marie JP (1995) P-glycoprotein in adult hematologic malignancies. *Hematol Oncol Clin North Am*, **9**, 239–49.
15. Georges E, Sharom FJ, Ling V (1990) Multidrug resistance and chemosensitization. Therapeutic implications for cancer chemotherapy. *Adv Pharmacol*, **21**, 185–220.
16. Cole SPC, Bhardwaj G, Gerlach JH, *et al.* (1992) Overexpression of a transporter gene in a multidrug-resistant human lung cancer cell line. *Science*, **258**, 1650–4.
17. Sognier MA, Zhang Y, Eberle RL, *et al.* (1994) Sequestration of doxorubicin in vesicles in a multidrug-resistant cell line. *Biochem Pharmacol*, **48**, 391–401.

18. Beck WT, Danks MK, Wolverton JS, *et al.* (1995) Resistance of mammalian tumor cells to inhibitors of DNA topoisomerase II. *Adv Pharmacol*, **29B**, 145–67.

19. Benchekroun MN, Pourquier P, Schott B, Robert J (1993) Doxorubicin-induced lipid peroxidation and glutathione peroxidase activity and expression in tumoral cell lines selected for resistance to doxorubicin. *Eur J Biochem*, **211**, 141–6.

20. Benjamin RS, Wiernik PH, Bachur NR (1974) Adriamycin chemotherapy: efficacy, safety, and pharmacologic basis of an intermittent single high-dose schedule. *Cancer*, **33**, 19–27.

21. Legha SJ, Benjamin RS, MacKay B, *et al.* (1982) Adriamycin therapy by continuous intravenous infusion in patients with metastatic breast cancer. *Cancer*, **49**, 1762–6.

22. Legha SJ, Benjamin RS, McKay B, *et al.* (1982) Reduction of doxorubicin cardiotoxicity by prolonged continuous infusion. *Ann Intern Med*, **96**, 133–9.

23. Baurain R, Deprez-De Campeneere D, Trouet A (1979) Rapid determination of doxorubicin and its fluorescent metabolites by high-pressure liquid chromatography. *Anal Biochem*, **94**, 112–16.

24. Robert J (1980) Extraction of anthracyclines from biological fluids for HPLC evaluation. *J Liquid Chromatogr*, **3**, 1561–72.

25. Israel M, Pegg WJ, Wilkinson M, Garnick MB (1978) Liquid chromatographic analysis of adriamycin and metabolites in biological fluids. *J Liquid Chromatogr*, **1**, 795–809.

26. Marie JP, Faussat-Suberville AM, Zhou D, Zittoun R (1993) Daunorubicin uptake by leukemic cells: correlations with treatment outcome and *MDR1* expression. *Leukemia*, **7**, 825–31.

27. Tarasiuk J, Garnier-Suillerot A (1992) Kinetic parameters for the uptake of anthracycline by drug-resistant and drug-sensitive K562 cells. *Eur J Biochem*, **204**, 693–8.

28. Felsted RL, Richter DR, Bachur NR (1977) Rat liver aldehyde reductase. *Biochem Pharmacol*, **26**, 1117–24.

29. Schott B, Robert J (1989) Comparative activity of anthracycline 13-dihydrometabolites against rat glioblastoma cells in culture. *Biochem Pharmacol*, **38**, 4069–74.

30. Olson RD, Mushlin PS, Brenner DE, *et al.* (1988) Doxorubicin cardiotoxicity may be caused by its metabolite, doxorubicinol. *Proc Natl Acad Sci USA*, **85**, 3585–9.

31. Asbell MA, Schwartzbach E, Bullock FJ, Yesair DW (1972) Daunomycin and adriamycin metabolism via reductive glycosidic cleavage. *J Pharmacol Exp Ther*, **182**, 63–9.

32. Weenen H, van Maanen JMS, de Planque MM, McVie JG, Pinedo HM (1984) Metabolism of 4′ modified analogs of doxorubicin. Unique glucuronidation pathway for 4′-epidoxorubicin. *Eur J Cancer Clin Oncol*, **20**, 919–26.

33. Robert J, Bui NB, Vrignaud P (1987) Pharmacokinetics of doxorubicin in sarcoma patients. *Eur J Clin Pharmacol*, **31**, 695–9.

34. Mross K, Maessen P, van der Vijgh WJF, Gall H, Boven E, Pinedo HM (1988) Pharmacokinetics and metabolism of epidoxorubicin and doxorubicin in humans. *J Clin Oncol*, **6**, 517–26.

35. Camaggi CM, Comparsi R, Strocchi E, Testoni F, Angelelli B, Pannuti F (1988) Epirubicin and doxorubicin comparative metabolism and pharmacokinetics. A crossover study. *Cancer Chemother Pharmacol*, **21**, 221–7.

36. Jacquet JM, Bressolle F, Galtier M, *et al.* (1990) Doxorubicin and doxorubicinol: intra and inter-individual variations of pharmacokinetic parameters. *Cancer Chemother Pharmacol*, **27**, 219–25.

37. Twelves CJ, Dobbs NA, Aldhous M, Harper PG, Rubens RD, Richards MA (1991) Comparative pharmacokinetics of doxorubicin given by three different schedules with equal dose intensity in patients with breast cancer. *Cancer Chemother Pharmacol*, **28**, 302–7.

38. Christen RD, McClay EF, Plaxe SC, Yen SSC, Kim S, Kimani S (1993) Phase I/pharmacokinetic study of high-dose progesterone and doxorubicin. *J Clin Oncol*, **11**, 2417–26.

39. Robert J, Hœrni B, Vrignaud P, Lagarde C (1983) Early-phase pharmacokinetics of doxorubicin in non-Hodgkin lymphoma patients. Dose-dependent and time-dependent pharmacokinetic parameters. *Cancer Chemother Pharmacol*, **10**, 115–19.

40. Bronchud MH, Margison JM, Howell A, Lind M, Lucas SB, Wilkinson PM (1990) Comparative pharmacokinetics of escalating doses of doxorubicin in patients with metastatic breast cancer. *Cancer Chemother Pharmacol*, **25**, 435–9.

41. Bugat R, Robert J, Herrera A, *et al.* (1989) Clinical and pharmacokinetic study of 96 h infusions of doxorubicin in advanced cancer patients. *Eur J Cancer Clin Oncol*, **25**, 505–11.

42. Muller C, Chatelut E, Guanalo V, *et al.* (1993) Cellular pharmacokinetics of doxorubicin in patients with chronic lymphocytic leukemia: comparison of bolus administration to continuous infusion. *Cancer Chemother Pharmacol*, **32**, 379–84.

43. Jakobsen P, Steiness E, Bastholt L, *et al.* (1991) Multiple dose pharmacokinetics of epirubicin at four different dose levels: studies in patients with metastatic breast cancer. *Cancer Chemother Pharmacol*, **28**, 63–8.

44. Robert J, Bui NB (1992) Pharmacokinetics and metabolism of epirubicin administered as i.v. bolus and 48h-infusion in patients with advanced soft tissue sarcoma. *Ann Oncol*, **3**, 651–6.

45. Camaggi CM, Strocchi E, Carisi P, Martoni A, Melotti B, Pannuti F (1993) Epirubicin metabolism and pharmacokinetics after conventional and high-dose intravenous administration: a cross-over study. *Cancer Chemother Pharmacol*, **32**, 301–9.

46. Eksborg S (1990) Anthracycline pharmacokinetics. Limited sampling model for plasma level monitoring with special reference to epirubicin. *Acta Oncol*, **29**, 339–42.

47. de Vries EGE, Greidanus J, Mulder NH, *et al.* (1987) A phase I and pharmacokinetic study with 21-day continuous infusion of epirubicin. *J Clin Oncol*, **5**, 1445–51.

48. Rahman A, Goodman A, Foo W, Harvey J, Smith FP, Schein PS (1984) Clinical pharmacology of daunorubicin in phase I patients with solid tumours: development of an analytical methodology for daunorubicin and its metabolites. *Semin Oncol*, 11, (Suppl 3), 36–44.

49. Speth PAJ, Linssen PCM, Boezeman JBM, Wessels HMC, Haanen C (1987) Leukemic cell and plasma daunomycin concentrations after bolus injection and 72-h infusion. *Cancer Chemother Pharmacol*, 20, 311–15.

50. Zanette L, Zucchetti M, Freshi A, Erranti D, Tirelli U, D'Incalci M (1990) Pharmacokinetics of 4-demethoxy-daunorubicin in cancer patients. *Cancer Chemother Pharmacol*, 25, 445–8.

51. Stewart DJ, Grewaal D, Green RM, *et al.* (1991) Bioavailability and pharmacology of oral idarubicin. *Cancer Chemother Pharmacol*, 27, 308–14.

52. Camaggi CM, Strocchi E, Carisi P, Martoni A, Tononi A, Guaraldi M. (1992) Idarubicin metabolism and pharmacokinetics after intravenous and oral administration in cancer patients: a crossover study. *Cancer Chemother Pharmacol*, 30, 307–16.

53. Robert J, Rigal-Huguet F, Harousseau JL, *et al.* (1987) Pharmacokinetics of idarubicin after daily intravenous administration in leukemic patients. *Leuk Res*, 11, 961–4.

54. Chassany O, Urien S, Claude-Pierre P, Bastian G, Tillement JP (1996) Comparative serum protein binding of anthracycline derivatives. *Cancer Chemother Pharmacol*, 38, 571–3.

55. Lee YN, Chan KK, Harris PA, Cohen JL (1980) Distribution of adriamycin in cancer patients: tissue uptakes, plasma concentration after i.v. and hepatic i.a. administration. *Cancer*, 45, 2231–9.

56. Speth PAJ, Linssen PCM, Boezeman JBM, Wessels HMC, Haanen C (1987) Cellular and plasma adriamycin concentrations in long-term infusion therapy of leukemia patients. *Cancer Chemother Pharmacol*, 20, 305–10.

57. Speth PAJ, Linssen PCM, Beex LVAM, Boezeman JBM, Haanen C (1986) Cellular and plasma pharmacokinetics of weekly 20-mg 4'-epiadriamycin bolus injection in patients with advanced breast carcinoma. *Cancer Chemother Pharmacol*, 18, 78–82.

58. Speth PAJ, van de Loo FAJ, Linssen PCM, Wessels HMC, Haanen C (1986) Plasma and human leukemic cell pharmacokinetics of oral and intravenous 4-demethoxy-daunorubicin. *Clin Pharmacol Ther*, 40, 643–9.

59. Reid JM, Pendergrass TW, Krailo MD, Hammond GD, Ames MM (1990) Plasma pharmacokinetics and cerebrospinal fluid concentrations of idarubicin and idarubicinol in pediatric leukemia patients: a childrens cancer study group report. *Cancer Res*, 50, 6525–8.

60. Takanashi S, Bachur NR (1976) Adriamycin metabolism in man. Evidence from urinary metabolites. *Drug Metab Dispos*, 4, 79–87.

61. Piscitelli SC, Rodvold KA, Rushing DA, Tewksbury DA (1993) Pharmacokinetics and pharmacodynamics of doxorubicin in patients with small-cell lung cancer. *Clin Pharmacol Ther*, 53, 555–61.

62. Camaggi CM, Strocchi E, Martoni A, Angelelli A, Comparsi R, Pannuti F (1985) Epirubicin plasma and blood pharmacokinetics after single i.v. bolus in advanced cancer patients. *Drugs Exp Clin Res*, 11, 285–94.

63. Twelves CJ, Dobbs NA, Michael Y, *et al.* (1992) Clinical pharmacokinetics of epirubicin: the importance of liver biochemistry tests. *Br J Cancer*, 66, 765–9.

64. Cummings J, Forrest GJ, Cunningham D, Gilchrist NL, Soukop M (1986) Influence of polysorbate 80 (Tween 80) and etoposide (VP-16213) on the pharmacokinetics and urinary excretion of adriamycin and its metabolites in cancer patients. *Cancer Chemother Pharmacol*, 17, 80–4.

65. Gianni L, Vigano L, Locatelli A, *et al.* (1997) Human pharmacokinetic characterization and *in vitro* study of the interaction between doxorubicin and paclitaxel in patients with breast cancer. *J Clin Oncol*, 15, 1906–15.

66. Rushing DA, Raber SR, Rodvold KA, Piscitelli SC, Plank GS, Tewksbury DA (1994) The effects of cyclosporine on the pharmacokinetics of doxorubicin in patients with small-cell lung cancer. *Cancer*, 74, 834–41.

67. Bartlett NL, Lum BL, Fisher GA, *et al.* (1994) Phase I trial of doxorubicin with cyclosporine as a modulator of multidrug resistance. *J Clin Oncol*, 12, 835–42.

68. Sikic BI (1997) Pharmacologic approaches to reversing multidrug resistance. *Semin Hematol*, 34, 40–7.

69. Hochster H, Liebes L, Wadler S, Oratz R, Wernz JC, Meyers M (1992) Pharmacokinetics of the cardioprotector ADR-529 (ICRF-187) in escalating doses combined with fixed-dose doxorubicin. *J Natl Cancer Inst*, 84, 1725–30.

70. Launay MC, Milano G, Iliadis A, Frenay M, Namer M (1989) A limited sampling procedure for estimating adriamycin pharmacokinetics in cancer patients. *Br J Cancer*, 60, 89–92.

71. Ratain MJ, Robert J, van der Vijgh, WJ (1991) Limited sampling models for doxorubicin pharmacokinetics. *J Clin Oncol*, 9, 871–6.

72. Bressolle F, Ray P, Jacquet JM, *et al.* (1991) Bayesian estimation of doxorubicin pharmacokinetic parameters. *Cancer Chemother Pharmacol*, 29, 53–60.

73. Jakobsen P, Bastholt L, Dalmark M, *et al.* (1991) A randomised study of epirubicin at four dose levels in advanced breast cancer. Feasibility of myelotoxicity prediction through single blood sample measurement. *Cancer Chemother Pharmacol*, 28, 465–9.

74. Wade JR, Kelman AW, Kerr DJ, Robert J, Whiting B (1992) Variability in the pharmacokinetics of epirubicin: a population analysis. *Cancer Chemother Pharmacol*, 29, 391–5.

75. Wheeler RH, Ensminger WD, Thrall JH, Anderson JL (1982) High-dose doxorubicin: an exploration of the dose-response curve in human neoplasia. *Cancer Treat Rep*, 66, 493–8.

76. Focan C, Andrien JM, Closon MT, Dicato M, Driesschaert P, Focan-Henrard D (1993) Dose-response relationship of epirubicin-based first-line chemotherapy for advanced breast cancer: a prospective randomized trial. *J Clin Oncol*, 11, 1253–63.

77. Robert J, Iliadis A, Hœrni B, Cano JP, Durand M, Lagarde C (1982) Pharmacokinetics of adriamycin in patients with breast cancer. Correlation between pharmacokinetic parameters and clinical short term response. *Eur J Cancer Clin Oncol*, **18**, 739–45.

7 8. Preisler HD, Gessner T, Azarnia N, *et al.* (1984) Relationship between plasma adriamycin levels and the outcome of remission induction therapy for acute non-lymphocytic leukemia. *Cancer Chemother Pharmacol*, **12**,125–30.

79. Ackland SP, Ratain MJ, Vogelzang NJ, Choi KE, Ruane M, Sinkule JA (1989) Pharmacokinetics and pharmacodynamics of long-term continuous infusion doxorubicin. *Clin Pharmacol Ther*, **45**, 340–7.

80. Galettis P, Boutagy J, Ma DDF (1994) Daunorubicin pharmacokinetics and the correlation with P-glycoprotein and response in patients with acute leukaemia. *Br J Cancer*, **70**, 324–9.

81. Elbaek K, Ebbehoj E, Jakobsen A, *et al.* (1989) Pharmacokinetics of oral idarubicin in breast cancer patients with reference to antitumor activity and side effects. *Clin Pharmacol Ther*, **45**, 627–34.

82. von Hoff D, Layard MD, Basa P, *et al.* (1979) Risk factors for doxorubicin-induced congestive heart failure. *Ann Intern Med*, **91**, 710–17.

83. Cummings J, Milstead R, Cunnigham D, Kaye S (1986) Marked interpatient variation in adriamycin biotransformation to 7-deoxyaglycones: evidence from metabolites identified in serum. *Eur J Cancer Clin Oncol*, **22**, 991–1001.

84. Basser RL, Green MD (1993) Strategies for prevention of anthracycline cardiotoxicity. *Cancer Treat Rev*, **19**, 57–77.

85. Didolkar MS, Kanter PM, Baffi RR *et al.* (1978) Comparison of regional versus systemic chemotherapy with adriamycin. *Ann Surg*, **187**, 332–6.

86. Pannuti F, Camaggi CM, Strocchi E, *et al.* (1986) Intrahepatic arterial administration of 4′-epidoxorubicin in advanced cancer patients. A pharmacokinetic study. *Eur J Cancer Clin Oncol*, **22**, 1309–14.

87. Raoul JL, Heresbach D, Bretagne JF, *et al.* (1992) Chemoembolization of hepatocellular carcinomas. A study of the biodistribution and pharmacokinetics of doxorubicin. *Cancer*, **70**, 585–90.

88. Ozols RF, Young RC, Speyer JL, *et al.* (1982) Phase I and pharmacological studies of adriamycin administered intraperitoneally to patients with ovarian cancer. *Cancer Res*, **42**, 4265–9.

89. Demicheli R, Bonciarelli G, Jirillo A, *et al.* (1985) Pharmacologic data and technical feasibility of intraperitoneal doxorubicin administration. *Tumori*, **71**, 63–8.

90. Chai M, Wientjes MG, Badalament RA, Burgers JK, Au JLS (1994) Pharmacokinetics of intravesical doxorubicin in superficial bladder cancer patients. *J Urol*, **152**, 374–8.

91. Mross K, Maessen P, van der Vijgh WJF, Bogdanowicz JF, Kurth KH, Pinedo HM (1987) Absorption of epi-doxorubicin after intravesical administration in patients with *in situ* transitional cell carcinoma of the bladder. *Eur J Cancer Clin Oncol*, **23**, 505–8.

92. Lau DHM, Duran GE, Lewis AD, Sikic BI (1994) Metabolic conversion of methoxymorpholinyl doxorubicin: from a DNA strand breaker to a DNA cross-linker. *Br J Cancer*, **70**, 79–84.

93. Vasey PA, Bissett D, Strolin-Benedetti M, *et al.* (1995) Phase I clinical and pharmacokinetic study of 3′-deamino-3′-(2-methoxy-4-morpholinyl)doxorubicin (FCE 23762). *Cancer Res*, **55**, 2090–6.

94. Arcamone F, Animati F, Capranico G, *et al.* (1997) New developments in antitumor anthracyclines. *Pharmacol Ther*, **76**, 117–24.

95. Gabizon A, Chisin R, Amselem S, *et al.* (1991) Pharmacokinetic and imaging studies in patients receiving a formulation of liposome-associated adriamycin. *Br J Cancer*, **64**, 1125–32.

96. Cowens JW, Creaven PJ, Greco WR, *et al.* (1993) Initial clinical (phase I) trial of TLC-99 (doxorubicin encapsulated in liposomes). *Cancer Res*, **53**, 2796–802.

97. Gabizon A, Catane R, Uziely B, *et al.* (1994) Prolonged circulation time and enhanced accumulation in malignant exsudates of doxorubicin encapsulate in polyethylene-glycol coated liposomes. *Cancer Res*, **54**, 987–92.

98. Gill PS, Espina BM, Muggia F, *et al.* (1995) Phase I/II clinical and pharmacokinetic evaluation of liposomal daunorubicin. *J Clin Oncol*, **13**, 996–1003.

99. Duncan R, Seymour LW, O'Hare KB, *et al.* (1992) Preclinical evaluation of polymer-bound doxorubicin. *J Control Release*, **19**, 331–46.

100. Seymour LW, Ulbrich K, Strohalm J, Kopecek J, Duncan R (1990) The pharmacokinetics of polymer-bound adriamycin. *Biochem Pharmacol*, **39**, 1125–31.

10 | Taxanes

Lucia Viganò, Alberta Locatelli, and Luca Gianni

Introduction

The taxanes paclitaxel (Taxol®) and docetaxel (Taxotere®) represent a novel class of antineoplastic drugs. They have very high activity in a spectrum of solid tumours that matches the combined spectrum of anthracyclines and platinating agents.

The discovery of the prototypic taxane (paclitaxel) dates back to 1960, when the drug was identified in a large screening programme of plant products evaluated for anticancer activity by the US National Cancer Institute. Paclitaxel was initially extracted from the bark of the Pacific yew (*Taxus brevifolia*). The procedure was laborious, gave a low yield of final product, and had deleterious long-term environmental consequences. The drug is now obtained by semisynthesis from 10-deacetylbaccatin III, which is extracted from the needles of the European yew (*Taxus baccata*). Docetaxel was obtained directly by semisynthesis from 10-deacetylbaccatin III.[1]

The two taxanes are structurally similar, but have different pharmacological characteristics. Paclitaxel and docetaxel share the same unique mechanism of

Summary

	Paclitaxel	Docetaxel
Brand name	Taxol®	Taxotere®
Molecular weight (Da)	853.9	807.9
Mechanism of action	Antimicrotubule	Same as paclitaxel
Cell-cycle specificity phase	G_2–M phase	S phase, less G_2–M phase
Route of administration	Intravenous	Same as paclitaxel
Protein binding (%)	>95	Same as paclitaxel
Metabolism	Yes, by 450 2C8, 3A4	Yes, by P-450 3A
Elimination	Biliary, renal	Same as paclitaxel
Terminal half-life (h)	18.7	11.2
Toxicities	Neutropenia, hypersensitivity, neuropathy, alopecia, cardiac toxicity	Same as paclitaxel plus fluid retention and skin and nail toxicity

action: they promote the assembly of microtubules and prevent their depolymerization, thus interfering with a number of normal cellular functions that depend on the physiological balance between tubulin and microtubules.

Clinical use

Paclitaxel has a very broad spectrum of antitumour activity in cancers of the ovary, breast, lung, head and neck, oesophagus, bladder, testis, and endometrium, and in some haematological and pediatric malignancies. Its activity in *ovarian cancer* is similar to that of cisplatin. In *breast cancer*, paclitaxel is the first major new drug since the introduction of doxorubicin in 1960s. The very good response reported after use of paclitaxel as a single agent has justified combination studies with several other anticancer drugs (anthracyclines, cisplatin, cyclophosphamide, 5-fluorouracil, mitoxantrone, and ifosfamide). The results are very encouraging for breast and ovarian cancer. Currently, sequential chemotherapy and polychemotherapy with paclitaxel are considered established therapeutic options not only in the metastatic setting but also for the treatment of early-stage breast cancer.[2,3]

In ovarian cancer the combination of paclitaxel with a platinating drug is more efficacious than the classical combination of cisplatin and cyclophosphamide.[4,5] In addition, two recently published large randomized trials have shown that *paclitaxel–carboplatin* achieved comparable efficacy with less toxicity than paclitaxel–cisplatin.[6,7]

Docetaxel has a similar broad spectrum of antitumour activity and notable effects in metastatic breast cancer as a first- and second-line treatment.[8] Of special note is the observation that response to docetaxel is independent of prior treatment with anthracyclines.[9] Like paclitaxel, docetaxel is now being studied in a number of combinations with other anticancer drugs to define new treatment options for common malignancies such as breast, lung, and ovarian cancer.

In ovarian cancer, docetaxel monotherapy has demonstrated good response in both paclitaxel and *platinum refractory* patients and the *docetaxel–carboplatin* combination appears to be a promising alternative to paclitaxel–carboplatin in terms of minimizing the incidence of severity of neurotoxicity, although bone marrow toxicity is far more pronounced.[10] In addition, combinations of docetaxel with the topoisomerase I inhibitors *CPT-11 and topotecan* has been successfully used as second-line therapy in patients with advanced ovarian cancer. Preliminary results also suggest good activity of the docetaxel–gemcitabine combination.[11] Like paclitaxel, docetaxel is under evaluation as an alternative to standard therapies in the adjuvant treatment of early-stage breast cancer. Early results suggest that docetaxel in combination with doxorubicin and cyclophosphamide results in improved disease-free and overall survival.[12,13]

Recent attempts to combine taxanes with new-generation drugs targeting specific cellular molecules involved in cell-cycle regulation, intracellular signal transduction, and apoptosis are also interesting.

Synergism between the anti-HER2 monoclonal antibody *trastuzumab (Herceptin®)* and paclitaxel has been shown *in vitro* and *in vivo*. In early experience, weekly administration of Herceptin and paclitaxel showed marked antitumour activity in metastatic[14] and anthracycline- and taxane-pretreated breast cancer.[15] Conclusive evidence for the value of combining paclitaxel with trastuzumab was obtained in a randomized phase III trial which indicated significant improvement in response rate and survival.[16]

Together with the known antimucrotubule effect, docetaxel potentially acts on a number of targets including apoptotic, angiogenic, and gene expression processes. These mechanisms provide a basis for combining docetaxel with a variety of novel anticancer agents. Promising clinical results have been obtained for combinations with trastuzumab, capecitabine, and cetuzimab in metastatic breast cancer and refractory/resistant advanced non-small-cell lung cancer.[17]

Chemistry

Paclitaxel (molecular weight, 853.9 Da) is classified as a taxane diterpenoid or taxoid. Like all known taxoids, it is isolated from plants of the *Taxaceae* family (bark of the Pacific yew *Taxus brevifoglia*). The structure (Fig. 10.1) is characterized by a taxane ring core, esterification at the C-13 position with a complex ester group (*N*-benzoylphenylisoserine), and an unusual fourth ring at the C-4,5 position. The last two structural features are necessary for its biological activity.[18] The docetaxel molecule (molecular weight, 807.9 Da) maintains the key structural elements required for the antimicrotubule activity of the taxoids, but it is different from paclitaxel in that it has a hydroxyl group instead of an acetyl group at the C-10 position, and a tert-butoxy moiety instead of a benzamide phenyl

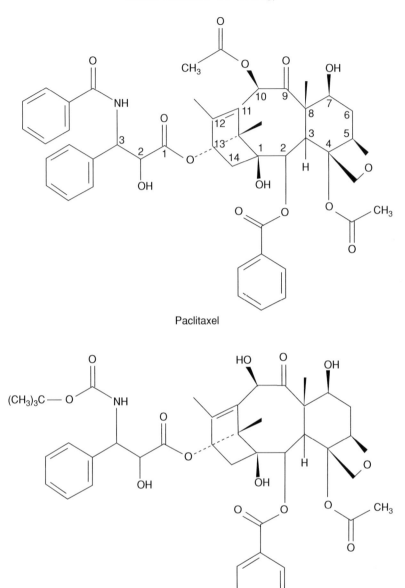

Figure 10.1. Chemical structures of paclitaxel and docetaxel.

group at the C-3' position on the C-13 side chain.[19] Paclitaxel and docetaxel are white crystalline powders that are virtually insoluble in water.

Paclitaxel and docetaxel are commercially available for intravenous administration. Because of their low solubility in water, both drugs are supplied in solution with surfactant agents. Paclitaxel is prepared as a 6 mg/ml solution in 50% polyoxyethylated castor oil (Cremophor EL®, CrEL) and 50% dehydrated ethanol USP. The appropriate dose must be diluted in normal saline or dextrose 5% to obtain a 0.3–1.2 mg/ml solution for infusion. Once diluted, paclitaxel is stable in solution for 27 h in daylight at 25°C. Docetaxel is also supplied as a concentrated solution, but the solvent is polysorbate 80 (Tween 80). Prior to use, docetaxel must be diluted in a solution of 13% ethanol in water, and then in normal saline or dextrose 5% to produce a final solution for infusion at 0.3–0.9 mg/ml. Several recent investigations have shown that CrEL and Tween 80 are not biologically and pharmacologically inert. Therefore the use of different solubilizing agents may be relevant to the pharmacological activity of the two drugs. For this reason in the past few years efforts have been made to find new formulations for taxanes or different ways of administering them. Work is in progress to develop Tween80- and CrEL-free formulations of docetaxel and paclitaxel based on pharmaceutical (e.g. albumin, nanoparticles, emulsions, and liposomes), chemical (e.g. polyglutamates, analogues and prodrugs), or biological (e.g. oral administration) strategies.[20]

Mechanism of action

The antitumour effect of the taxanes has been attributed to their ability to interfere with microtubule function. *Microtubules* are involved in many normal cell functions including mitotic spindle formation during cell division, maintenance of cellular shape, motility, signal transduction, intracellular transport, hormonal secretion, and membrane association of receptor.[1,21] Microtubules are tubulin polymers which are in dynamic equilibrium with tubulin heterodimers composed of α-and β-subunits (Fig. 10.2). Energy in the form of guanosine triphosphate (GTP) is required for microtubule formation. Unlike other antimicrotubule drugs, such as vinca alkaloids, which prevent the polymerization of tubulin, taxanes promote the assembly of tubulin in extraordinarily stable and dysfunctional microtubules even in absence of GTP, in the presence of Ca^{2+}, and at +4°C.[19,22] The final consequence is the disruption of the normal microtubule dynamics that is required for cell division and vital processes during interphase. Both taxanes bind to the β-subunit of *tubulin*, rather than to tubulin dimers, and they bind to a specific site which is different from the binding site of GTP, colchicine, vinblastine, and podophyllotoxin.[1,21] Docetaxel has a 1.9-fold higher affinity for the site than paclitaxel, and induces tubulin polymerization at a 2.1-fold lower critical tubulin concentration.[1] In addition, the mean diameter of microtubules stabilized from docetaxel is larger than that of microtubules induced by paclitaxel.[23]

Docetaxel has been found to be two to four times more potent than paclitaxel in several tumour cell lines, probably because of its larger intracellular uptake, slower efflux from tumoral cells, and higher affinity for the tubulin target compared with paclitaxel. Docetaxel is 3.7 times more cytotoxic against human haematopoietic bone marrow stem cells at concentrations similar to those measured in human plasma after administration of recommended doses.[24] This may explain why dose-limiting neutropenia is more common with docetaxel than with paclitaxel.

Even though a clear mechanistic explanation is missing, the two taxoids have a different effect on the cell cycle. Paclitaxel inhibits the cell-cycle traverse at the G_2–M phase junction,[25] while docetaxel produces its maximum cell-killing effect against cells in the S phase.[26] The G_2–M phase-specific activity of paclitaxel is in keeping with preclinical observations indicating greater cytotoxicity for long exposure than for short exposure. In MCF-7 breast cancer cells, the paclitaxel exposure causing 50% inhibition of colony formation

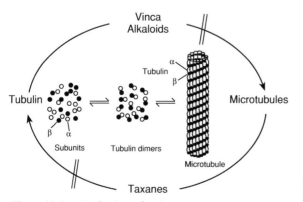

Figure 10.2. Mechanism of action.

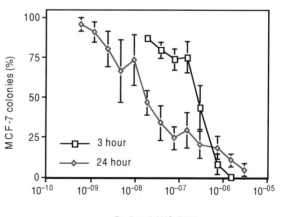

Figure 10.3. Toxicity of paclitaxel versus different times of exposure (AUC) in MCF-7 cell line. Reproduced from G. Capri *et al.* (1996) *Semin Oncol*, **23** (Suppl 2), 68–75.

(AUC$_{50}$) is about 10 times lower for 24 h exposure than for 3 h treatment. (L.Gianni and A.Locatelli, unpublished data) (Fig. 10.3).

A recent study that examined the relationship between treatment duration, concentration, and effect of paclitaxel on six human epithelial cancer cell lines may shed some light on the duration of exposure and cytotoxicity.[27] An 'immediate effect' was measurable immediately after treatment and increased with treatment duration and drug concentration, and a 'delayed effect' was observed after removing the drug from the culture medium. The delayed effect was attributed to the slow manifestation of apoptosis and the significant amount of drug retained intracellularly. The apoptotic effect of low accumulation of paclitaxel has also been described by other investigators. After a phase-specific proliferation arrest, cell death occurs with morphological features and patterns of DNA fragmentation that are typical of *apoptosis*.[28]

These observations support the use of paclitaxel with long duration of infusion in clinical application.

Paclitaxel enhances the cytotoxic effects of *ionizing radiation in vitro*, possibly via the cell-cycle arrest in the G$_2$ and M phases that are the most radiosensitive phases of the cell cycle.[29] A radiation sensitivity effect has also been demonstrated for docetaxel in HL-60 cells, although the drug exerts the maximum activity in the S phase.[30]

Recently, other potential antitumour effects not directly associated with the classical anti-microtubule action have been reported for the taxoids. Paclitaxel- and docetaxel-induced apoptosis is associated with enhanced phosphorylation of *bcl-2*. Phosphorylated *bcl-2* is unable to form heterodimers with the *bax* protein, shifting the equilibrium to the formation of *bax* homodimers which are components of the signal transduction cascade leading to apoptosis.[31] Interestingly, cancer cell lines that are *bcl-2* negative are also insensitive to the apoptotic effect of paclitaxel[31] (see also the section on mechanism of resistance). Docetaxel is capable of inducing *bcl-2* phosphorylation at 100-fold lower concentrations than paclitaxel.[32]

Paclitaxel mimics two effects normally induced by bacterial lipopolysaccharides on macrophages by inducing release of *tumour necrosis factor-α (TNF-α)* and a decrease in expression of TNF receptors.[33] In particular, specific structural changes in the molecule do not alter the antimicrotubule effects of paclitaxel, whereas they prevent the induction of TNF-α gene expression.[34]

In endothelial cell lines, treatment with paclitaxel causes inhibition of the chemotaxis and chemo-

invasiveness that is normally triggered by tumour-derived angiogenic factors such as basic fibroblast growth factor (*bFGF*) and vascular endothelial growth factor (*VEGF*).[35] This activity has been attributed to the drug-induced stabilization of microtubules that affects the motility of several cell types. The inhibition of motility occurs at concentrations that do not cause cytotoxicity. Paclitaxel is able to inhibit tumour-induced angiogenesis in murine models *in vivo*.[36]

In vitro studies have shown a sequence-dependent synergism or antagonism between paclitaxel and other drugs *used in combination*.[37,38] Significant differences in cytotoxicity have been noted in treatments in which paclitaxel was administered over 24 h before and after cisplatin, doxorubicin, cyclophosphamide, antimetabolites, and other antineoplastic drugs. In all cases, with the exception of cyclophosphamide, the sequence effects noted *in vitro* have a corresponding pharmacokinetic interference between paclitaxel and combined drugs in humans. Sequence-dependent drug interactions have also been shown for docetaxel *in vitro*.[39]

When considering the *in vivo* effects of paclitaxel, an important source of pharmacological/pharmacokinetic interference with other drugs is the vehicle of the taxane's clinical formulation. *In vitro*, CrEl can reverse *P-glycoprotein*-mediated multidrug resistance (MDR) at concentrations similar to those reached in plasma during a 3 h infusion in humans,[40] suggesting a possible enhancement of paclitaxel activity in MDR-expressing tumours. However, CrEL has a volume of distribution (3.7 ± 0.49 l/m^2) equal to the central plasma compartment and very limited tissue distribution, so that the concentrations required to reverse the MDR phenotype (0.3–1μl/ml) are probably not reached in solid tumours.[41] In addition, CrEL is responsible for the non-linear pharmacokinetics of paclitaxel in plasma, as demonstrated by animal studies in which paclitaxel has been administered with and without the vehicle of the clinical formulation[42] (see section on pharmacokinetics).

The clinical observation that patients with breast cancer over-expressing the human epidermal growth factor 2 (HER 2) are more sensitive to treatment with paclitaxel and doxorubicin than patients with HER2-negative tumours has no mechanistic explanation as yet.[43] HER2 is a tyrosine kinase receptor over-expressed in 25–30% of patients with breast cancer and is a marker of poor prognosis. Recently, a recombinant humanized anti-p185 HER2 antibody *(Herceptin)* has been developed and has already shown clinical activity against HER2-positive *breast cancer*. In preclinical studies *in vitro* and *in vivo*, the combination between rhuMAb HER2 and paclitaxel or doxorubicin resulted in an enhancement of the cytotoxic activity of the drugs. The better results in tumour growth inhibition and tumour rate regression are obtained with the association of rhuMAb HER2 and paclitaxel.[44]

Mechanism of resistance

Two major mechanisms of acquired resistance to the taxanes have been characterized *in vitro*. The first one involves altered forms of tubulin α and β that have an impaired ability to polymerize into microtubules.[21,45]

The second mechanism of resistance is associated with the amplification (over-expression) of the membrane P-glycoprotein which is responsible for the increased efflux of many anticancer drugs and is encoded by the multidrug resistance *mdr*1 gene in humans.[1,46,47]

The clinical relevance of these mechanisms of resistance is not known. According to studies in breast cancer, there is a lack of complete clinical cross-resistance between the taxanes and anthracyclines.[48] Resistance to the latter class of drugs is mainly attributed to the MDR mechanism, even though the direct transfer of laboratory observations to the clinical setting is very difficult.[49] If resistance to anthracyclines is due to MDR in humans, the observation of activity of both taxanes in patients who failed prior treatment with doxorubicin or epirubicin indicates that MDR is not a clinically relevant mechanism of resistance to paclitaxel and docetaxel.[50]

Taxane resistance has also been related to the expression of bcl-2[31] and Bcl-xL,[51] the upregulation of caveolin-1 expression,[52] the inhibition of caspase activity and associated multimininucleation,[53] and other mechanisms that are unrelated to MDR. However, the effects on these targets need a paclitaxel concentration much higher than the typical concentrations reached in patients so that these mechanisms of resistance are not clinically relevant.

No cross-resistance between paclitaxel and docetaxel has been observed in several *in vitro* and *in vivo* studies in cell lines made resistant to paclitaxel.[54] A recent clinical study, aimed at evaluation of the efficacy of docetaxel in patients with paclitaxel-resistant metastatic breast cancer, is in possible agreement with the concept that there is only a 'partial' cross-resistance between the two taxanes.[55]

Analytical methodology

Several high-pressure liquid chromatography (HPLC) methods have been described for the determination of paclitaxel in biological fluids and tissues. The more sensitive assays are based on liquid–liquid extraction (LLE) or solid phase extraction (SPE) of biological samples followed by reverse phase HPLC separation and UV detection at a wavelength of 227 nm. The sensibility is between 5 and 10 ng/ml and the simultaneous detection of major metabolites is possible. Higher sensibility (2.5–5 ng/ml) is obtained by a time-saving method in which SPE of plasma and urine samples is carried out on column automatically switched on-line with the chromatographic separation system.[56]

Similar methods with LLE, SPE, automated column switching,[57] and HPLC separation are applicable to docetaxel measurement with similar sensitivity. Recently, methods have been developed for paclitaxel analysis using HPLC–ion-spray single mass spectrometry (ISP–MS) or tandem mass spectrometry (ISP–MS/MS).[58] Capillary electrophoresis affords a higher sensibility (0.1–0.4 ng/ml).[59]

Pharmacokinetics and protein binding

The pharmacokinetic characterization of paclitaxel and docetaxel has been the subject of several investigations in humans. The two drugs share some pharmacokinetic characteristics: a large volume of distribution, a rapid uptake by most tissues, long terminal half-lives of elimination from plasma, and a substantial hepatic metabolism.[1] The plasma disposition and elimination of both drugs can be fitted by a three-compartment model. The relative pharmacokinetic parameters of both agents, administered at the recommended dose and schedule (175 mg/m^2 palitaxel infused over 3 h, and 100 mg/m^2 docetaxel infused over 1 h), are summarized in Table 10.1.

Tissue distribution

Paclitaxel has volumes of distribution V_{dc} and V_{dss} that are significantly larger than the volume of total body water, indicating an extensive protein binding and substantial sequestration by other tissue components.[1] Drug penetration into classical sanctuary sites, such as testis and central nervous system, is low.[60]

Table 10.1   Main pharmacokinetic parameters of taxanes

Parameter	Paclitaxel (175 mg/m^2)[70,72]	Docetaxel (100 mg/m^2)[69]
$t_{1/2\alpha}$ (h)	0.27	0.1
$t_{1/2\beta}$ (h)	2.34	0.6
$t_{1/2\gamma}$ (h)	18.7	11.2
CL (l/h/m^2)	11.4	21
C_{max} (μM)	5.9	4.7
AUC (μM h)	18.5	5.69
V_{ss} (l/m^2)	99.2	67.3

$t_{1/2\alpha}$ $t_{1/2\beta}$, distribution phase half-lives; $t_{1/2\gamma}$, terminal plasma half-life;
CL, total body clearance; C_{max}, peak plasma concentration;
AUC, area under the plasma concentration–time curve;
V_{SS}, volume of distribution at steady state.

Interestingly, in a phase I study in humans, paclitaxel was measured in brain tumours but not in adjacent normal brain tissue.[61]

The tissue distribution of docetaxel is similar to that of paclitaxel, with a rapid and high uptake in almost all tissues, including fetal tissues and milk, except the brain. Levels in reproductive organs are higher in females than in males. In tumour tissue the drug exposure is fivefold higher than in plasma and other tissues owing to a longer terminal elimination from the tumour.[62]

Metabolism and elimination

The major pathway of paclitaxel and docetaxel elimination is hepatic metabolism and biliary excretion. Although the cytochrome P-450 system is implicated in the metabolism of both drugs, the specific enzymes and products are different. Paclitaxel undergoes hydroxylation leading to the formation of three major metabolites: 6α-hydroxy-paclitaxel, 3′-*p*-hydroxy paclitaxel,

and 6α,3′-*p*-hydroxy-paclitaxel. Cytochromes P-450 2C8, P-450 3A4, and P-450 3A3 are implicated. Docetaxel has four major metabolites produced by stepwise oxidation of the tert-butyl ester group in the side chain at C13 by cytochrome P-450 3A. The metabolites of both taxanes are inactive or less cytotoxic than the parent compounds, and represent an important detoxification pathway. Several drugs, such as corticosteroids and selected anti-H$_2$ histamine receptors acting as specific substrates of cytochrome P-450 enzymes, may interfere with the metabolism and possibly with the toxicity and antitumour activity of the taxanes.[63] To date, no clear indication of any such metabolic interference is apparent from the literature on the clinical use of the two compounds.

Enhanced toxicity has been reported in patients with liver alterations due to changes in drug disposition. Guidelines for dose modification in the presence of altered liver enzymes have been defined for paclitaxel[64] and docetaxel.[65]

The major route of elimination for taxanes and their metabolites is the biliary excretion that accounts for about 70% of the total dose in 48 h.[1] Urinary excretion is minimal for both taxanes (< 10% of the injected dose in 48 h) and is in the form of the parent drug.

Protein binding

The paclitaxel binding to plasma proteins is very extensive (95–97%), independent of paclitaxel concentration in the therapeutic range, and reversible, indicating non-specific hydrophobic binding. Human serum albumin and α$_1$-acid glycoprotein are equally involved in the binding, with a minor contribution from lipoproteins.[66]

Table 10.2   Main pharmacological features of taxanes

Paclitaxel	Docetaxel
Preclinical	
Phase-specific (G$_2$–M)	Phase-specific (S)
MDR drug	MDR drug
Schedules/sequence-dependent synergy or antagonism with some antineoplastic drugs	Higher affinity for microtubules; intracellular accumulation and potency
Clinical	
Non-linear pharmacokinetics	Linear pharmacokinetics
Formulated in Cremophor EL	Formulated in polysorbate 80
PK interference with anthracyclines and CDDP	PK interference with anthracyclines
Threshold-linked pharmacodynamics (neutropenia)	AUC, Cl, and threshold-linked pharmacodynamics
Liver metabolism and biliary elimination	Liver metabolism and biliary elimination

Similarly to paclitaxel, 98% of docetaxel binds to human plasma albumin, α_1-acid glycoprotein and lipoproteins.[67] Altered levels of α_1-acid glycoprotein have been shown to interfere with docetaxel plasma clearance and may be responsible for the increased toxicity of standard doses.[68] None of drugs commonly co-administered with paclitaxel and docetaxel (cisplatin, doxorubicin, 5-fluorouracil, dexamethasone, etc.) altered the protein binding of the two taxanes.[66,69]

Paclitaxel

Some differences in the pharmacokinetics of paclitaxel and docetaxel have relevant pharmacological and clinical implications (Table 10.2).

The pharmacokinetics of paclitaxel was characterized as linear in early studies in humans. However, later studies comparing the disposition of paclitaxel administered at similar doses over 3 or 24 h of infusion revealed inconsistencies that could only be reconciled by non-linear drug disposition. Non-linearity of paclitaxel plasma disappearance has been demonstrated by different investigators, showing that the drug has saturable distribution, saturable metabolism, and saturable elimination in humans.[70–73] The pharmacokinetic model developed for paclitaxel and 6α-hydroxypaclitaxel[70] is shown in Figure 10.4. The non-linear behaviour of paclitaxel disposition is related to the co-administration of CrEL in mice.[42] Therefore it is likely that the non-linear pharmacokinetics of paclitaxel in humans is due to its pharmaceutical formulation and not to an intrinsic property of the drug. Additional investigations demonstrated that *CrEL* alters the blood distribution of paclitaxel as a result of entrapment of the compound in circulating CrEL micelles, thereby reducing the free fraction available for cellular partitioning.[74] Based on this finding, the non-linear kinetics of paclitaxel would not be due to saturable tissue binding or elimination, but to the time- and dose-dependent concentration of CrEL in the central compartment.[75]

The non-linear behaviour of paclitaxel pharmacokinetics is more pronounced when the drug is administered via an infusion of short duration, when the plasma maximal concentration C_{max} and the area under the plasma concentration–time curve (AUC) are not proportional to the administered dose. The same lack of proportionality is less evident in the 24 h schedule of administration, as expected in the presence of a saturable elimination system in which low plasma concentrations are cleared faster than high concentrations. The schedule dependence of the paclitaxel disposition has an important clinical consequence because changes in the administered dose or in the duration of infusion can lead to unpredictable changes in plasma concentrations and total exposure to the drug and to unpredictable pharmacodynamic effects.

As previously mentioned, the combination of paclitaxel with other drugs is associated *in vitro* with cytotoxic synergism or antagonism depending on the sequence of administration. In humans, sequence-dependent effects have pharmacokinetic and pharmacodynamic counterparts (Table 10.3). In patients, the use of *paclitaxel and cisplatin* was associated with a 25% reduction of paclitaxel clearance when cisplatin preceded paclitaxel.[76] In the case of the paclitaxel–*doxorubicin* combination, several investigators found a consistent decrease in doxorubicin clearance when paclitaxel was given before doxorubicin.[77] The involvement of CrEL in the alterations of anthracycline pharmacokinetics and in the unexpected high cardiotoxicity of the combination has been postulated. When paclitaxel, as clinically formulated in CrEL, and doxorubicin are administered simultaneously, the taxane is

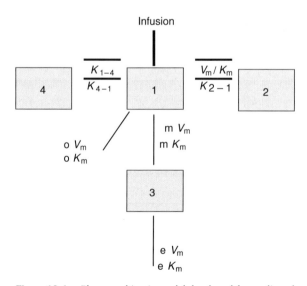

Figure 10.4. Pharmacokinetic model developed for paclitaxel and 6α-hydroxypaclitaxel: 1, paclitaxel central compartment; 2, first peripheral paclitaxel compartment; 3, 6α-hydroxypaclitaxel compartment; 4, second peripheral compartment of paclitaxel; V_m, K_m, mV_m, mK_m, eV_m, eK_m, Michaelis–Menten constants estimate for the saturable distribution of paclitaxel and the formation and elimination of 6α-hydroxylpaclitaxel, respectively; oV_m, oK_m, parameters for central elimination. Modified from L. Gianni *et al.* (1995) *J Clin Oncol*, **13**, 180–90.

Table 10.3   Main interactions of taxanes with other anticancer drugs in humans

Drug	Sequence	PK interactions	PD effects	Comment	Reference
Paclitaxel (PTX) plus CDDP	PTX last	25% reduction in PTX clearance	Increase in neutropenia	Effect on cytochrome P-450	76
DOXO	PTX first (24 h infusion)	32% reduction in DOXO clearance; 70% increase in DOXO C_{max}	Increase in neutropenia and stomatitis		77
DOXO	PTX first (3 h infusion)	Increase in DOXO C_{max}	No		78
DOXO	Concomitant	30% increase in DOXO AUC; 100% increase in Doxolo AUC	Increase in cardiotoxicity over DOXO cumulative dose of 360-380 mg/ m^2	Implication of CrEL; competition for biliary excretion	78
EPI	Concomitant	Increase in EPI detoxification	Reduction in toxic effects		80
CYT	PTX last	No	Reduction in toxic effects		88
CBDCA	Indifferent	No	Reduction in CBDCA-induced thrombocytopenia		87
Capecitabine		No	Increase in activity	Upregulation of dThdPase	91
Docetaxel (DTX) plus CDDP	DTX first	No	Reduction in CDDP–DNA adducts in WBCs		94
DOXO	Indifferent	Increase in DTX AUC	Increase in clinical efficacy; reduction in cardiotoxicity	Interference with cytochrome P-450	84
Ifo	DTX first	Increase in Ifo clearance Decrease in Ifo AUC	Reduction in toxicity		95
	DTX last		Increase in toxicity		95

PTX, paclitaxel; CDDP, cisplatin; DOXO, doxorubicin; EPI, epirubicin; CYT, cyclophosphamide; CBDCA, carboplatin; Ifo, ifosfamide.

responsible for a non-linear disposition of the anthracycline and for increased plasma AUCs of doxorubicin (30%) and its major metabolite doxorubicinol (more than 100%).[78] Conflicting results are reported for the interference between *paclitaxel and epirubicin*. While a pharmacokinetic investigation conducted during a dose-finding study reported a reduction of epirubicinol plasma levels,[79] other studies showed a doubling of the plasma AUC of epirubicinol and strong interference with the elimination of the glucuronated forms of epirubicin (EPI-glu) and its metabolite (EOL-glu),[80] indicating a global increase of epirubicin detoxification.[79]

Docetaxel

The pharmacokinetics of docetaxel have been characterized by Bruno and coworkers during phase I and phase II studies of the drug. This characterization is a model of how pharmacokinetic studies should be conducted in order to produce information during early clinical evaluation of a new drug.[65,81] The approach has allowed rapid definition of a limited-sampling strategy for docetaxel, and the characterization of several important observations on some pharmacokinetic–pharmacodynamic relationships. Docetaxel pharmacokinetics are well described by linear processes, as shown by the proportional increase of the plasma AUC with dose and the independence of total body clearance from the administered dose.[82] It should be noted that the use of a limited-sampling strategy, the administration of docetaxel by the same schedule (infusion over 1 h), and the restricted range of the doses given with concomitant pharmacokinetic analysis do not allow for an ideal setting to explore non-linear disposition. Indeed, some investigators have detected subtle non-linear characteristics of docetaxel disposition.[83] However, this non-linearity does not appear to have major clinical relevance at the recommended dose and schedule of docetaxel. Few pharmacokinetic interactions have been detected in combinations of docetaxel with cisplatin, vinorelbine, ifosfamide, and 5-fluorouracil.

When docetaxel is combined with doxorubicin, a higher taxane AUC was measured using different schedules of administration.[84] This effect was attributed to interference at the liver microsomal system level (CYP). These authors did not observe any alteration in the pharmacokinetics of doxorubicin caused by docetaxel.

Pharmacodynamics

The pharmacokinetic–pharmacodynamic relationships of paclitaxel used as a single agent have been investigated in many studies. Key information was provided by a phase II clinical study in which two different doses of paclitaxel (135 and 175 mg/m²) were administered by infusion for either 3 or 24 h.[70,72] The pharmacodynamic consequences of the non-linear disposition of paclitaxel are counter-intuitive. No correlation was found between C_{max}, AUC, or dose of paclitaxel and the limiting toxicity neutropenia, which is more frequent and severe when the drug is given as an infusion for 24 h. However, a good relationship was shown between the percentage decrease of white blood cells (WBCs) or neutrophils (ANC) and the time (T) during

which the plasma concentration of paclitaxel was above the threshold concentration of 0.05 μM.[70] This parameter was higher for the 24 h infusion ($T \geq 24$ h) of the same dose than for the 3 h infusion ($T \leq 24$h), justifying the significantly higher neutropenia associated with the longer 24 h schedule (75% of patients showed grade 3 or 4 neutropenia compared with 15% of patients in the 3 h schedule) (Fig. 10.5).[70] Other investigators found a similar relationship using a paclitaxel concentration of 0.1 μM as the threshold level.[72] However, the 0.05 μM threshold can be applied to basically all schedules of paclitaxel, including those with infusion durations of 96 h during which plasma concentrations of 0.1 μM are almost never reached.[85] For toxicity other than neutropenia, the pharmacokinetic–pharmacodynamic relationship is less clear, with the exception of neurotoxicity which has been linked to paclitaxel AUC.[86]

Combination therapies of paclitaxel and *carboplatin* showed pharmacodynamic interference without measurable pharmacokinetic or sequence-dependent alterations. In several studies paclitaxel had a significant protective effect on carboplatin-induced thrombocytopenia.[87] No mechanistic explanation for this observation is available. The sequence of *cisplatin* before paclitaxel, which has less antitumour activity *in vitro*, induced more neutropenia than the opposite sequence and was associated with a reduction of paclitaxel clearance.[76] In combination with *cyclophosphamide*, administration of paclitaxel before cyclophosphamide resulted in more toxicity than the opposite sequence but no mechanistic or pharmacokinetic explanation was advanced.[88] The combination of paclitaxel with *capecitabine* is of interest in view of favourable preclinical observations of a TNF-α dependent upregulation of thymidine phosphorilase (dThdPase) induced by paclitaxel and docetaxel treatment in *in vivo* experiments.[89] dThdPase is the key enzyme for the activation of capecitabine and its intermediate metabolite to 5-fluorouracil in tumours.[90] Studies in humans evaluating the paclitaxel–capecitabine combination demonstrated no pharmacokinetic interaction and prominent antitumour activity supporting the preclinical observations.[91] Finally, for the combination of paclitaxel and *doxorubicin*, haematological and mucosal toxic effects were worse in the sequence paclitaxel (infused over 24 h) followed by doxorubicin (infused over 48 h).[77] In this sequence, the doxorubicin C_{max} was 70% higher and clearance was 32% lower than in the opposite sequence. Other investigators did not find any effects of the sequence on the tolerability of the combination

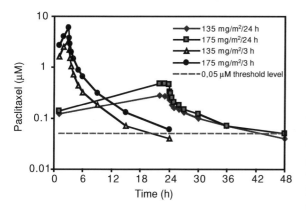

Figure 10.5. Pharmacokinetics of paclitaxel at different doses and times of administration. The threshold at 0.05 μM is shown as a broken line.

when paclitaxel was administered over 3 h before or after a doxorubicin bolus.[78] This absence of sequence effects can be attributed to the short interval between the two drugs. The combination is significantly more effective than single-agent therapy in breast cancer patients, but it also causes a high incidence of reversible congestive heart failure.[92]

The population pharmacokinetic–pharmacodynamic analysis for docetaxel, carried out by Bruno *et al.*,[93] explored the correlation between pharmacokinetic data measured at first course with pharmacodynamic observations in a large number of patients (640) treated in 24 phase II studies using logistic and Cox multivariate regression. AUC, clearance, and duration of exposure to 0.2 μM correlated with toxicity, neutropenia, and fluid retention. CL was strongly dependent on α_1-acid glycoprotein level (AAG), hepatic function, and body surface area. Age and plasma albumin level had significant but minor influence. Of clinical relevance, the decrease in docetaxel CL (27%) observed in patients with altered *liver transaminases* and alkaline phosphatase was the basis for the definition of guidelines for dose reduction in patients. AUC resulted in a significant predictor of time to progression in patients with non-small-cell lung cancer, but not in cases of *breast cancer*. A retrospective validation study[81] demonstrated the good performance (bias and precision) of the limited-sampling method based on three samples for patients.

Fewer pharmacodynamic drug interactions have been shown for docetaxel in combination with other antineoplastic drugs. The schedule of docetaxel before cisplatin caused lower levels of *cisplatin*–DNA adducts in peripheral WBCs in patients even in the absence of significant pharmacokinetic interference.[94] The sequence of docetaxel before *ifosfamide* was better tolerated than the opposite sequence.[95] The *capecitabine*–docetaxel combination resulted in significantly superior efficacy in time to disease progression and overall survival than single-agent docetaxel[96] in agreement with the docetaxel-mediated upregulation of dThdPase.[97] Finally, the increment of docetaxel AUC when combined with *doxorubicin* could explain both the high antitumour activity and the high haematological toxicity of the combination.[84]

Toxicity

Data from phase I and II studies established that paclitaxel and docetaxel share many toxic effects including hypersensitivity reactions, neutropenia, alopecia, peripheral neuropathy, and skin toxicity.[71] (Table 10.4).

Hypersensitivity reactions are probably due to the vehicle in which the drugs are formulated for clinical use, and they are characterized by dyspnea, bronchospasm, urticaria, and hypotension of various degrees of severity. Their occurrence is controlled or prevented by use of prophylactic medication with corticosteroids and histamine H_1 and H_2 receptor antagonists.[1]

Neutropenia is the dose-limiting toxicity of both drugs and, in the case of paclitaxel (40–70% of cases have an ANC count <500/μl), is schedule related, with longer infusions producing more neutropenia than short infusions. Docetaxel causes more frequent episodes of severe neutropenia at the recommended dose of 100 mg/m² infused over 1 h every 3 weeks (70–80% of patients have ANC counts <500/μl at nadir, and about 10% have episodes of febrile neutropenia).[1,93] The schedule dependence of paclitaxel toxicity also

Table 10.4 Main toxicities of taxanes (toxicity is **dose** and **schedule** dependent)

Type	Paclitaxel	Docetaxel
Hypersensitivity reactions (type I)	1–2.3% severe with premedication	2% severe without premedication
Neutropenia	40–70% at <500 ANC/μl	70–80% at <500 ANC/μl
Febrile neutropenia	5%	10–15%
Peripheral neuropathy	20–40% grade II or III	6–10% grade II or III
Stomatitis/mucositis	0–10% grade II or III	10–20% grade II or III
Total body alopecia	Universal	Universal
Diarrhoea	No	Up to 10% grade III–IV
Skin and nail toxicity	No	0–12% at grade III
Cumulative dose-dependent toxicity	No	Median dose to toxicity is 400 mg/m² (800 mg/m² with co-administration of steroids)

applies to peripheral neuropathy and stomatitis, which are more frequent and severe with the 3 h schedule of infusion than with the 24 h schedule.

Stomatitis, total-body alopecia (reversible and dose dependent), and peripheral neuropathy are side effects common to both taxanes. Peripheral neuropathy is less frequent and less severe for docetaxel than for paclitaxel,[1] making this drug an alternative to paclitaxel for inclusion in platinum-based regimens for the management of ovarian cancer.[98]

Adverse effects that are unique to the individual drug are also known. Paclitaxel may induce disturbances of cardiac conduction in the form of asymptomatic bradycardia that is rarely associated with haemodynamic changes. Myocardial ischaemia, atrial arrhythmias, and ventricular tachycardia have also been reported.[1] A greater than expected incidence of congestive heart failure has been reported when paclitaxel infused over 3 h is combined with bolus doxorubicin.[92] A recent reappraisal of the overall experience with anthracyclines and paclitaxel showed that the risk of cardiac events is similar to that expected with single-agent doxorubicin when the combination is given for a maximum total dose of doxorubicin of 360–380 mg/m^2. After this cumulative dose, the risk appears significantly larger than expected, reaching an incidence of more than 20% of congestive heart failure at doses of 480 mg/m^2 of doxorubicin.[95,99]

Two observations taken together could provide an explanation for the pathogenesis of the severe cardiotoxicity demonstrated by the paclitaxel–doxorubicin combination.[100] First, the pharmacokinetic interactions between drugs, due to the clinical formulation of paclitaxel or to competition for the same route of biliary elimination, lead to higher concentrations of doxorubicin in plasma and, consequently, in cardiac tissue. *Paclitaxel* is able to stimulate the metabolism of *doxorubicin* to toxic species, such as doxorubicinol and doxorubicinol–aglicone, inside cardiomyocytes as indicated in recent work.[101]

Docetaxel shares the same ability to stimulate doxorubicinol and doxorubicinol–aglicone synthesis in human cardiomyocytes, but within a narrow range of enzymatic activity, thus limiting enhancement of the cardiotoxicity of the anthracycline.[102] Two unusual types of toxicity are unique to docetaxel. The first is a syndrome of fluid retention characterized by edema (localized, pulmonary, peripheral, or generalized) and is related to the cumulative administered dose of docetaxel. *Fluid retention* appears in 50% of patients after a total dose of 400 mg/m^2 of docetaxel. Recent studies

showed that in patients who received dexamethasone premedication there was a modest increase in the median cumulative dose given before the development of peripheral edema.[9] The second unusual side effect of docetaxel is a skin and nail toxicity, consisting of erythroderma, erythrodysestesia, and progressive thickening, discoloration, and loss of nails, that appears unpredictably in some patients.

As with other anticancer drugs, paclitaxel and docetaxel have been administered in 3-weekly cycles. Recently, the weekly administration of both taxanes demonstrated an efficacy level comparable with the standard 21-day administration and with a better toxicity profile.[103–105] The weekly schedule allows for prolonged treatment to high cumulative doses with minimal myelotoxicity and tolerable neuropathy. The rationale for this dose-dense approch is that the more frequent delivery of moderate doses may inhibit tumour regrowth between cycles and limit the emergence of a malignant cell population resistant to chemotherapy.[106] The minimal side effects make this approach very interesting for treatment of elderly or bone-marrow-depleted patients and for combination therapy with other drugs as well as with new biological agents such as anti-HER2 and anti-EGFR molecules.[107]

References

1. Rowinsky EK (1997) The development and clinical utility of the taxane class of antimicrotubule chemotherapy agents. *Annu Rev Med*, 48, 353–74.
2. Bishop JF, Dewar J, Toner GC, et al. (1999) Initial paclitaxel improves outcome compared with CMFP combination chemotherapy as front-line therapy in untreated metastatic breast cancer. *J Clin Oncol*, 17, 2355–64.
3. Henderson IC, Berry DA, Demetri GD, et al. (2003) Improved outcomes from adding sequential paclitaxel but not from escalating doxorubicin dose in an adjuvant chemotherapy regimen for patients with node-positive primary breast cancer. *J Clin Oncol*, 21, 976–83.
4. McGuire WP, Hoskins WJ, Brady MF, et al. (1996) Cyclophosphamide and cisplatin versus paclitaxel and cisplatin: a phase III randomized trial in patients with suboptimal stage III/IV ovarian cancer (from the Gynecologic Oncology Group). *Semin Oncol*, 23, 40–7.
5. Piccart, MJ, Bertelsen K, James K, et al. (2000) Randomized intergroup trial of cisplatin–paclitaxel versus cisplatin–cyclophosphamide in women with advanced epithelial ovarian cancer: three-year results. *J Natl Cancer Inst*, 92, 699–708.
6. du Bois A, Luck HJ, Meier W, et al. (2003) A randomized clinical trial of cisplatin/paclitaxel versus carboplatin/paclitaxel as first-line treatment of ovarian cancer. *J Natl Cancer Inst*, 95, 1320–9.

7. Ozols RF, Bundy BN, Greer BE, *et al.* (2003) Phase III trial of carboplatin and paclitaxel compared with cisplatin and paclitaxel in patients with optimally resected stage III ovarian cancer: a Gynecologic Oncology Group study. *J Clin Oncol*, **21**, 3194–200.

8. Fulton B, Spencer CM (1996) Docetaxel. A review of its pharmacodynamic and pharmacokinetic properties and therapeutic efficacy in the management of metastatic breast cancer. *Drugs*, **51**, 1075–92.

9. Ravdin PM, Burris HA, Cook G (1995) Phase II trial of docetaxel in advanced anthracycline-resistant or anthracenedione-resistant breast cancer. *J Clin Oncol*, **13**, 2879–85.

10. Vasey PA (2003) Role of docetaxel in the treatment of newly diagnosed advanced ovarian cancer. *J Clin Oncol*, **21**, 136–44.

11. Maenpaa JU (2003) Docetaxel: promising and novel combinations in ovarian cancer. *B J Cancer*, **89**, S29–34.

12. Piccart M (2003) The role of taxanes in the adjuvant treatment of early stage breast cancer. *Breast Cancer Res Treat*, **79**, S25–34.

13. Nabholtz JM, Vannetzel JM, Llory JF, Bouffette P (2003) Advances in the use of taxanes in the adjuvant therapy of breast cancer. *Clin Breast Cancer*, **4**, 187–92.

14. Seidman AD, Fornier MN, Esteva FJ, *et al.* (2001) Weekly trastuzumab and paclitaxel therapy for metastatic breast cancer with analysis of efficacy by HER2 immunophenotype and gene amplification. *J Clin Oncol*, **19**, 2587–95.

15. Gori S, Colozza M, Mosconi AM, *et al.* (2004) Phase II study of weekly paclitaxel and trastuzumab in anthracycline—and taxane—pretreated patients with HER2-overexpressing metastatic breast cancer. *B J Cancer*, **90**, 36–40.

16. Slamon, DJ, Leyland-Jones B, Shak S, *et al.* (2001).Use of chemotherapy plus a monoclonal antibody against HER2 for metastatic breast cancer that overexpresses HER2. *N Engl J Med*, **344**, 783–92.

17. Herbst RS, Khuri FR (2003) Mode of action of docetaxel—a basis for combination with novel anticancer agents. *Cancer Treat Rev*, **29**, 407–15.

18. Kingston, DGI (1995) History and chemistry. In McGuire WP, Rowinsky EK (eds) *Paclitaxel in Cancer Treatment*. New York: Marcel Dekker, 1–33.

19. Ringel I, Horwitz SB (1991) Studies with RP 56976 (Taxotere): a semisynthetic analogue of Taxol. *J Natl Cancer Inst*, **83**, 288–91.

20. ten Tije AJ, Verweij J, Loos WJ, Sparreboom A (2003) Pharmacological effects of formulation vehicles: implications for cancer chemotherapy. *Clin Pharmacokinet*, **42**, 665–85.

21. Orr GA, Verdier-Pinard P, McDaid H, Horwitz SB (2003) Mechanisms of Taxol resistance related to microtubules. *Oncogene*, **22**, 7280–95.

22. Diaz JF, Andreu JM (1993) Assembly of purified GDP–tubulin into microtubules induced by Taxol and Taxotere: reversibility, ligand stoichiometry, and competition. *Biochemistry*, **32**, 2747–55.

23. Andreu JM, Diaz JF, Gil R, *et al.* (1994) Solution structure of Taxotere-induced microtubules to 3-nm resolution. The change in protofilament number is linked to the binding of the Taxol side chain. *J Biol Chem*, **269**, 31785–92.

24. Braakhuis BJ, Hill BT, Dietel M, *et al.* (1994) *In vitro* antiproliferative activity of docetaxel (Taxotere), paclitaxel (Taxol) and cisplatin against human tumour and normal bone marrow cells. *Anticancer Res*, **14**, 205–8.

25. Dorr RT (1997) Pharmacology of the taxanes. *Pharmacotherapy*, **17**, 96S–104S.

26. Hennequin C, Giocanti N, Favaudon V (1995) S-phase specificity of cell killing by docetaxel (Taxotere) in synchronized HeLa cells. *Br J Cancer*, **71**, 1194–8.

27. Au JL, Li D, Gan Y, *et al.* (1998) Pharmacodynamics of immediate and delayed effects of paclitaxel: role of slow apoptosis and intracellular drug retention. *Cancer Res*, **58**, 2141–8.

28. Jordon MA, Wenkell K, Gardiner S (1996) Mitotic block induced in HeLa cells by low concentrations of paclitaxel (Taxol) results in abnormal mitotic exit and apoptotic cell death. *Cancer Res*, **56**, 816–25.

29. Schiff PB, Gubits R, Kashimawo S, Geard CR (1995) Paclitaxel with ionizing radiation. In McGuire WP, Rowinsky EK (eds) *Paclitaxel in Cancer Treatment*. New York: Marcel Dekker, 81–90.

30. Choy H, Rodriguez F, Wilcox B, Koester SK, Degen D (1992) Radiation sensitizing effects of Taxotere (RP56976) *Proc Am Assoc Cancer Res*, **33**, 500 (abstract).

31. Haldar S, Chintapalli J, Croce CM (1996) Taxol induces *bcl–2* phosphorylation and death of prostate cancer cells. *Cancer Res*, **56**, 1253–5.

32. Haldar S, Basu A, Croce CM (1997) Bcl2 is the guardian of microtubule integrity. *Cancer Res*, **57**, 229–33.

33. Ding AH, Porteu F, Sanchez E, Nathan CF (1990) Shared actions of endotoxin and Taxol on TNF receptors and TNF release. *Science*, **248**, 370–2.

34. Burkhart CA, Berman JW, Swindell CS, Horwitz SB (1994) Relationship between the structure of Taxol and other taxanes on induction of tumor necrosis factor–alpha gene expression and cytotoxicity. *Cancer Res*, **54**, 5779–82.

35. Belotti D, Vergani V, Drudis T, *et al.* (1996) The microtubule-affecting drug paclitaxel has anti-angiogenic activity. *Clin Cancer Res*, **2**, 1843–9.

36. Klauber N, Parangi S, Flynn E, Hamel E, D'Amato RJ (1997) Inhibition of angiogenesis and breast cancer in mice by the microtubule inhibitors 2–methoxyestradiol and Taxol. *Cancer Res*, **57**, 81–6.

37. Rose WC, Fairchild CR (1995) Combination with other agents: preclinical data . In McGuire WP, Rowinsky EK (eds) *Paclitaxel in Cancer Treatment*. New York: Marcel Dekker, 55–79.

38. Vigano L, Locatelli A, Grasselli G, Gianni L (2001) Drug interactions of paclitaxel and docetaxel and their relevance for the design of combination therapy. *Invest New Drugs*, **19**, 179–96.

39. Chou TC, Otter GN, Sirotnak FM (1993) Combined effects of edatrexate with Taxol and Taxotere against breast cancer cell growth. *Proc Am Assoc Cancer Res* , **34**, 300 (abstract).

40. Chervinsky DS, Brecher ML, Hoelcle MJ (1993) Cremophor–EL enhances Taxol efficacy in a multi-drug

resistant C1300 neuroblastoma cell line. *Anticancer Res*, 13, 93–6.

41. Sparreboom A, Verweij J, van der Burg ME, *et al.* (1998) Disposition of Cremophor EL in humans limits the potential for modulation of the multidrug resistance phenotype *in vivo. Clin Cancer Res*, 4, 1937–42.

42. Sparreboom A, van Tellingen O, Nooijen WJ, Beijnen JH (1996) Nonlinear pharmacokinetics of paclitaxel in mice results from the pharmaceutical vehicle Cremophor EL. *Cancer Res*, 56, 2112–15.

43. Gianni L, Capri G, Mezzelani A, *et al.* (1997) Her2/Neu (HER2) amplification and response to doxorubicin/paclitaxel (AT) on women with metastatic breast cancer. *Proc Am Soc Clin Oncol*, 16, 139 (abstract).

44. Baselga J, Norton L, Albanell J, Kim YM, Mendelsohn J (1998) Recombinant humanized anti–HER2 antibody (Herceptin) enhances the antitumor activity of paclitaxel and doxorubicin against HER2/neu overexpressing human breast cancer xenografts. *Cancer Res*, 58, 2825–31.

45. Cabral F, Barlow SB (1991) Resistance to antimitotic agents as genetic probes of microtubule structure and function. *Pharmacol Ther*, 52, 159–71.

46. Kelland LR, Abel G (1992) Comparative *in vitro* cytotoxicity of Taxol and Taxotere against cisplatin-sensitive and -resistant human ovarian carcinoma cell lines. *Cancer Chemother Pharmacol*, 30, 444–450.

47. Gottesman MM (2002) Mechanisms of cancer drug resistance. *Annu Rev Med*, 53, 615–27.

48. Ravdin PM (1995) Taxoids: effective agents in anthracycline-resistant breast cancer. *Semin Oncol*, 22, 29–34.

49. Gianni L (1997) Future directions of paclitaxel-based therapy of breast cancer. *Semin Oncol*, 24, S17-91–6.

50. Gianni L, Munzone E, Capri G, *et al.* (1995) Paclitaxel in metastatic breast cancer: a trial of two doses by a 3-hour infusion in patients with disease recurrence after prior therapy with anthracyclines [see comments]. *J Natl Cancer Inst*, 87, 1169–75.

51. Blagosklonny MV, Fojo T (1999) Molecular effects of paclitaxel: myths and reality (a critical review). *Int J Cancer*, 83, 151–6.

52. Yang CP, Galbiati F, Volonte D, Horwitz SB, Lisanti MP (1998) Upregulation of caveolin-1 and caveolae organelles in Taxol-resistant A549 cells. *FEBS Lett*, 439, 368–72.

53. Panvichian R, Orth K, Day ML, Day KC, Pilat MJ, Pienta KJ (1998) Paclitaxel-associated multimininucleation is permitted by the inhibition of caspase activation: a potential early step in drug resistance. *Cancer Res*, 58, 4667–72.

54. Lavelle F, Bissery MC, Combeau C, Riou JF, Vrignaud P, Andre S (1995) Preclinical evaluation of docetaxel (Taxotere). *Semin Oncol*, 22, 3–16.

55. Valero V, Jones SE, Von Hoff DD, *et al.* (1998) A phase II study of docetaxel in patients with paclitaxel-resistant metastatic breast cancer. *J Clin Oncol*, 16, 3362–8.

56. Song D, Au JL (1995) Isocratic high-performance liquid chromatographic assay of Taxol in biological fluids and tissues using automated column switching. *J Chromatogr B Biomed Appl*, 663, 337–344.

57. Rouini MR, Lotfolahi A, Stewart DJ, *et al.* (1998) A rapid reversed phase high performance liquid chromatographic method for the determination of docetaxel (Taxotere) in human plasma using a column switching technique [In Process Citation]. *J Pharm. Biomed Anal*, 17, 1243–7.

58. Sottani C, Minoia C, D'Incalci M, Paganini M, Zucchetti M (1998) High-performance liquid chromatography tandem mass spectrometry procedure with automated solid phase extraction sample preparation for the quantitative determination of paclitaxel (Taxol) in human plasma. *Rapid Commun Mass Spectrom*, 12, 251–5.

59. Hempel G, Lehmkuhl D, Krumpelmann S, Blaschke G, Boos J (1996) Determination of paclitaxel in biological fluids by micellar electrokinetic chromatography. *J Chromatogr A*, 745, 173–9.

60. Klecker RW, Jamis-Dow CA, Egorin MJ, *et al.* (1994) Effect of cimetidine, probenecid, and ketoconazole on the distribution, biliary secretion, and metabolism of [3H]Taxol in the Sprague–Dawley rat. *Drug Metab Dispos*, 22, 254–8.

61. Hilmans JJ, Vermorken JB, Wolbers JG *et al.* (1994) Paclitaxel (Taxol) concentrations in brain tumour tissue. *Ann Oncol*, 5, 951–3.

62. Bissery MC, Renard A, Montay G, Bayssas M, Lavelle F (1991) Taxotere: antitumor activity and pharmacokinetics in mice. *Proc Am Assoc Cancer Res*, 32, 401 (abstract).

63. Crommentuyn KM, Schellens JH, van den Berg JD, Beijnen JH (1998) *In-vitro* metabolism of anti-cancer drugs, methods and applications: paclitaxel, docetaxel, tamoxifen and ifosfamide [In Process Citation]. *Cancer Treat Rev*, 24, 345–66.

64. Venook AP, Egorin M, Brown TD, *et al.* (1994) Paclitaxel (Taxol) in patients with liver dysfunction (CALGB9264) *Proc Am Soc Clin Oncol*, 13, 139 (abstract).

65. Bruno R, Hille D, Thomas L (1995) Population pharmacokinetics/pharmacodynamics of docetaxel (Taxotere) *Proc Am Assoc Cancer Res*, 14, 457 (abstract).

66. Kumar GN, Walle UK, Bhalla KN, Walle T (1993) Binding of Taxol to human plasma, albumin and alpha 1-acid glycoprotein. *Res Commun Chem Pathol Pharmacol*, 80, 337–44.

67. Bissery MC, Nohynek G, Sanderink GJ, Lavelle F (1995) Docetaxel (Taxotere): a review of preclinical and clinical experience. Part I: Preclinical experience. *Anticancer Drugs*, 6, 339–55, 363–8.

68. Urien S, Barre J, Morin C, Paccaly A, Montay G, Tillement JP (1996) Docetaxel serum protein binding with high affinity to alpha 1-acid glycoprotein. *Investig New Drugs*, 14, 147–51.

69. Monsarrat B, Royer I, Wright M *et al.* (1997) Biotransformation of taxoids by human cytochromes P450: Structure-activity relationship. *Bull Cancer*, 84, 125–33.

70. Gianni L, Kearns CM, Giani A, *et al.* (1995) Nonlinear pharmacokinetics and metabolism of paclitaxel and its pharmacokinetic/pharmacodynamic relationships in humans. *J Clin Oncol*, 13, 180–90.

71. Eisenhauer EA, Vermorken JB (1998) The taxoids. Comparative clinical pharmacology and therapeutic potential. *Drugs*, 55, 5–30.

72. Huizing MT, Keung AC, Rosing H., *et al.* (1993) Pharmacokinetics of paclitaxel and metabolites in a randomized comparative study in platinum-pretreated ovarian cancer patients. *J Clin Oncol*, **11**, 2127–35.

73. Ohtsu T, Sasaki Y, Tamura T, *et al.* (1995) Clinical pharmacokinet and pharmacodynamics of paclitaxel: a 3-hour infusion versus a 24-hour infusion. *Clin Cancer Res*, **1**, 599–606.

74. Capri G, Tarenzi E, Fulfaro F, Gianni L (1996) The role of taxanes in the treatment of breast cancer. *Semin Oncol*, **23** (Suppl 2), 68–75.

75. Gianni L, Kearns CM, Gianni A, *et al.* (1995) Non-linear pharmcokinetics and metabolism of paclitaxel and its pharmacokinetic/pharmacodynamic relationships in humans. *J Clin Oncol*, **13**, 180–90.

76. Rowinsky EK, Gilbert MR, McGuire WP, *et al.* (1991) Sequences of Taxol and cisplatin: a phase I and pharmacologic study. *J Clin Oncol*, **9**, 1691–1703.

77. Holmes FA, Madden T, Newman RA, *et al.* (1996) Sequence-dependent alteration of doxorubicin pharmacokinetics by paclitaxel in a phase I study of paclitaxel and doxorubicin in patients with metastatic breast cancer. *J Clin Oncol*, **14**, 2713–21.

78. Gianni L, Vigano L, Locatelli A, *et al.* (1997) Human pharmacokinetic characterization and *in vitro* study of the interaction between doxorubicin and paclitaxel in patients with breast cancer. *J Clin Oncol*, **15**, 1906–15.

79. Conte PF, Baldini E, Gennari A, *et al.* (1997) Dose-finding study and pharmacokinetics of epirubicin and paclitaxel over 3 hours: a regimen with high activity and low cardiotoxicity in advanced breast cancer. *J Clin Oncol*, **15**, 2510–17.

80. Gianni L, Vigano L, Locatelli A, *et al.* (1997) Different interference of paclitaxel (PTX) on human pharmacokinetics of doxorubicin (DOX) and epirubicin (EPI) *Proc Am Soc Clin Oncol*, **16**, 224 (abstract).

81. Bruno R, Vivler N, Vergniol JC, De Phillips SL, Montay G, Sheiner LB (1996) A population pharmacokinetic model for docetaxel (Taxotere): model building and validation. *J Pharmacokinet Biopharm*, **24**, 153–72.

82. McLeod HL, Kearns CM, Kuhn JG, Bruno R (1998) Evaluation of the linearity of docetaxel pharmacokinetics. *Cancer Chemother Pharmacol*, **42**, 155–9.

83. Kearns CM (1997) Pharmacokinetics of the taxanes. *Pharmacotherapy*, **17**, 105S–9S.

84. D'Incalci M, Schuller J, Colombo T, Zucchetti M, Riva A (1998) Taxoids in combination with anthracyclines and other agents: pharmacokinetic considerations. *Semin Oncol*, **25**, 16–20.

85. Seidman AD, Hochhauser D, Gollub M, *et al.* (1996) Ninety-six-hour paclitaxel infusion after progression during short taxane exposure: a phase II pharmacokinetic and pharmacodynamic study in metastatic breast cancer. *J Clin Oncol*, **14**, 1877–84.

86. Sonnichsen DS, Hurwitz CA, Pratt CB, Shuster JJ, Relling MV (1994) Saturable pharmacokinetics and paclitaxel pharmacodynamics in children with solid tumors. *J Clin Oncol*, **12**, 532–8.

87. Kearns CM, Egorin MJ (1997) Considerations regarding the less-than-expected thrombocytopenia encountered with combination paclitaxel/carboplatin chemotherapy. *Semin Oncol*, **24**, S2-91–6.

88. Kennedy MJ, Zahurak ML, Donehower RC, *et al.* (1996) Phase I and pharmacologic study of sequences of paclitaxel and cyclophosphamide supported by granulocyte colony-stimulating factor in women with previously treated metastatic breast cancer. *J Clin Oncol*, **14**, 783–91.

89. Sawada N, Ishikawa T, Fukase Y, Nishida M, Yoshikubo T, Ishitsuka H (1998) Induction of thymidine phosphorylase activity and enhancement of capecitabine efficacy by Taxol/Taxotere in human cancer xenografts. *Clin Cancer Res*, **4**, 1013–19.

90. Eda H, Fujimoto K, Watanabe S, *et al.* (1993) Cytokines induce thymidine phosphorylase expression in tumor cells and make them more susceptible to 5′-deoxy-5-fluorouridine. *Cancer Chemother Pharmacol*, **32**, 333–8.

91. Villalona-Calero MA, Weiss GR, Burris HA, *et al.* (1999) Phase I and pharmacokinetic study of the oral fluoropyrimidine capecitabine in combination with paclitaxel in patients with advanced solid malignancies. *J Clin Oncol*, **17**, 1915–25.

92. Gianni L, Munzone E, Capri G, *et al.* (1995) Paclitaxel by 3-h infusion in combination with bolus doxorubicin in women with untreated metastatic breast cancer: high antitumor efficacy and cardiac effects in a dose-finding and sequence-finding study [see comments]. *J Clin Oncol*, **13**, 2688–99.

93. Bruno R, Hille D, Riva A, *et al.* (1998) Population pharmacokinetics/pharmacodynamics of docetaxel in phase II studies in patients with cancer. *J Clin Oncol*, **16**, 187–96.

94. Schellens JHM, Ma J, Bruno R, *et al.* (1994) Pharmacokinetics of cisplatin and Taxotere (docetaxel) and WBC DNA–adduct formation of cisplatin in the sequence Taxotere/cisplatin and cisplatin/Taxotere in a phase II study in solid tumor patients. *Proc Am Soc Clin Oncol*, **13**, 132 (abstract).

95. Pronk LC, Schrijvers D, Schellens JH, *et al.* (1998) Docetaxel and ifosfamide in patients with advanced solid tumors: results of a phase I study. *Semin Oncol*, **25**, 23–8.

96. O'Shaughnessy J, Miles D, Vukelja S, *et al.* (2002) Superior survival with capecitabine plus docetaxel combination therapy in anthracycline-pretreated patients with advanced breast cancer: phase III trial results. *J Clin Oncol*, **20**, 2812–23.

97. Nadella P, Shapiro C, Otterson GA, *et al.* (2002) Pharmacobiologically based scheduling of capecitabine and docetaxel results in antitumor activity in resistant human malignancies. *J Clin Oncol*, **20**, 2616–23.

98. Katsumata N (2003) Docetaxel: an alternative taxane in ovarian cancer. *Br J Cancer*, **89**, S9–15.

99. Gianni L, Dombernowsky P, Sledge G, *et al.* (1998) Cardiac function following combination therapy with Taxol (T) and Doxorubicin (A) for advanced breast cancer (ABC). *Proc Am Soc Clin Oncol*, **17**, 115a (abstract).

100. Perotti A, Cresta S, Grasselli G, Capri G, Minotti G, Gianni L (2003) Cardiotoxic effects of anthracycline–taxane combinations. *Expert Opin Drug Safety*, **2**, 59–71.

101. Minotti G, Cairo G, Monti E (1999) Role of iron in anthracycline cardiotoxicity: new tunes for an old song? *FASEB J*, **13**,199–212.

102. Minotti G, Saponiero A, Licata S, *et al.* (2001) Paclitaxel and docetaxel enhance the metabolism of doxorubicin to toxic species in human myocardium. *Clin Cancer Res*, 7, 1511–15.

103. Marchetti P, Urien S, Cappellini GA, Ronzino G, Ficorella C (2002) Weekly administration of paclitaxel: theoretical and clinical basis. *Crit Rev Oncol Hematol*, **44**, S3–13.

104. Baselga J, Tabernero JM (2001) Weekly docetaxel in breast cancer: applying clinical data to patient therapy. *Oncologist*, **6** (Suppl 3), 26–9.

105. Kuroi K, Bando H, Saji S, Toi M (2003) Weekly schedule of docetaxel in breast cancer: evaluation of response and toxicity. *Breast Cancer*, **10**, 10–14.

106. Seidman AD, Hudis CA, Albanel J, *et al.* (1998) Dose-dense therapy with weekly 1-hour paclitaxel infusions in the treatment of metastatic breast cancer. *J Clin Oncol*, **16**, 3353–61.

107. Zimatore M, Danova M, Vassallo E, *et al.* (2002) Weekly taxanes in metastatic breast cancer (review) *Oncol Rep*, **9**, 1047–52.

11 | *Vinca alkaloids*

Timothy W. Synold

Introduction

The periwinkle plant (*Cantharantus roseus*; *Vinca rosea L.*), originally indigenous to Madagascar but now cultivated all over the world, has a long and colourful history of medicinal uses for the treatment of such widely dissimilar conditions as haemorrhage, scurvy, toothache, wound healing, and diabetes. Research into the compounds responsible for the therapeutic effects of the periwinkle led to the discovery of the antitumour vinca alkaloids, vincristine and vinblastine.[1,2] These cytotoxic vinca alkaloids act by binding to tubulin, thereby preventing the polymerization of microtubules essential for many cellular

Summary

	Vincristine	Vinblastine	Vindesine	Vinorelbine
Brand names	Oncovin, Vincasar, Kyocristine, Vincosid, Vincrex	Exal, Velban, Velbe, Velsar	Eldisine, Fildesin	Navelbine
Previous name	Leurocristine	Vincaleukoblastine		
Molecular weight (Da)	825 (base) 923 (sulphate salt)	811 (base) 909 (sulphate salt)	754 (base) 852 (sulphate salt)	779 (base) 1079 (ditartrate salt)
Mechanism of action	Binds tubulin and prevents polymerization of mitotic spindles	Same as vincristine	Same as vincristine	Same as vincristine
Cell-cycle specificity	Blocks cells in mitosis	Same as vincristine	Same as vincristine	Same as vincristine
Route of administration	Intravenous only	Intravenous only	Intravenous only	Intravenous, oral
Protein binding (%)	>99	>99	NA	87
Metabolism	Yes, predominantly P450 IIIA	Same as vincristine	Same as vincristine	Same as vincristine
Elimination	Biliary/faecal	Biliary/faecal	Biliary/faecal	Biliary/faecal
Terminal half-life (h)	85 (range 19–155)	25 (range 7–47)	24 (range 12–42)	33 (range 14–44)
Toxicities	Neuromuscular	Bone marrow suppression	Bone marrow suppression	Bone marrow suppression

processes, including cell division. Since their clinical introduction in the 1960s, the naturally occurring vinca alkaloids have become an important part of many potentially curative regimens used in the treatment of leukaemia, lymphoma, and testicular cancer. The semisynthetic analogues vindesine and vinorelbine have demonstrated significant clinical activity in lung, ovarian, and breast tumours, highlighting the fact that small modifications of these complex molecular structures can lead to large differences in both the pharmacology and clinical activity of these important agents.

Clinical use

The vinca alkaloids are among the most widely used and broadly active of available anticancer agents.[3] Vincristine, vinblastine, and vindesine have been used as a part curative therapy, as well as palliative treatment in such malignancies as Hodgkin's disease, acute lymphocytic leukaemia, breast carcinoma, Wilms' tumour, Ewing's sarcoma, neuroblastoma, hepatoblastoma, rhabdomyosarcoma, testicular cancer, and small-cell lung cancer. The semisynthetic analogue vinorelbine has demonstrated significant single-agent activity in non-small-cell lung cancer, breast cancer, ovarian cancer, and Hodgkin's disease. Vincristine is an important part of front-line combination chemotherapy for the treatment of acute lymphocytic leukaemia, while vinblastine is used in combination with other agents in the front-line therapy of Hodgkin's disease and testicular cancer. Vindesine is indicated for the treatment of vincristine-resistant acute lymphocytic leukaemia and non-small lung cancer. Vinorelbine is currently used as either second- or third-line therapy for non-small-cell lung cancer.

Vincristine sulphate is commercially available as an intravenous formulation (1 mg/ml) supplied in either prefilled syringes (1 and 2 mg) or in single- and multidose vials. Vinblastine and vindesine are supplied as lyophilized powders in 10 mg and 5 mg vials, respectively, that are reconstituted for intravenous injection with sterile sodium chloride to a final concentration of 1 mg/ml. Solutions of vincristine sulphate contain 100 mg/ml mannitol, while solutions of vindesine contain 5 mg/ml mannitol. Although preparations of vincristine, vinblastine, and vindesine are stable in NaCl 0.9% and dextrose 5%, it is recommended that these agents be injected either into a large vein or into the tubing of a running intravenous solution.

Vincristine, vinblastine, and vindesine are strong vesicants, and extreme caution should be taken to prevent leakage into surrounding tissue. Therefore it is recommended that administration of these agents be completed within 1 min to minimize the risk of extravasation. Vinorelbine is supplied as a colourless to pale yellow solution of 10 mg/ml in water. Preparations of vinorelbine in NaCl 0.9% or dextrose 5% are stable at 0.5–2 mg/ml for up to 24 h. Unlike the other vinca alkaloids, vinorelbine is not an irritant and can be given by the oral route. Investigational trials of orally administered vinorelbine have used liquid-filled soft gelatin capsules (40 mg).

Mechanism of action

The principle mechanism of action of the vinca alkaloids is disruption of mitotic spindle assembly through the interaction with tubulin.[4–6] Although the vinca alkaloids have been shown to interfere with amino acid metabolism,[7] calmodulin-dependent Ca^{2+} ATPase activity,[8] and nucleic acid synthesis,[9] these pharmacological effects occur at drug concentrations much higher than those achievable *in vivo*. Vinca alkaloids kill actively dividing cells by inhibiting progression through mitosis. As a result, cytotoxicity is highly dependent on the duration of exposure.

Tubulin is a heterodimeric protein with a molecular weight of 110 kDa. Under normal physiological conditions, tubulin polymerizes to form microtubules, which are essential for such cellular processes as morphology, mitosis, meiosis, secretion, and axonal transport.[10] The processes of polymerization and depolymerization of tubulin are complex and well controlled, involving the binding of guanosine 5-triphosphate (GTP) and tubulin.[11] All the vinca alkaloids have a high affinity for tubulin, and, by binding to the protein, they both prevent polymerization and promote depolymerization of the microtubules. It has been shown that the binding of vincristine to tubulin is two- to threefold higher in the presence of GTP than in its absence, suggesting that tissue levels of GTP may play an important role in the activity of these agents.[12] Tubulin binding constants for vincristine, vinblastine, vindesine, and vinorelbine are 8.0×10^6 mol/l, 6.0×10^6 mol/l, 3.3×10^6 mol/l, and 5.4×10^6 mol/l, respectively.[13,14] Because of the similarities in their binding affinities, it has been suggested that the differences in the relative potencies of these agents are related to their intracellular retention, and more specifically, to the stability of the drug–tubulin complexes.[14–16]

Although vinorelbine, vincristine, and vinblastine have been shown to cause microtubule depolymerization and subsequent metaphase blockade at equivalent concentrations in most tissues, vincristine is a much more potent inhibitor of axonal microtubule formation than either vinorelbine or vinblastine.[17] These tissue-specific effects may help to explain differences in toxicity profiles. Vinorelbine is a relatively weak inhibitor of axonal microtubule function and spiralization, and has the least neurotoxic potential and largest therapeutic window of all the vinca alkaloids.

While disruption of microtubule assembly and function results in metaphase blockade, the terminal event in the cytotoxic pathway of the vinca alkaloids is the initiation of programmed cell death.[18–21] *In vitro* investigations carried out in multiple cell lines have identified these agents as potent inducers of apoptosis through both p53-dependent and p53-independent pathways.[22–24] Tumour cells exposed to these microtubule poisons display dose- and time-dependent morphological and molecular changes characteristic of apoptosis.

Mechanisms of resistance

As with other chemotherapeutic agents, resistance to the vinca alkaloids is multifactorial. By far the most widely recognized mechanism is via the multidrug resistance (MDR) associated P-glycoprotein (P-gp)[25] and the multidrug resistance protein (MRP).[26] Although changes in tubulin binding,[27–29] alterations in heat-shock response,[29] and disruption in apoptotic signalling[21,30,31] have also been identified as mechanisms of vinca alkaloid resistance, MDR has been most commonly described. Both P-gp and MRP are central to a well-characterized biochemical pathway that describes the mechanism of resistance to a variety of structurally and mechanistically dissimilar anti-cancer agents (as detailed in Chapter 1). These multidrug resistance associated proteins are transmembrane transporters, which have been shown to facilitate the rapid efflux of intracellular chemotherapeutic agents. Over-expression of either of these proteins in mammalian cells is associated with reduced intracellular accumulation of vinca alkaloids, and corresponding reductions in cytotoxicity. The cross-resistance profiles of cells that over-express MRP or P-gp are similar but

not identical. There also appear to be differences in the mechanisms by which the two proteins transport drugs. P-gp-enriched membrane vesicles have been shown to transport several chemotherapeutic drugs directly, whereas vincristine transport by MRP-enriched membrane vesicles is demonstrable only in the presence of reduced glutathione.[26]

Programmed cell death, or apoptosis, is initiated after exposure to vinca alkaloids and occurs through a complex signalling pathway involving activation of c-Jun and stress-activated protein kinase.[22] Several pro- and anti-apoptotic effectors which regulate various steps in the apoptotic pathway have previously been identified. Anti-apoptotic genes like Bcl-2 and its homologue Bcl-XL are expressed in a variety of tumours, and their expression modulates the sensitivity of cells to a wide spectrum of chemotherapeutic agents. Both Bcl-XL and Bcl-2 over-expression provide protection to vincristine and vinblastine in the absence of P-gp or other drug resistance associated genes.[32,33]

Chemistry

The vinca alkaloids are dimeric asymmetrical compounds consisting of two multi-ringed subunits, vindoline and catharantine, linked by a carbon–carbon bridge (Fig. 11.1).[34] Vincristine and vinblastine differ from one another in the R1 position of the vindoline subunit, while vinblastine and vindesine differ in the R2 and R3 positions. Vinorelbine is a semisynthetic derivative of vinblastine, differing in the catharanthine subunit of the molecule. In general, modifications to the catharantine moiety have a negative effect on activity, while changes to the vindoline portion have a minor impact.[35] As illustrated by the four clinically approved agents in this class, relatively small modifications to the complex vinca skeleton can result in significant changes in the spectrum of activity and toxicity.

Analytical methodology

Radioactive assays

The dose-limiting toxicities of vincristine, vinblastine, and vindesine occur following administration of fairly modest doses. Relatively low plasma concentrations of these agents are achieved *in vivo* at the doses used

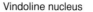

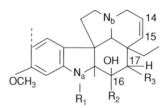

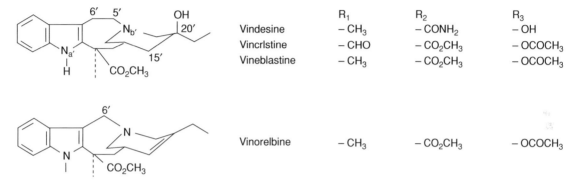

Figure 11.1. Chemical structures of the vinca alkaloids. Reproduced with permission from Zhou and Rahmani (1992) *Drugs*, 44 (Suppl 4), 1–16.

clinically, and as a result very sensitive analytical methodologies are required. Early pharmacological investigations in animals relied on administration of radiolabelled drugs and used liquid scintillation counting.[36–40] These assays, while simple to perform, are unable to discriminate between parent drug and metabolites. Figure 11.2 illustrates the different results for vinorelbine obtained when measuring total plasma radioactivity versus radio-immunological (RIA) measurements.[41] As can be seen in the figure, the concentrations of vinorelbine determined by scintillation counting are systematically higher than those measured by RIA, probably reflecting the non-specificity of radioactivity determinations. Combined use of radiolabelled drugs with either thin-layer or high-performance liquid chromatography allows separation of parent drug and metabolites; however, plasma pharmacokinetics are difficult to characterize as levels of radioactivity decline rapidly to undetectable levels.[38,42]

With the advent of RIA and enzyme-linked immunosorbent assay (ELISA), plasma levels of the vinca alkaloids can be monitored for up to 72–96 h following a dose. These immunological methods offer advantages over scintillation counting with respect to selectivity and sensitivity; however, cross-reactivity with unknown

metabolites and breakdown products remains a concern. The antibodies used in these assays have specificity directed at the catharantine moiety of the molecule and are unable to detect changes in the vindole subunit, particularly at the 2, 3, and 4 positions.[43] RIA and ELISA methods exist for vincristine, vinblastine, and vindesine, and have been applied to multiple human pharmacokinetic trials. Limits of detection for these assays range from 0.05 to 0.5 ng/ml in plasma, allowing for prolonged pharmacokinetic monitoring. While quantitation of circulating drug levels during the apparent terminal elimination phase is possible using these immunological methods, cross-reactivity with metabolites cannot be excluded.[35]

High-performance liquid chromatography

Concern about assay cross-reactivity and improvements in detection capabilities has fuelled the development of a number of high-performance liquid chromatography (HPLC) methods for detection of vinca alkaloids in human plasma. Using a variety of sample pretreatment methods and both normal and reverse phase separation, selective and sensitive HPLC assays now exist for all of the vinca alkaloids, as well

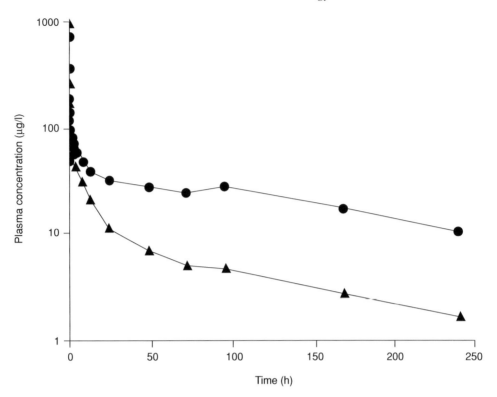

Figure 11.2.   Plasma levels of vinorelbine in a patient receiving 30 mg/m² of [³H]vinorelbine. Solid circles, data from direct counts of radioactivity; solid triangles, data from radio-immunoassay. Reproduced with permission from Bore, *et al.* (1989) *Cancer Chemother Pharmacol,* **23**, 247–51.

as for some metabolites. Most of these assays rely on ultraviolet, electrochemical, or fluorescence detection, and have limits of detection as low as 0.5 ng/ml. Mass spectrometry has also recently been combined with liquid chromatography, resulting in a highly selective and sensitive assay for vincristine, vinblastine, and desacetylvinblastine.[44] Owing to the need for highly sensitive assays for determination of these drugs in clinical specimens, adequate sample clean-up prior to HPLC analysis is critical. While both liquid–liquid and solid phase extraction methods have been described, liquid extraction has the advantage of being more flexible and is amenable to analysis of drug in virtually all sample matrixes including tissues and faeces.[35] Although studies using radiolabelled compounds and RIAs have provided insight into the pharmacokinetics of the vinca alkaloids, the use of these highly selective and sensitive HPLC assays has provided a better understanding of the disposition of parent drug and metabolites in humans.

Pharmacokinetics

Absorption

Owing to the strong vesicant properties and unreliable gastrointestinal absorption of the other vinca alkaloids, only vinorelbine has been thoroughly investigated by the oral route. Oral absorption of vinorelbine is rapid, with maximal drug concentrations reached in 1–2 h. The absolute bioavailability of vinorelbine given in soft gelatin capsules in adult cancer patients is approximately 27%, with a range of 10–60%.[45] The oral clearance of vinorelbine is high and approaches hepatic flow values (0.8 l/h/kg), suggesting a significant first-pass effect. Rahmani *et al.*[40] studied the oral absorption of radiolabelled vinorelbine in two patients, and reported large differences between the results obtained by radioactivity counting and by radio-immunological determinations, suggesting significant bioconversion of absorbed drug. As a result of this first-pass effect, vinorelbine doses of 80–100 mg/m² are required orally to give comparable systemic exposures to the standard intravenous dose of 30 mg/m².

The oral bioavailability of vinorelbine decreases by 22% when taken with food, most likely due to a delay in gastric emptying. The time to reach maximum plasma vinorelbine concentrations doubles when the dose is taken with food compared with when it is taken in the fasting state.[46] The bioavailability of vinorelbine also declines by 16% when administered in divided doses. The lack of dose proportionality in AUC and the high oral clearance further indicates that there is a large first-pass effect, and that it may be saturable above single doses of 120 mg/m².

To date, studies of orally administered vinorelbine have only been conducted in the context of closely supervised clinical trials. Patients enrolled in these trials have been selected for features such as good hepatic function and performance status. The pharmacokinetics of oral vinorelbine have not yet been determined in the wide range of patients seen in routine clinical practice. It is expected that other factors, such as concomitant medications, age, liver function, and genetic polymorphisms, will increase the already large inter- and intra-patient variability in bioavailability.

Protein binding

Vincristine, vinblastine, vindesine, and vinorelbine are significantly protein bound. The vinca alkaloids bind to several plasma proteins, including α1-acid glycoprotein, albumin, and lipoproteins.[47] The predominant binding protein for the vinca alkaloids in human plasma is α1-acid glycoprotein, with an approximately 10-fold higher affinity for these drugs than albumin.[48,49] Binding of the vincas to α1-acid glycoprotein is best described by a two-class model, with both higher- and lower-affinity sites in similar numbers. At concentrations in the range of 10^{-6} M *in vitro*, unbound fractions in plasma range from 13 to 40%. However, at drug concentrations similar to those achieved *in vivo*, protein binding of vincristine and vinblastine is greater than 99%, suggesting that the number of available binding sites in plasma is saturable.[50] The protein binding of vinorelbine determined *in vivo* is 87%, with a range of 80–91%.[47]

In addition to protein binding, the vinca alkaloids are rapidly and extensively bound to platelets and lymphocytes following intravenous administration.[47,51] Similar findings have been reported for all these drugs, indicating that platelets are the predominant cellular carriers of drug in whole blood. The platelet compartment accounts for approximately 80% of blood-bound drug, while lymphocytes account for an additional 5%. Owing to the significant partitioning of vinorelbine into platelets and lymphocytes, while the free fraction in plasma is approximately 13%, the unbound fraction in whole blood is less than 2%. The distribution of drug into platelets and lymphocytes is complete within 30 min for vinorelbine, 1 h for vinblastine, and 3 h for vincristine.[47,51,52] Drug binding to platelets is a reversible process and release is much slower for vincristine than for either vinblastine or vinorelbine, which may help to explain the differences in terminal elimination half-lives (Table 11.1).

Tissue distribution

Animal studies using radiolabelled drugs show that, following intravenous administration, the vinca alkaloids are widely and rapidly distributed throughout the body.[38,42,53–56] For vincristine, vinblastine, and vindesine, high amounts of radioactivity concentrate in the spleen, liver, kidney, lymph nodes, and thymus. Moderate amounts of these agents are found in lung, heart, and skeletal muscles, and relatively low amounts are present in fat and brain. Although vinorelbine also accumulates in spleen, liver, and kidney, very high levels of drug are found in lung. Measurement of radioactive drug uptake in human lung tissue has shown that vinorelbine is present in up to 300-

Table 11.1 Summary of the disposition of vinca alkaloids by bolus injection in patients with normal organ function: pooled values (range) from multiple studies

	Clearance (l/h/kg)	Volume of distribution (l/kg)	Elimination half-life (h)	Faecal clearance (%)	Renal clearance (%)
Vincristine	0.16 (0.1–0.3)	7.2 (3.1–11.0)	45.1 (8.2–144)	69	4–13.5
Vinblastine	0.79 (0.7–0.9)	24.7 (17.3–35.1)	25.6 (19.6–29.2)	25–41	5.5–34
Vindesine	0.22 (0.1–0.3)	8.6 (6.8–10.5)	23.6 (19.0–34.8)	ND	4–19
Vinorelbine	0.95 (0.8–1.3)	54.3 (44.7–75.6)	41.2 (31.2–62.4)	40–58	3.3–24.6

Some clearance and volume of distribution results were converted by assuming that 1.73 m² = 70 kg. For more detailed evaluation see van Tellingen *et al.*[35]

fold greater concentrations in lung tissue than in serum.[57] Therefore the patterns of tissue distribution for the different vinca alkaloids correlate with their spectrum of clinical activity, since vincristine, vinblastine, and vindesine are particularly active lymphatic malignancies and vinorelbine is an active agent in the treatment of non-small-cell lung cancer.

Central nervous system penetration

The vinca alkaloids do not significantly distribute into the central nervous system (CNS). In the rhesus monkey model CNS levels of vincristine are detectable but low (4–5 ng/ml) up to 24 h after an intravenous dose,[58] while in humans penetration of vincristine and its products into the cerebrospinal fluid after intravenous bolus injection is very poor.[59] Despite the relatively high lipophilicity of these agents, their large size and significant platelet and protein binding prevent them from crossing the blood–brain barrier. In addition, P-gp in the

brain capillary endothelium has been identified as a functional component of the barrier,[60] and, as previously stated, the vinca alkaloids are substrates for P-gp. Unidirectional transport of vincristine from the basal side to the apical side of the epithelial membrane by P-gp has been demonstrated. Mice lacking constitutive expression of P-gp have a 22-fold higher accumulation of vinblastine in brain tissue than wild-type mice.[61] In addition, CNS uptake of vinblastine can be enhanced ninefold by co-administration of an inhibitor of P-gp,[62] further indicating the importance of this transport protein in the function of the blood–brain barrier.

Metabolism

Uptake and accumulation of the vinca alkaloids by human hepatocytes has been shown to increase with increasing lipophilicity.[63,64] Vinorelbine, the most lipid soluble of the available vinca alkaloids, is most rapidly and extensively taken up by the liver.[63] The *in vitro*

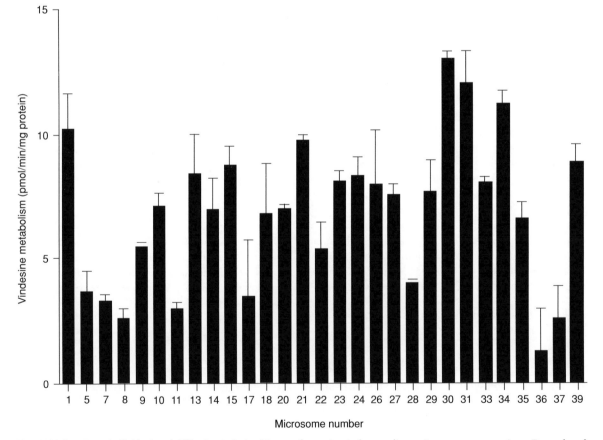

Figure 11.3. Inter-individual variability in vindesine biotransformation in human liver microsome preparations. Reproduced with permission from Owellen RJ, *et al.* (1977) *Cancer Res*, **37**, 2597–602.

metabolism of the vinca alkaloids has been investigated in freshly isolated human and animal hepatocytes and in human microsomal subcellular fractions.[55,56,65] After incubation in suspensions of hepatocytes, vincristine, vinblastine, vindesine, and vinorelbine are almost completely converted into several water-soluble metabolites which are excreted into the extracellular fluid. Remaining intracellular drug is predominantly unchanged, presumably bound to tubulin. While most vinca alkaloid metabolites remain uncharacterized, deacetylated vinblastine and vinorelbine have been detected in the faeces, urine, and tissues of animals, although at relatively low concentrations.[66,67] Only desactyl-vinorelbine has been measured in the urine of patients, and although evidence suggests that desacetyl-vinorelbine is roughly equipotent to vinorelbine, it is probably of limited clinical significance since the appearance of this metabolite in urine represents only 0.25% of the administered dose.[67]

The metabolism of the vinca alkaloids by human liver microsomes shows considerable inter-patient variability (Fig. 11.3). Several different lines of evidence have identified cytochrome P450 3A as the principle isoform responsible for their conversion.[65,68] First, biotransformation of vinblastine and vindesine by human microsomes is inhibited by co-incubation with drugs that are known substrates for P450 3A.[65,68] Moreover, a significant correlation exists between erythromycin N-demethylase activity and vinca alkaloid metabolism.[65,68] In addition, polyclonal anti-P450 3A antibodies prevent the hepatic microsomal conversion of vinblastine and vindesine.[65,68] Finally, individual vinca alkaloids inhibit the biotransformation of one another, indicating that their metabolic pathways are similar. The characterization of the metabolic conversion of the vinca alkaloids is significant with respect to potential drug interactions, since many agents used clinically are substrates for cytochrome P450 3A.

Elimination

The vinca alkaloids are primarily metabolized and excreted via the hepatobiliary system. While only a limited number of clinical studies provide data on the faecal elimination of these agents, these data are in good agreement with preclinical investigations.[42,53,69] In two patients treated with [³H]vinorelbine, faecal drug excretion accounted for between 34% and 58.4% of the administered radioactivity, while approximately 21% was eliminated in the urine.[55] Similar studies with other radiolabelled vinca alkaloids have demonstrated that urinary excretion accounts for between 10% and

13% of the administered dose, with the majority of the radioactivity detected in faeces.[37,39,70] Urinary clearance of vinorelbine determined using HPLC detection methods has been reported to be only 11% of the administered dose.[67] While the major route of elimination is biliary, with a small but significant renal component, the total recovery of vinca alkaloids following a dose is incomplete. The incomplete recovery is most likely due to intracellular protein binding and prolonged tissue retention, leading to the delayed elimination of undetectable levels of drug.

Pharmacokinetic drug interactions

As previously stated, the vinca alkaloids are substrates for cytochrome P450 3A, and therefore it is anticipated that drugs which share this detoxification pathway will interfere with their metabolism. Drugs such as quinidine, erythromycin, cyclosporin, and nifedipine are P450 3A substrates that have been shown to inhibit conversion of vindesine by human liver microsomes *in vitro*.[65] *In vivo*, the plasma clearance of vincristine decreases by 69% when it is used in combination with nifedipine.[71] Moreover, although detailed pharmacokinetic studies have not been performed, patients receiving vinblastine in combination with cyclosporin and erythromycin experience much greater vinblastine-associated toxicity than would be expected with vinblastine alone.[72,73] Similarly, vincristine-associated peripheral neuropathy is significantly worse when vincristine is given in combination with *etoposide*, another substrate for cytochrome P450 3A4.[74] Conversely, as with other agents which are extensively metabolized in the liver, it is possible that drugs which induce hepatic enzymes (e.g. phenytoin and phenobarbital) could increase the metabolic clearance and tolerance to the vinca alkaloids. In one particular trial in children with acute leukaemia, vincristine plasma clearance in a child receiving concomitant phenobarbital was significantly higher than in the other children studied.[75] In addition, in this same trial, children treated with ranitidine and cimetidine, known inhibitors of cytochrome P450 enzymes, had lower than expected clearances.

Alterations with disease or age

Owing to the importance of hepatobiliary excretion in the systemic clearance of vinca alkaloids, it is recommended that the dosage of all these agents is reduced in patients with evidence of hepatic insufficiency. Despite this recommendation, there are no clear guidelines for

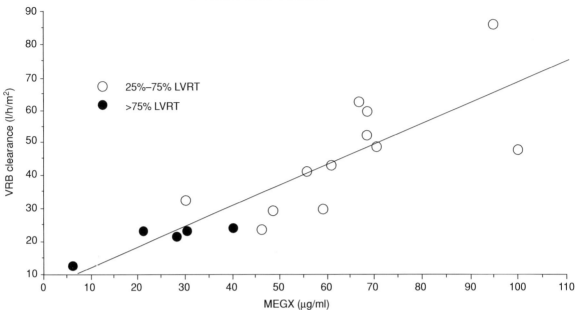

y = .631x + 5.645. R–squared: .7

Figure 11.4. Correlation between vinorelbine (VRB) plasma clearance and monoethylglycinexylidide (MEGX) test in patients with liver metastases (*n* = 17). %LVRT, percentage of liver volume replaced by tumour. Reproduced with permission from Robieux I, *et al.* (1996) *Clin Pharmacol Ther*, **59**, 32–40.

dose modifications. Patients with elevated serum alkaline phosphatase levels receiving vincristine have been determined to have significantly longer elimination half-lives and higher AUCs than patients with normal laboratory values.[76] Likewise, serum albumin concentrations in patients receiving vinblastine have been shown to correlate positively with clearance.[77] In a study of women with metastatic breast cancer, vinorelbine clearance was twice as slow in patients with more than 75% of their liver replaced by tumour than in women without liver involvement. In addition, there was good correlation between vinorelbine clearance and liver function assessed by the MEGX test (Fig. 11.4).[78]

As illustrated in Figure 11.3, there is a greater than 10-fold inter-patient variability in human microsomal biotransformation of vindesine under *in vitro* conditions. In the clinical setting, it is expected that other factors such as liver blood flow and drug interactions will increase this variability in drug metabolism significantly. As a result, additional studies are needed to describe further the disposition of the vinca alkaloids in patients with varying degrees of liver dysfunction, with special attention paid to the use of model substrates as predictors of clearance a priori.

Hepatic clearance of some anticancer agents has been shown to decrease with increasing age. Given the exten-

sive metabolism of the vinca alkaloids, it has been hypothesized that the clearance of these agents will also vary with age. Pharmacokinetic studies in very young children and adolescents suggest an effect of age on systemic clearance of vincristine.[75] While these studies have used historical controls for adult comparisons, vincristine clearance normalized to either weight or body surface area has been reported to be roughly twice as fast in children (Fig. 11.5). There have been no prospectively controlled trials of vincristine pharmacokinetics in patients spanning a wide range of ages. However, one trial of vinorelbine in elderly patients suggested that there is no effect of age on drug clearance when compared with historical controls under the age of 65.[79,80] Similar pharmacokinetic studies of vinorelbine have not yet been performed in very young children.

Pharmacokinetic models

Both compartmental and non-compartmental pharmacokinetic modelling methods have been applied to the vinca alkaloids. The majority of human pharmacokinetic investigations of vinca alkaloids have concluded that the plasma concentration–time profiles display a tri-exponential pattern of decay.[81–85] All the vinca alka-

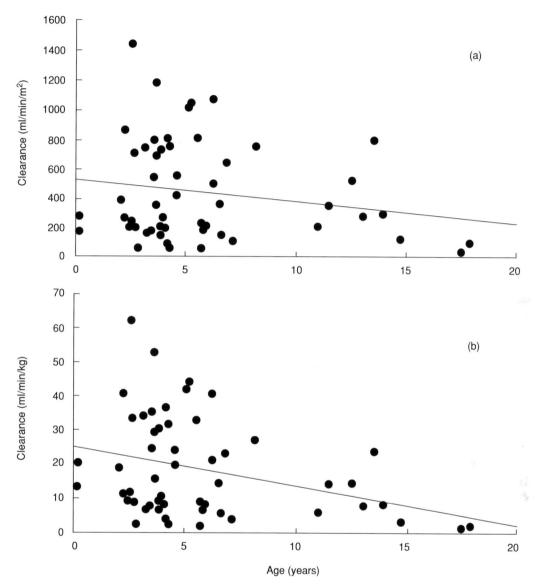

Figure 11.5. Vincristine clearance plotted versus age. Clearance is normalized to (a) body surface area and (b) body weight. Regression lines for both relationships are shown ($R^2 = 3.1\%$, $p = 0.206$ for body surface area; $R^2 = 9.5\%$, $p = 0.023$ for body weight). Reproduced with permission from Crom, *et al.* (1994) *J Pediatr*, **125**, 642–9.

loids share in common the features of rapid distribution into large tissue pools, followed by delayed elimination. Furthermore, large inter-patient variability in the pharmacokinetic parameters of the vinca alkaloids has been observed.[81,83] While the initial distribution half-lives of these drugs are similar, the terminal half-lives differ markedly, ranging from 24 h for vindesine to 85 h for vincristine. As illustrated in Figure 11.6, differences in terminal elimination half-lives and systemic clearances are closely related to the maximum tolerated clinical

doses of the vincas. As shown in the figure, vincristine has the slowest clearance (0.11 l/h/kg) and the lowest maximum tolerated weekly dose (1.4 mg/m²),[86] while vinorelbine has the fastest clearance (1.3 l/h/kg) and highest weekly dose (30 mg/m²).[87]

Despite many years of clinical use and pharmacokinetic investigation of the vinca alkaloids, there have been few attempts to simplify their plasma level monitoring. One such trial of vinblastine has been reported using linear regression analysis to predict the AUC

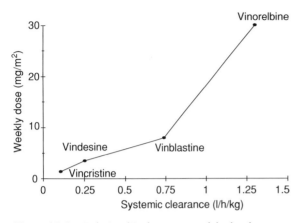

Figure 11.6. Relationship between total body clearances and clinically tolerated weekly doses of the individual vinca alkaloids.

following a single intravenous bolus dose.[88] A linear regression model, using sampling times of 10 and 36 h following the dose, was developed using a training dataset of 15 intensively sampled patients and was subsequently validated in a second cohort of 15 patients. Although the model performed well in the validation subset, it has never been applied and confirmed in a larger study set. In any event, it is predicted that such limited sampling methods, particularly those using only two sampling time points, are not sufficiently accurate to predict the exposure to agents with complex tri-exponential plasma decay and long terminal elimination half-lives. Bayesian estimation should provide the most effective means of pharmacokinetic monitoring for agents such as the vincas; however no such studies have been reported to date. The paucity of limited sampling strategies for vinca alkaloids may be a result of the relative lack of previously described pharmacodynamic relationships.

Pharmacodynamics

Despite over 30 years of clinical use, the pharmacodynamics of the vinca alkaloids have not been well described. A significant relationship between plasma vincristine AUC and the maximum grade of neurotoxicity has been described.[76] Patients with higher plasma AUCs were more likely to have grade 2 or 3 neurotoxic effects in the 2 month observation period following the assessment of vincristine pharmacokinetics. In addition, elevated serum alkaline phosphatase concentrations were associated with both higher vincristine AUCs and greater neurotoxicity, presumably due to impaired liver function and delayed vincristine clearance.

Other investigators have reported pharmacodynamic relationships in patients receiving continuous infusions of vinblastine. In three separate trials using a continuous infusion schedule, it was shown that vinblastine pharmacokinetics correlated with the degree of leukopenia,[89] the severity of non-haematological toxicity,[91] or the clinical response.[90] In one such study, patients who had higher steady-state plasma vinblastine concentrations were more likely to experience dose-limiting myelosuppression.[89] In another trial of continuous infusion vinblastine a positive correlation between mean steady-state vinblastine concentrations and the severity of non-haematological toxicity was found in patients with testicular cancer.[91] However, no relationship could be identified between vinblastine pharmacokinetics and the occurrence of haematological toxicity since all patients experienced severe myelosuppression at the doses used in the trial. Finally, patients with breast cancer who had slower vinblastine clearance had a better clinical response than those who cleared the drug more quickly.[90]

The extensive tissue distribution of the vinca alkaloids means that the plasma drug compartment may not be the most informative. For these agents with large volumes of distribution, plasma concentrations reflect only a small part of total drug in the body. In the case of vinorelbine, there is significant drug binding to platelets and lymphocytes. As a result, whole-blood or platelet vinorelbine levels may provide more information than plasma concentrations. Because of the methodological and pharmacological limitations, there is still much to learn about the pharmacodynamics of these potentially curative chemotherapeutic agents.

References

1. Cutts JH, Beer CT, Noble RT (1960) Biological properties of vincaleukoblastine, an alkaloid in *Vinca Rosea Linn.*, with reference to its antitumor action. *Cancer Res*, **20**, 1023–31.
2. Johnson IS, Armstrong JG, Gorman M, Burnett JF (1963) The vinca alkaloids: a new class of oncolytic agents. *Cancer Res*, **23**, 1390–1427.
3. Chabner BA (1992) Mitotic inhibitors. *Cancer Chemother Biol Response Modif*, **13**, 69–74.
4. Na GC, Timasheff SN (1982) *In vitro* vinblastine-induced tubulin paracrystals. *J Biol Chem*, **257**, 10387–91.
5. Himes RH (1991) Interactions of the catharanthus (Vinca) alkaloids with tubulin and microtubules. *Pharmacol Ther*, **51**, 257–67.
6. Lobert S, Vulevic B, Correia JJ (1996) Interaction of vinca alkaloids with tubulin: a comparison of vinblastine, vincristine, and vinorelbine. *Biochemistry*, **35**, 6806–14.

7. Cline MJ (1968) Effects of vincristine on synthesis of ribonucleic acid and protein in leukemic leucocytes. *Br J Haematol*, **14**, 21–9.

8. Watanabe K, West WL (1982) Calmodulin, activated cyclic nucleotide phosphodiesterase, microtubules and vinca alkaloids. *Fed Proc*, **41**, 2292–9.

9. Creasy WA (1968) Modifications in biochemical pathways produced by vinca alkaloids. *Cancer Chemother Rep*, **52**, 501–7.

10. Luduena RF, Shooter EM, Wilson L (1977) Structure of the tubulin dimer. *J Biol Chem*, **252**, 7006–14.

11. Mitchison TJ (1993) Localization of an exchangeable GTP binding site at the plus end of microtubules. *Science*, **261**, 1044–7.

12. Houghton PJ, Houghton JA, Bowman LC, Hazelton BJ (1987) Therapeutic selectivity of vinca alkaloids: a role for guanosine 5'- triphosphate? *Anticancer Drug Des*, **2**, 165–79.

13. Owellen RJ, Hartke CA, Dickerson RM, Hains FO (1976) Inhibition of tubulin-microtubule polymerization by drugs of the vinca alkaloid class. *Cancer Res*, **36**, 1499–1502.

14. Lobert S, Vulevic B, Correia JJ (1996) Interaction of vinca alkaloids with tubulin: a comparison of vinblastine, vincristine, and vinorelbine. *Biochemistry*, **35**, 6806–14.

15. Wierzba K, Sugiyama Y, Okudaira K, Iga T, Hanano M (1987) Tubulin as a major determinant of tissue distribution of vincristine. *J Pharm Sci*, **76**, 872–5.

16. Singer WD, Himes RH (1992) Cellular uptake and tubulin binding properties of four vinca alkaloids. *Biochem Pharmacol*, **43**, 545–51.

17. Binet S, Chaineau E, Fellous A, *et al.* (1990) Immunofluorescence study of the action of navelbine, vincristine and vinblastine on mitotic and axonal microtubules. *Int J Cancer*, **46**, 262–6.

18. Tsukidate K, Yamamoto K, Snyder JW, Farber JL (1993) Microtubule antagonists activate programmed cell death (apoptosis) in cultured rat hepatocytes. *Am J Pathol*, **143**, 918–25.

19. Huschtscha LI, Bartier WA, Ross CE, Tattersall MH (1996) Characteristics of cancer cell death after exposure to cytotoxic drugs *in vitro*. *Br J Cancer*, **73**, 54–60.

20. Harmon BV, Takano YS, Winterford CM, Potten CS (1992) Cell death induced by vincristine in the intestinal crypts of mice and in a human Burkitt's lymphoma cell line. *Cell Prolif*, **25**, 523–36.

21. Srivastava RK, Srivastava AR, Korsmeyer SJ, Nesterova M, Cho-Chung YS, Longo DL (1998) Involvement of microtubules in the regulation of Bc12 phosphorylation and apoptosis through cyclic AMP-dependent protein kinase. *Mol Cell Biol*, **18**, 3509–17.

22. Yu K, Ravera CP, Chen YN, McMahon G (1997) Regulation of Myc-dependent apoptosis by p53, c-Jun N-terminal kinases/stress-activated protein kinases, and Mdm-2. *Cell Growth Differ*, **8**, 731–42.

23. Li G, Tang L, Zhou X, Tron V, Ho V (1998) Chemotherapy-induced apoptosis in melanoma cells is p53 dependent. *Melanoma Res*, **8**, 17–23.

24. Fan S, Cherney B, Reinhold W, Rucker K, O'Connor PM (1998) Disruption of p53 function in immortalized human cells does not affect survival or apoptosis after taxol or vincristine treatment. *Clin Cancer Res*, **4**, 1047–54.

25. Sikic BI, Fisher GA, Lum BL, Halsey J, Beketic-Oreskovic L, Chen G (1997) Modulation and prevention of multidrug resistance by inhibitors of P-glycoprotein. *Cancer Chemother Pharmacol*, **40** (Suppl), S13–19.

26. Lautier D, Canitrot Y, Deeley RG, Cole SP (1996) Multidrug resistance mediated by the multidrug resistance protein (MRP) gene. *Biochem Pharmacol*, **52**, 967–77.

27. Pain J, Sirotnak FM, Barrueco JR, Yang CH, Biedler JL (1988) Altered molecular properties of tubulin in a multidrug-resistant variant of Chinese hamster cells selected for resistance to vinca alkaloids. *J Cell Physiol*, **136**, 341–7.

28. Geyp M, Ireland CM, Pittman SM (1996) Resistance to apoptotic cell death in a drug resistant T cell leukaemia cell line. *Leukemia*, **10**, 447–55.

29. Lee WC, Lin KY, Chen KD, Lai YK (1992) Induction of HSP70 is associated with vincristine resistance in heat-shocked 9L rat brain tumour cells. *Br J Cancer*, **66**, 653–9.

30. Jia L, Allen PD, Macey MG, Grahn MF, Newland AC, Kelsey SM (1997) Mitochondrial electron transport chain activity, but not ATP synthesis, is required for drug-induced apoptosis in human leukaemic cells: a possible novel mechanism of regulating drug resistance. *Br J Haematol*, **98**, 686–98.

31. Kern MA, Helmbach H, Artuc M, Karmann D, Jurgovsky K, Schadendorf D (1997) Human melanoma cell lines selected *in vitro* displaying various levels of drug resistance against cisplatin, fotemustine, vindesine or etoposide: modulation of proto-oncogene expression. *Anticancer Res*, **17**, 4359–70.

32. Zhang J, Alter N, Reed JC, Borner C, Obeid LM, Hannun YA (1996) Bcl-2 interrupts the ceramide-mediated pathway of cell death. *Proc Natl Acad Sci USA*, **93**, 5325–8.

33. Simonian PL, Grillot DA, Nunez G (1997) Bcl-2 and Bcl-XL can differentially block chemotherapy-induced cell death. *Blood*, **90**, 1208–16.

34. Zhou XJ, Rahmani R (1992) Preclinical and clinical pharmacology of vinca alkaloids. *Drugs*, **44** (Suppl 4), 1–16.

35. van Tellingen O, Sips JH, Beijnen JH, Bult A, Nooijen WJ (1992) Pharmacology, bio-analysis and pharmacokinetics of the vinca alkaloids and semi-synthetic derivatives (review). *Anticancer Res*, **12**, 1699–1715

36. van Tellingen O, Beijnen JH, Nooyen WJ (1991) Analytical methods for the determination of vinca alkaloids in biological specimens: a survey of the literature. *J Pharm Biomed Anal*, **9**, 1077–82.

37. Bender RA, Castle MC, Margileth DA, Oliverio VT (1977) The pharmacokinetics of [³H]-vincristine in man. *Clin Pharmacol Ther*, **22**, 430–5.

38. El Dareer SM, White VM, Chen FP, Mellet LB, Hill DL (1977) Distribution and metabolism of vincristine in mice, rats, dogs, and monkeys. *Cancer Treat Rep*, **61**, 1269–77.

39. Owellen RJ, Hartke CA (1975) The pharmacokinetics of 4-acetyl tritium vinblastine in two patients. *Cancer Res*, **35**, 975–80.

40. Rahmani R, Zhou XJ, Bore P, van Cantfort J, Focan C, Cano JP (1991) Oral administration of [^{3}H]navelbine in patients: comparative pharmacokinetics using radioactive and radioimmunologic determination methods. *Anticancer Drugs*, **2**, 405–10.

41. Bore P, Rahmani R, van Cantfort J, Focan C, Cano JP (1989) Pharmacokinetics of a new anticancer drug, navelbine, in patients. Comparative study of radioimmunologic and radioactive determination methods. *Cancer Chemother Pharmacol*, **23**, 247–51.

42. Castle MC, Margileth DA, Oliverio VT (1976) Distribution and excretion of (^{3}H) vincristine in the rat and the dog. *Cancer Res*, **36**, 3684–9.

43. Rahmani R, Barbet J, Cano JP (1983) A 125I-radiolabelled probe for vinblastine and vindesine radioimmunoassays: applications to measurements of vindesine plasma levels in man after intravenous injections and long-term infusions. *Clin Chim Acta*, **129**, 57–69.

44. Ramirez J, Ogan K, Ratain MJ (1997) Determination of vinca alkaloids in human plasma by liquid chromatography/atmospheric pressure chemical ionization mass spectrometry. *Cancer Chemother Pharmacol*, **39**, 286–90.

45. Rowinsky EK, Noe DA, Trump DL, *et al.* (1994) Pharmacokinetic, bioavailability, and feasibility study of oral vinorelbine in patients with solid tumors. *J Clin Oncol*, **12**, 1754–63.

46. Rowinsky EK, Lucas VS, Hsieh AL, *et al.* (1996) The effects of food and divided dosing on the bioavailability of oral vinorelbine. *Cancer Chemother Pharmacol*, **39**, 9–16.

47. Urien S, Bree F, Breillout F, Bastian G, Krikorian A, Tillement JP (1993) Vinorelbine high-affinity binding to human platelets and lymphocytes: distribution in human blood. *Cancer Chemother Pharmacol*, **32**, 231–4.

48. Fitos I, Visy J, Simonyi M (1991) Binding of vinca alkaloid analogues to human serum albumin and to alpha 1-acid glycoprotein. *Biochem Pharmacol*, **41**, 377–83.

49. Steele WH, Haughton DJ, Barber HE (1982) Binding of vinblastine to recrystallized human alpha 1-acid glycoprotein. *Cancer Chemother Pharmacol*, **10**, 40–2.

50. Steele WH, King DJ, Barber HE, Hawksworth GM, Dawson AA, Petrie JC (1983) The protein binding of vinblastine in the serum of normal subjects and patients with Hodgkin's disease. *Eur J Clin Pharmacol*, **24**, 683–7.

51. Gout PW, Wijcik LL, Beer CT (1978) Differences between vinblastine and vincristine in distribution in the blood of rats and binding by platelets and malignant cells. *Eur J Cancer*, **14**, 1167–78.

52. Gout PW, Wijcik LL, Beer CT (1978) Differences between vinblastine and vincristine in distribution in the blood of rats and binding by platelets and malignant cells. *Eur J Cancer*, **14**, 1167–78.

53. Culp HW, Daniels WD, McMahon RE (1977) Disposition and tissue levels of [^{3}H]vindesine in rats. *Cancer Res*, **37**, 3053–6.

54. Castle MC, Mead JA (1978) Investigation of the metabolic fate of tritiated vincristine in the rat by high-pressure liquid chromatography. *Biochem Pharmacol*, **27**, 37–44.

55. Rahmani R, Zhou XJ, Placidi M, Martin M, Cano JP (1990) *In vivo* and *in vitro* pharmacokinetics and metabolism of vincaalkaloids in rat. I. Vindesine (4-deacetyl-vinblastine 3- carboxyamide). *Eur J Drug Metab Pharmacokinet*, **15**, 49–55.

56. Zhou XJ, Martin M, Placidi M, Cano JP, Rahmani R (1990) *In vivo* and *in vitro* pharmacokinetics and metabolism of vincaalkaloids in rat. II. Vinblastine and vincristine. *Eur J Drug Metab Pharmacokinet*, **15**, 323–32.

57. Leveque D, Quoix E, Dumont P, *et al.* (1993) Pulmonary distribution of vinorelbine in patients with non-small-cell lung cancer. *Cancer Chemother Pharmacol*, **33**, 176–8.

58. Jackson DVJ, Castle MC, Poplack DG, Bender RA (1980) Pharmacokinetics of vincristine in the cerebrospinal fluid of subhuman primates. *Cancer Res*, **40**, 722–4.

59. Jackson DVJ, Sethi VS, Spurr CL, McWhorter JM (1981) Pharmacokinetics of vincristine in the cerebrospinal fluid of humans. *Cancer Res*, **41**, 1466–8.

60. Tatsuta T, Naito M, Oh-Hara T, Sugawara I, Tsuruo T (1992) Functional involvement of P-glycoprotein in blood–brain barrier. *J Biol Chem*, **267**, 20383–91.

61. van Asperen J, Schinkel AH, Beijnen JH, Nooijen WJ, Borst P, van Tellingen O (1996) Altered pharmacokinetics of vinblastine in Mdr1a P-glycoprotein- deficient mice. *J Natl Cancer Inst*, **88**, 994–9.

62. Drion N, Lemaire M, Lefauconnier JM, Scherrmann JM (1996) Role of P-glycoprotein in the blood–brain transport of colchicine and vinblastine. *J Neurochem*, **67**, 1688–93.

63. Zhou XJ, Placidi M, Rahmani R (1994) Uptake and metabolism of vinca alkaloids by freshly isolated human hepatocytes in suspension. *Anticancer Res*, **14**, 1017–22.

64. Rahmani-Jourdheuil D, Coloma F, Placidi M, Rahmani R (1994) Human hepatic uptake of two vinca alkaloids: navelbine and vincristine. *J Pharm Sci*, **83**, 468–71.

65. Zhou-Pan XR, Seree E, Zhou XJ, *et al.* (1993) Involvement of human liver cytochrome P450 3A in vinblastine metabolism: drug interactions. *Cancer Res*, **53**, 5121–6.

66. Owellen RJ, Hartke CA, Hains FO (1977) Pharmacokinetics and metabolism of vinblastine in humans. *Cancer Res*, **37**, 2597–602.

67. Jehl F, Quoix E, Leveque D, *et al.* (1991) Pharmacokinetic and preliminary metabolic fate of navelbine in humans as determined by high performance liquid chromatography. *Cancer Res*, **51**, 2073–6.

68. Zhou XJ, Zhou-Pan XR, Gauthier T, Placidi M, Maurel P, Rahmani R (1993) Human liver microsomal cytochrome P450 3A isozymes mediated vindesine biotransformation. Metabolic drug interactions. *Biochem Pharmacol*, **45**, 853–61.

69. Leveque D, Merle-Melet M, Bresler L, *et al.* (1993) Biliary elimination and pharmacokinetics of vinorelbine in micropigs. *Cancer Chemother Pharmacol*, **32**, 487–90.

70. Owellen RJ, Root MA, Hains FO (1977) Pharmacokinetics of vindesine and vincristine in humans. *Cancer Res*, **37**, 2603–7.

71. Fedeli L, Colozza M, Boschetti E, *et al.* (1989) Pharmacokinetics of vincristine in cancer patients treated with nifedipine. *Cancer*, **64**, 1805–11.

72. Tobe SW, Siu LL, Jamal SA, Skorecki KL, Murphy GF, Warner E (1995) Vinblastine and erythromycin: an

unrecognized serious drug interaction [see comments]. *Cancer Chemother Pharmacol*, **35**, 188–90.

73. Samuels BL, Mick R, Vogelzang NJ, *et al.* (1993) Modulation of vinblastine resistance with cyclosporine: a phase I study. *Clin Pharmacol Ther*, **54**, 421–9.

74. Thant M, Hawley RJ, Smith MT, *et al.* (1982) Possible enhancement of vincristine neuropathy by VP-16. *Cancer*, **49**, 859–64.

75. Crom WR, de Graaf SS, Synold T, *et al.* (1994) Pharmacokinetics of vincristine in children and adolescents with acute lymphocytic leukemia. *J Pediatr*, **125**, 642–9.

76. Van den Berg HW, Desai ZR, Wilson R, Kennedy G, Bridges JM, Shanks RG (1982) The pharmacokinetics of vincristine in man: reduced drug clearance associated with raised serum alkaline phosphatase and dose-limited elimination. *Cancer Chemother Pharmacol*, **8**, 215–19.

77. Ratain MJ, Vogelzang NJ, Sinkule JA (1987) Interpatient and intrapatient variability in vinblastine pharmacokinetics. *Clin Pharmacol Ther*, **41**, 61–7.

78. Robieux I, Sorio R, Borsatti E, *et al.* (1996) Pharmacokinetics of vinorelbine in patients with liver metastases. *Clin Pharmacol Ther*, **59**, 32–40.

79. Egorin MJ (1993) Cancer pharmacology in the elderly. *Semin Oncol*, **20**, 43–9.

80. Sorio R, Robieux I, Galligioni E, *et al.* (1997) Pharmacokinetics and tolerance of vinorelbine in elderly patients with metastatic breast cancer. *Eur J Cancer*, **33**, 301–3.

81. van Tellingen O (1994) Bioanalysis and pharmacokinetics of (investigational) vinca alkaloids. *Pharm World Sci*, **16**, 164–6.

82. Nelson RL (1982) The comparative clinical pharmacology and pharmacokinetics of vindesine, vincristine, and vinblastine in human patients with cancer. *Med Pediatr Oncol*, **10**, 115–27.

83. Rahmani R, Zhou XJ (1993) Pharmacokinetics and metabolism of vinca alkaloids. *Cancer Surv*, **17**, 269–81.

84. Mooberry SL, Taoka CR, Busquets L (1996) Cryptophycin 1 binds to tubulin at a site distinct from the colchicine binding site and at a site that may overlap the vinca binding site. *Cancer Lett*, **107**, 53–7.

85. Marquet P, Lachatre G, Debord J, Eichler B, Bonnaud F, Nicot G (1992) Pharmacokinetics of vinorelbine in man. *Eur J Clin Pharmacol*, **42**, 545–7.

86. Nelson RL, Dyke RW, Root MA (1980) Comparative pharmacokinetics of vindesine, vincristine and vinblastine in patients with cancer. *Cancer Treat Rev*, **7** (Suppl 1), 17–24.

87. Jehl F, Debs J, Herlin C, Quoix E, Gallion C, Monteil H (1990) Determination of navelbine and desacetyl-navelbine in biological fluids by high-performance liquid chromatography. *J Chromatogr*, **525**, 225–33.

88. Ratain MJ, Vogelzang NJ (1987) Limited sampling model for vinblastine pharmacokinetics. *Cancer Treat Rep*, **71**, 935–9.

89. Ratain MJ, Vogelzang NJ (1986) Phase I and pharmacological study of vinblastine by prolonged continuous infusion. *Cancer Res*, **46**, 4827–30.

90. Chong CD, Logothetis CJ, Savaraj N, Fritsche HA, Gietner AM, Samuels ML (1988) The correlation of vinblastine pharmacokinetics to toxicity in testicular cancer patients. *J Clin Pharmacol*, **28**, 714–18.

91. Lu K, Yap HY, Loo TL (1983) Clinical pharmacokinetics of vinblastine by continuous intravenous infusion. *Cancer Res*, **43**, 1405–8.

12 | Topoisomerase I targeting agents

Eric K. Rowinsky and Sharyn D. Baker

Introduction and historical survey

An extensive National Cancer Institute programme to screen natural products during the 1950s led to the isolation of an extract of the Chinese tree *Camptotheca acuminata* which had cytotoxic activity against a wide variety of leukaemia and solid tumours, including drug-refractory malignancies. Subsequent studies by Wall *et al.*[1] in 1966 demonstrated that camptothecin (CPT) (Fig.12.1) was the active constituent of the extract, and initial studies of the mechanism of action of this compound suggested that cytotoxicity might be due to inhibitory effects on both DNA and RNA synthesis.[2–5] However, the precise mechanism of CPT was not delineated until approximately two decades later when it was demonstrated to stabilize covalent adducts between genomic DNA and the nuclear enzyme topoisomerase I (topo I). Unfortunately, the characterization of the precise cytotoxic mechanisms and structure–activity relationships for CPT did not occur until after initial clinical trials of the drug in the early 1970s.

Owing to the aqueous insolubility of the active closed-ring lactone form of CPT, the agent was formulated as a ring-opened sodium carboxylate salt which was active only by virtue of lactone ring closure that preferentially occurred in acidic pH.[6–9] Although antitumour activity was observed with sodium CPT in patients with colorectal, gastric, small bowel, and non-small-cell lung carcinomas, and malignant melanoma in phase I and II studies, a high rate of severe and unpredictable toxicities, including haemorrhagic cystitis and gastrointestinal effects, which in retrospect were most likely due to the lactone ring closure and direct mucosal toxicity in these acidic tissues, led to discontinuation of the development of CPT.[6–12] Recognition by several laboratories of the novel mechanism of CPT as an inhibitor of topo I resulted in renewed interest in developing CPT derivatives 20 years later.

In 1996, two CPT analogues received regulatory approval for use in patients with solid malignancies: topotecan (TPT, Hycamtin) for previously treated patients with advanced ovarian cancer, and irinotecan (CPT-11, Camptosar) for patients with advanced colorectal carcinoma who previously received 5-fluorouracil. Irinotecan is the first new therapeutic agent in over 30 years to receive regulatory approval for metastatic colorectal cancer, which is the second most common cause of death due to cancer. Several other CPT analogues and non-CPT inhibitors of topo I are in earlier stages of clinical development. In this chapter, the following topics are discussed: the chemistry and structure–function relationships of CPT and CPT derivatives, the proposed mechanisms of cytotoxicity and resistance of these agents, the clinical pharmacology of CPT, topotecan, and irinotecan, which were the first CPT analogues to undergo extensive clinical evaluations, and finally other novel inhibitors of topo I.

Chemistry and structure–activity relationships of CPT analogues

The structures of the CPT derivatives that are currently undergoing extensive preclinical and clinical evalu-

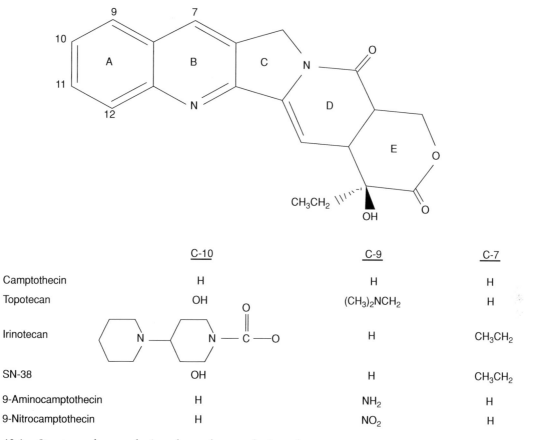

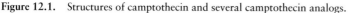

	C-10	C-9	C-7
Camptothecin	H	H	H
Topotecan	OH	$(CH_3)_2NCH_2$	H
Irinotecan	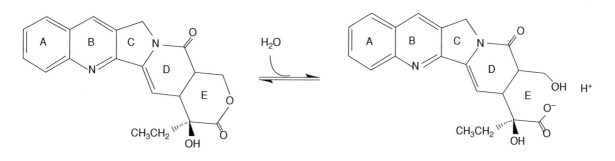	H	CH_3CH_2
SN-38	OH	H	CH_3CH_2
9-Aminocamptothecin	H	NH_2	H
9-Nitrocamptothecin	H	NO_2	H

Figure 12.1. Structures of camptothecin and several camptothecin analogs.

ations are shown in Figure 12.1. CPT and all CPT derivatives have a basic five-ring (A–E) structure with a chiral centre located at the 20 position in the terminal E ring.[12,13] Since CPT is relative insoluble in aqueous solutions, initial attempts to synthesize CPT derivatives involved defining features of the molecule that are essential for cytotoxicity and producing derivatives with increased solubility under physiological conditions.[13] Reversible pH-dependent non-enzymatic hydrolysis of the lactone ring of all CPT derivatives

Figure 12.2. The lactone form of CPT undergoes E-ring opening to form the carboxylate. A basic pH favours lactone E-ring opening.

results in an open-ring carboxylate, as shown Figure 12.2. These two species are in equilibrium in aqueous buffers. As discussed in the previous section, the sodium salt of the CPT carboxylate was evaluated in early clinical trials of CPT because of the difficulty in formulating the parent compound and the increased aqueous solubility of the hydroxy acid derivative.[6-12]

For all CPTs, the active lactone predominates at acidic pH, whereas the carboxylate predominates at neutral or basic pH (including physiological pH). In addition, the carboxylate acid is a less potent inhibitor of topo I and a much less potent antitumour agent.[12-15] Thus E-ring closure is required for topo I targeting activity. Consistent with this conclusion, replacement of the ring oxygen with sulphur or nitrogen has been shown to abolish the activity of CPT.[16,17] In addition, the a-hydroxyl group at position 20 on the E ring is essential for cytotoxicity, although several ester linkages at the 20(S) a-hydroxyl CPT position appear to stabilize the E-ring lactone.[17] In contrast, CPT retains activity with many diverse structural modifications of the A and B rings. For example, several substitutions at the 9 or 10 positions of the A ring can enhance water solubility without interfering with activity, though substitutions at the 12 position result in compounds devoid of activity.[12,13] The 9 and 10 positions of topotecan are substituted with dimethylaminomethyl and hydroxyl groups, respectively, which enhance aqueous solubility.[12,13,15,18] In contrast, the addition of an amino group at the 9 position results in analogues with enhanced activity; however, the insolubility of these compound, [e.g. 9-aminoCPT (9-AC)] in aqueous solutions made them difficult to formulate for intravenous administration until recently.[13] The prodrug irinotecan is unique among the CPT derivatives because of the bulky piperidino side chain at the 10 position, which is cleaved enzymatically by a carboxylesterase-converting enzyme to generate the much more biologically active, albeit water-insoluble, metabolite SN-38 (7-ethyl-10-hydroxyCPT).[12,13]

Likewise, addition of a 10,11-methylenedioxy group on the A ring results in hydrophobic compounds with substantially greater potencies.[16] In addition, several types of substitutions at the 7 position result in 'alkylating' CPT analogues that form irreversible complexes with topo I and DNA.[18,19]

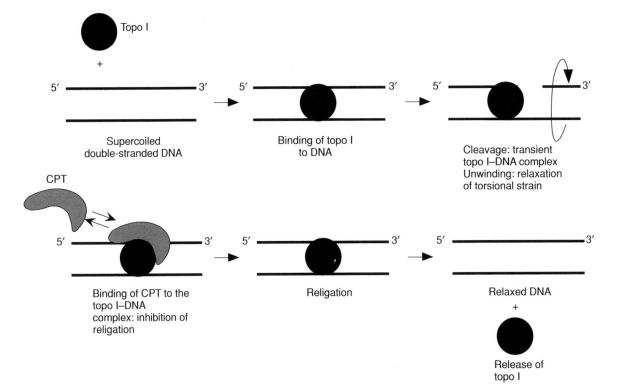

Figure 12.3. The effect of CPT and its derivatives on the catalytic cycle of topo I.

Mechanism of action

The cellular target of topotecan, irinotecan, and other CPT derivatives is DNA topo I, a ubiquitous nuclear enzyme that is primarily localized in the nucleolus.[20] Topo I catalyses the relaxation of supercoiled DNA during the processes of replication, transcription, and recombination.[21] During the catalytic cycle, topo I binds to double-stranded DNA, and cleaves and religates one strand of the duplex DNA (Fig.12.3).[21,22] This involves a nucleophilic attack by a catalytic tyrosine residue on the phosphodiester backbone of DNA which results in the formation of a covalent bond between topo I and the 3' end of the broken strand and a short-lived topo I–DNA complex.[21-24]

Topotecan, irinotecan, and other CPT derivatives cause DNA damage by interfering with the catalytic cycle of topo I. These agents reversibly bind to the topo I–DNA complex, inhibit the religation step, and thus stabilize the topo I–DNA complex and prolong the duration of the single-strand intermediates (Fig. 12.3).[12,25-29] *In vitro*, drug-induced increases in the number of topo I–DNA complexes have been correlated with the cytotoxicity of CPT and derivatives.[12,30-32] An increase in the number of these complexes has been measured in peripheral blood mononuclear cells, gastric and lung adenocarcinomas, and normal tissue counterparts in patients receiving topotecan, which supports this mechanism of action *in vivo*.[33-35] However, the complexes are reversible and decrease rapidly following removal of the drug,[30,36] which suggests that steps subsequent to complex stabilization are also involved in cytotoxicity. It has been proposed that the single-strand DNA breaks are converted to double-strand breaks by collision of advancing replication forks with the topo I–DNA complex.[12,37] This model for the mechanism of action supports the selective toxicity of CPT and derivatives to cells in the S phase of the cell cycle.[12]

These agents may also have mechanisms of cytotoxicity that involve other phases of the cell cycle. For instance, CPT is active in tumours with relatively low S-phase fractions,[38,39] and *in vitro* cytotoxicity studies with CPT have not observed a correlation between the S-phase fraction of the cell population and cytotoxicity.[40-42] The nature of the S-phase-independent CPT-induced cytotoxicity is unknown, but it may be related to inhibition of transcription.[43,44] In addition, the composition of the extracellular matrix, which contains factors that affect cell adhesion, may play a role in the cytotoxicity of topotecan and other CPT derivatives.[45]

Mechanisms of resistance

Although little is known about the mechanisms of resistance to CPT and its derivatives in human tumours, possible cellular mechanisms of resistance which may have relevance in the clinical setting have been described.[12,46,47] These can be separated into factors that affect the stabilization of the topo I–DNA complex, and cellular alterations after DNA damage occurs. In the former category, decreased drug accumulation, decreased activation of the prodrug, decreased cellular content and activity of topo I, and mutations of the topo I enzyme have the potential to alter the stabilization of topo I–DNA complexes.

The multidrug resistance (MDR) associated with P-glycoprotein (P-gp) is accompanied by a decrease in the intracellular concentration and cytotoxicity of topotecan in cultured cells, although the degree to which MDR-associated resistance affects topotecan is much less than that for other high-affinity P-gp substrates.[12,48,49] Similarly, cells expressing high levels of P-gp confer low-level resistance to irinotecan, SN-38, and 9-AC.[12,48-50] Resistance to topotecan and SN-38 is also caused by reduced cellular accumulation that is to be mediated by a novel mechanism, possibly related to impaired energy-dependent uptake.[51,52] This mechanism is enhanced cellular efflux by the membrane band ABC transporter BCRP (ABCG2).[53-55]

Few of the CPT derivatives require metabolism to generate the topo I targeting moiety. Irinotecan is unique in that it is a relatively poor topo I inhibitor and requires metabolism to SN-38 by carboxylesterases for antitumour activity.[47,56,57] Reduced expression of these carboxylesterases may play a role in resistance to irinotecan. Indeed, decreased expression of carboxylesterase activity and reduced activation of irinotecan has been observed in cell lines selected for resistance to irinotecan,[47,58,59] and expression of a cDNA encoding a rabbit liver carboxylesterase in cultured cells dramatically increased the sensitivity of the cells to irinotecan.[60] Recently, human butyrylcholinesterase was identified as an enzyme that efficiently converts irinotecan to SN-38.[61] Future studies will determine whether differences in expression of this specific esterase in various tissues and tumour play a role in irinotecan resistance. Another mechanism of resistance to CPT-11 may involve increased inactivation of SN-38 by catabolism to SN-38 glucuronide.[62] 9-Nitro-CPT is partially metabolized *in vivo* to 9-amino-CPT which has activity as a topo I inhibitor.[63,64]

However, the relevance of this conversion step in resistance to 9-nitro-CPT is unknown.

Several other well-recognized mechanisms of resistance have been characterized in cell lines that were selected for resistance in the presence of drug. Reduced cellular amount and activity of topo I enzyme have been shown to confer low-level resistance to CPT and derivatives.[12,47] In contrast, mutations in topo I enzyme confer high-level resistance to CPT without affecting protein levels or catalytic activity.[12,65–70] These mutations are located in the core and C-terminal domains of topo I and presumably identify residues important for drug binding.[24,71] However, studies have now demonstrated that, in cell lines exhibiting natural differences in sensitivity to the CPT, topo I protein content, enzyme activity, and the number DNA-topo I complexes do not consistently predict cytotoxicity to the CPT analogues.[41,42,44]

Another possible cellular determinant of drug sensitivity to the CPT analogues involves the rate and extent of drug-induced subcellular redistribution of topo I. Treatment of cultured cells with topotecan induces the relocalization of topo I from the nucleolus to the nucleoplasm and cytoplasm,[67,68,72–74] and much higher topotecan concentrations are required to induce the redistribution of topo I in resistant cells compared with the parent cell line.[69] In cells with inherent sensitivity to topotecan, the maximum redistribution of topo I occurs within 30–60 min,[72] whereas the maximum number of topo I–DNA complexes occurs 5–15 min after treatment with a similar concentration of topotecan in the same cell line.[70] Combined, these results indicate that the decline in the number of complexes seen after 15 min may be due to redistribution of this enzyme away from optimal sites for DNA binding. Differences in the rate and amount of drug-induced topo I redistribution within the tumour may be a mechanism of resistance for these agents when they are given on virtually all routes and schedules of administration including daily short infusions, daily oral doses, or weekly or chronic administration schedules.

Several mechanisms of resistance occurring downstream from CPT-induced stabilization of topo I–DNA complexes have been described *in vitro*. These include decreased CPT-induced DNA double-strand breaks,[73] misrepair of damaged replicons,[44] alterations in DNA damage checkpoints,[44,75–77] and altered apoptotic pathways.[74,78]

To examine factors that may affect sensitivity to CPT and its derivatives in the clinical setting, several investigators have measured topo I content and topo I–DNA complexes in tumour specimens from patients receiving topotecan in conjunction with phase I and II trials. Measurement of baseline topo I in marrow leukaemic blasts revealed substantial inter-individual variation in topo I content.[79,80] Similarly, measurement of topotecan-stabilized topo I–DNA complexes in circulating leukaemic cells at baseline,[81] and in gastric and lung adenocarcinoma tumour tissue during a 30 min infusion of topotecan,[35] has also shown wide variability in the number of complexes. Inter-individual variability in the amount of topo I content and topo I–DNA complexes might represent potential mechanisms for differential sensitivity to topotecan in patients receiving this drug, although correlations between these parameters and tumour response have not been observed, possibly due to the small patient numbers. Examination of these topo I parameters in larger clinical trials and the use of assays to detect topo I redistribution, apoptosis, and other potential markers of CPT sensitivity may identify mechanisms of resistance in the clinic.

Topoisomerase I targeting agents approved as cancer therapeutics

Topotecan

Topotecan was the first camptothecin analogue and topo I targeting agent that received regulatory approval. It was selected as the lead compound for development by SmithKline Beecham following extensive structure–function studies.[12,13,18] Topotecan was synthesized by the introduction of a basic side chain at the 9 position of the 10-hydroxycamptothecin ring (Fig. 12.1), which enabled topotecan to retain its water solubility in the lactone form.[12,18] In addition, topotecan was not a prodrug and demonstrated broad and superior antitumour activity to that of CPT in preclinical studies.[18] As predicted, neutropenia is the principal toxicity of topotecan in cancer patients.[12,18,82–84] Other infrequent and less severe toxicities of topotecan at clinically relevant doses include thrombocytopenia, anaemia, and alopecia. Severe nausea, vomiting, and diarrhoea are uncommon at clinically relevant doses. Although a broad range of dosing schedules have been evaluated, topotecan has primarily been developed and approved for use as a 30 min infusion administered daily for 5 days every 3 weeks. However, the relative merits of alternate dosing schedules have not been evaluated prospectively in randomized trials.

Initially, topotecan received regulatory approval for use in patients with recurrent or refractory ovarian epithelial malignancies, and more recently it was approved for patients with recurrent or refractory small-cell lung carcinoma. Notable preliminary results have also been observed in patients with non-small-cell lung carcinoma, myelodysplastic syndrome, acute non-lymphocytic leukaemia, non-Hodgkin's lymphoma, and other malignancies, and clinical evaluations are ongoing to define the role of topotecan in these tumour types.[79,80]

Clinical pharmacology

Pharmacokinetics

The intravenous route has been the most common for the administration of topotecan. However, there is increasing interest and experience with oral formulations; this has largely been due to the results of preclinical studies indicating that protracted drug exposure produces greater topo I–DNA complex formation and superior cytotoxicity as well as preliminary antitumour activity associated with prolonged intravenous administration schedules in clinical studies.[34,79,80,85]

Like CPT, the topotecan lactone is unstable in aqueous solutions and physiological conditions, and undergoes reversible pH-dependent hydrolysis to the open-ring carboxylate.[79,80,86,87] The half-life of this reaction in human plasma (pH 7.4 and 37°C) is 50–70 min.[79,88] Because of the instability of the topotecan lactone, plasma samples must be processed rapidly prior to assay. The most common assays are high-performance liquid chromatography (HPLC) methods that enable detection of both the parent compound (topotecan lactone) and total drug (topotecan lactone plus carboxylate species).[84]

Following ether intravenous or oral administration, the lactone ring undergoes relatively rapid hydrolysis to generate the carboxylate form; however, characterizing the pharmacokinetics of topotecan is complicated by hydrolysis of the lactone ring even prior to intravenous administration.[89] The extent of this reaction is dependent on the pH of the infusate. For example, intravenous preparations of topotecan in dextrose 5% (pH 4.5) result in hydrolysis of as much as 16% of the drug, with a half-life of 30 min, and an even greater extent of hydrolysis may occur when topotecan is administered in normal saline which has a higher pH than dextrose.

Table 12.1 displays the principal pharmacokinetic parameters that have been reported with topotecan administered as a 30 min intravenous infusion. Less than 1 h after the start of the infusion, the carboxylate constitutes the majority of circulating drug in plasma, and it predominates thereafter. Following intravenous administration, the pharmacokinetic behaviour of topotecan appears linear at dosages ranging from 0.5 to 22.5 mg/m^2/day.[85–90] The ratio of the area under the concentration–time curve (AUC) for the topotecan lactone to that of total topotecan averages 28%.[85,90–92] The range of values for the AUC and other pertinent pharmacokinetic parameters for both the topotecan lactone and total topotecan is large in individual patients treated at the same dose level.[85–88,93]

Topotecan lactone plasma concentration data have generally been described using a linear two-compartment pharmacokinetic model.[85–89,94] The lactone has a short terminal phase half-life, averaging 2.5 h (range, 1.7–3.4), whereas the mean half-life for total drug is 3.6 h (range 2.9–4.3).[85–87,89] The mean clearance of the topotecan lactone is 77.3 ± 53.7 l/h/m^2, while the clearance for total topotecan averages 19.3 ± 10.8 l/h/m^2. Studies comparing pharmacokinetic parameters over 5 days of intravenous dosing have not demonstrated changes in drug clearance during this period.[88,89] In general, the pharmacokinetics of topotecan in children and adults are similar, with overlapping values reported for terminal half-lives, clearance, and steady-state volume of distribution (V_{ss}) at all dose levels and schedules evaluated to date.[95–99]

Absorption: oral and intraperitoneal administration

Several oral formulations of topotecan have also been evaluated on daily oral dosing schedules ranging from

Table 12.1   Pharmacokinetic parameters for topotecan[85,90]

	Terminal half-life (h)	Clearance (l/h/m^2)	V_{ss} (l/m^2)	Urinary excretion (%)	Ratio of AUC lactone to AUC total (%)
Topotecan lactone	2.5 ± 0.9	77.3 ± 53.7	76.3 ± 77.0	–	28.1 ± 8.5
Topotecan total	3.6 ± 0.7	19.3 ± 10.8	50.6 ± 32.5	36.3± 5.5	–

Data are mean values ± standard deviation from referenced studies of topotecan administered as a 30 min intravenous infusion.

5 to 21 consecutive days since the MTD was demonstrated to be no greater than 1.7-fold that of parenteral administration in preclinical studies in mice.[100–104] The bioavailability of oral topotecan has been reported to range from 32% to 44%.[96,97] Plasma concentrations peak approximately 45 min after oral administration. The preliminary results of clinical studies have demonstrated clinical activity with oral topotecan comparable to that of parenteral administration.[100]

The impressive clinical antitumour activity of topotecan in patients with recurrent and refractory ovarian cancer also served as the impetus to evaluate the feasibility of administering topotecan directly into the intraperitoneal cavity.[105,106] In phase I studies evaluating intraperitoneal administration of topotecan, minimal local toxicity has been reported and extremely high intracavitary topotecan concentrations with biologically-relevant plasma concentrations have been achieved.

Protein binding

The topotecan lactone distributes widely, with V_{ss} values averaging 76.3 ± 77.0 l/m^2, whereas the mean V_{ss} for total drug is 50.6 ± 77.0 l/m^2.[85–87,89] Higher values for V_{ss} have been reported in studies using topotecan at higher doses ranging from 4.2 to 10.5 mg/m^2/day.[89,107] The plasma protein binding of topotecan is relatively low, with values of <20% to 35% reported.[108] Both the lactone and carboxylate species associate well with serum albumin. In contrast with CPT, in which there is preferential binding of the CPT carboxylate to human serum albumin which may shift the equilibrium towards lactone ring opening, there does not seem to be preferential binding of the topotecan carboxylate form to human serum albumin.[104,109] *In vitro* studies with MCF-7 and HL-60 human tumour cell lines demonstrated that there is no difference in the cytotoxic activity of topotecan in the presence or absence of human serum albumin, further supporting the notion that the low protein binding of topotecan and the lack of differential protein binding between the carboxylate and lactone make it unlikely that albumin affects topotecan pharmacokinetics and pharmacodynamics in clinical situations.[104,105]

Cerebrospinal fluid penetration

In rhesus monkeys treated with intravenous topotecan, drug concentrations in cerebrospinal fluid (CSF) were approximately 32% of simultaneous plasma levels, and the clearance rates of drug from these compartments were similar.[110,111] Interestingly, the penetration of CPT into the CSF of primates was reported to be negligible, perhaps due to the higher protein binding of CPT relative to topotecan. A similar degree of topotecan penetration into the CSF has also been noted in children who received topotecan by 24 or 72 h continuous intravenous infusion.[95,107,112] The median percentages of plasma concentrations of the topotecan lactone and total drug in the CSF relative to plasma concentrations are 29% (range 10%–59%) and 50% (range 11%–97%), respectively. The penetration of drug into the CSF, which may approximate drug penetration into the central nervous system, might have many important ramifications with regard to treating patients with leukaemia, small-cell lung cancer, and other malignancies that frequently involve the central nervous system.

Metabolism

Topotecan undergoes negligible metabolism. A desmethyl metabolite has been identified in the urine and plasma of patients, but the maximal metabolite concentration is approximately 0.7% of the concentration of total topotecan.[113]

Elimination

The hydrolysis of the lactone is the dominant process with regard to the clearance of topotecan *in vivo*. Renal mechanisms also play a principal role in the elimination of topotecan. The percentage of an administered dose of topotecan that is excreted into the urine averages 30–70%.[85–90] Although the precise mechanism for the renal excretion of the lactone and carboxylate forms of TPT is not known, the carboxylate may undergo renal tubular secretion. This is based, in part, on the significant reduction in topotecan clearance and consequential increase in topotecan AUC when it is administered with probenecid, which is probably due to competitive inhibition of these agents for renal tubular secretion since both the topotecan carboxylate and probenicid are weak acids.[114] In a phase I study of topotecan given as a 30 min infusion daily for 5 days to patients with varying degrees of renal impairment, there were strong relationships between the clearance of both total topotecan and lactone with creatinine clearance (Spearman's rank correlation of 0.65 for both).[115] The systemic clearance of topotecan was significantly reduced, and dose-limiting toxicities were noted more frequently in patients with moderate renal dysfunction (creatinine clearance, 20–39 ml/min) than those with mild renal dysfunction (creatinine clearance, 40–59 ml/min) and normal renal function. Based on the results of the study, a starting topotecan dose of 0.75 mg/m²/day was recommended for patients with moderate renal dysfunction and 1.5 mg/m²/day for patients with creatinine clearances >39 ml/min. No dosing recommendations were made for patients with creatinine clearance <20 ml/min because of the lack of data for this group. These results suggest that patients with recurrent or refractory ovarian cancer may have an increased risk for developing toxicity on the basis of subclinical renal impairment due to prior treatment with platinum compounds, and this may not be appreciated by strictly utilizing the serum creatinine concentration alone to assess renal dysfunction.

Topotecan has been demonstrated to be concentrated in the bile, with biliary concentrations approximately 1.5-fold higher than simultaneous plasma concentrations.[86] However, a prospective phase I study of topotecan as a 30 min infusion every 3 weeks in patients with varying degrees of hepatic impairment indicated that its pharmacokinetic profile was not altered by liver dysfunction, and patients with hepatic dysfunction tolerated topotecan at doses up to 1.5 mg/m²/day, which was the recommended dose on this schedule.[111] Therefore dose modifications do not appear necessary for patients with hepatic dysfunction.

Pharmacokinetic drug interactions

There has been considerable interest in evaluating regimens of topotecan combined with platinating agents, alkylating agents, and radiation, since synergistic cytotoxic interactions have been consistently reported with such combinations in preclinical studies.[12] The results with alkylating and platinating agents, and possibly radiation, might reflect an effect of topo I directed drugs on the repair of DNA damage caused by these other cytotoxic modalities. Alternatively, the modalities might promote unscheduled DNA synthesis and thereby provide replication forks that can interact with topo I–DNA adducts. Based on preclinical evaluations demonstrating sequence-dependent antitumour activity between *topotecan and cisplatin*, with greater antitumour activity when treatment with cisplatin precedes that with topotecan, the potential for sequence-dependent drug interactions has been studied in phase I studies of cisplatin combined with topotecan administered either intravenously or orally.[116,117] In one study, alternating sequences of topotecan were administered to the same subjects.[112] Topotecan was administered as a 30 min infusion daily for 5 days, and cisplatin was given either before topotecan on day 1 or after topotecan on day 5. Paired analysis of the toxicological

data revealed that the sequence of cisplatin before topotecan induced significantly greater haematological toxicity than the alternate sequence. Although it was felt that these sequence-dependent toxicological differences were principally due to the mechanisms discussed above, the results of pharmacokinetic studies suggested that they were due in part to progressively lower topotecan clearance and greater drug exposure (AUC) from days 1 to 5 when treatment with cisplatin precedes topotecan, possibly because of the subclinical renal tubular toxicity induced by cisplatin.

There have also been reports of pharmacokinetic interactions between topotecan and other medications. Phenytoin has been demonstrated to increase topotecan clearance by 30%, largely due to the induction of topotecan metabolism to form *N*-desmethyl topotecan,[118] but drug interactions have not been consistently reported in large population studies.

Pharmacodynamics

The majority of pharmacodyamic studies performed in both adults and children have demonstrated that the relationship between topotecan (lactone and total) systemic exposure and haematological effects, particularly effects on neutrophils, are described by sigmoidal E_{max} (maximal response) models (Table 12.2).[76,77,85,89,91,92,94,98,119–122] Systemic exposure has been measured as either AUC or steady-state plasma concentrations (C_{ss}). Toxicity has been measured as either the percentage decrease in absolute neutrophil count (the dose-limiting toxicity for topotecan administered either intravenously or orally daily for 5 days) or as the NCI grade of mucositis (the dose-limiting toxicity of topotecan administered as a 120 h continuous infusion in patients with relapsed or refractory leukaemia).[76] A sigmoidal E_{max} model has been used to describe the relationship between topotecan C_{ss} and clinical antileukaemic effects in children with relapsed leukaemia.[92,95] In one study, the proportion of courses associated with an oncolytic effect (defined as a reduction of >75% in circulating blast count or a complete or partial response) increased as C_{ss} increased, albeit at concentrations below those associated with severe toxicity.[95] These results suggest that pharmacological monitoring of topotecan may provide benefit in improving tumour response and ecreasing toxicity.

Thus far, investigations of the pharmacodynamic behaviour have been limited to phase I studies with small numbers of patients. Recently, limited-sampling models for the AUC of the lactone and total forms

Table 12.2   Pharmacodynamics of topotecan in adult and pediatric patients with solid tumours and leukaemia

Regimen	Pharmacokinetic parameters	Drug effect measured	Pharmacodynamic relationship
Adult patients			
30 min infusion daily × 5 days[85,116]	Dose, AUC (total)	% decrease in ANC	Sigmoidal E_{max} model
	Dose, AUC (total), time lactone >10 nM	% decrease in ANC	Sigmoidal E_{max} model
24 h continuous infusion weekly[117]	AUC (lactone and total), C_{ss} (lactone and total), dose	% decrease in ANC	Sigmoidal E_{max} model
24 h continuous infusion[118]	AUC (total), C_{ss} (total),	% decrease in ANC	Sigmoidal E_{max} model
120 h continuous infusion (leukaemia)[76]	Dose, C_{ss} (total)	NCI grade of mucositis	Higher dose and AUC significantly associated with higher-grade toxicity
Oral twice daily for 21 days[98]	AUC (total)	% decrease in WBC	Sigmoidal E_{max} model
Pediatric patients			
30 min infusion daily × 5 days[94]	AUC (lactone and total)	% decrease in ANC	Sigmoidal E_{max} model
72 h continuous infusion[92]	AUC (lactone and total), C_{ss} (lactone and total)	% decrease in ANC and platelets	Sigmoidal E_{max} model
120 h continuous infusion[95]	C_{ss} (lactone)	NCI grade of mucositis and oncolytic response	Sigmoidal E_{max} model

ANC, absolute neutrophil count; AUC, area under plasma concentration–time curve; C_{ss}, plasma concentration at steady state; E_{max}, maximal effect model; WBC, white blood cells.

have been developed.[123,124] These models, which require as few as one or two plasma samples, make it feasible to evaluate the relationship between topotecan exposure and tumour response, survival, and toxicity in multi-institutional studies.

Irinotecan (CPT-11)

Irinotecan (CPT-11, Camptosar) is a water-soluble CPT analogue that was synthesized by Yokokura and coworkers at Yakult Central Institute, Tokyo, Japan. Irinotecan (7-ethyl-10-[4-[1-piperidino]-1-piperidino] carbonyloxyCPT; molecular weight 587 Da) was synthesized by the introduction of an ethyl group at the 7 position of CPT and a hydroxyl group at the 10 position, forming an ester linkage with a biperidon carbonyl group. Unlike CPT and topotecan, irinotecan has little inherent antitumour activity *in vitro*.[53,121] Rather, it is a prodrug that undergoes de-esterification *in vivo* to yield SN-38 (7-ethyl-10-hydroxyCPT), a water-insoluble metabolite that is 1000-fold more potent than the parent compound *in vitro*.[53,125] Irinotecan became available commercially in Japan in 1994 for treating patients with non-small-cell and small-cell lung, cervi-

cal, and ovarian carcinomas. The agent subsequently received regulatory approval in the United States and elsewhere for patients with metastatic colorectal carcinoma who previously received 5-fluorouracil.

Irinotecan is administered over 30–90 min every 3 weeks, weekly for 4 weeks every 6 weeks, weekly without treatment breaks, or every other week. In North America, irinotecan was granted regulatory approval as a 90 min infusion weekly for 4 weeks every 6 weeks.[126–136] In addition, an oral formulation of irinotecan is currently in clinical development. Neutropenia and diarrhoea are the most common toxicities of irinotecan on these administration schedules. Thrombocytopenia, alopecia, nausea, vomiting, anaemia, fatigue, mucositis, and elevations of hepatic transaminases are less common. Pulmonary toxicity has also been described as a rare complication, particularly in patients with non-small-cell lung cancer.[132,137] Diarrhoea, which occurs in two forms, is more common with repeated dosing or on weekly schedules. The less common form of diarrhoea occurs in the peritreatment period and is dose related. This acute form of diarrhoea is usually associated with abdominal cramping, vomiting, flushing, visual (accommodation) disturbances, lacrimation, salivation, bradycardia, and diaphoresis. These effects appear to be due to the cholinergic actions of irinotecan, which is a non-competitive inhibitor of acetocholinesterase *in vitro*, and can be successfully managed with atropine.[115,138] The more common form, a delayed-onset diarrhoea, usually occurs after the second or third dose of irinotecan, particularly on weekly treatment schedules, and appears to be caused by a secretory mechanism with an exudative component.[139] The diarrhoea can be managed successfully by promptly initiating treatment with loperamide 4 mg initially followed by 2 mg every 2 h (4 mg every 4 h during the night) until it has resolved for at least 12 h.[135]

Clinical pharmacology

Pharmacokinetics

The lactone and carboxylate (open-ring) forms of irinotecan and SN-38 have been measured in plasma using HPLC methods with fluorimetric detection.[136] Following intravenous administration, both the closed-ring lactone and the open-ring carboxylate forms of irinotecan and SN-38 circulate in plasma.[126,128,140,141] However, approximately 1 h after drug treatment, SN-38 concentrations are about 50–100 times lower than irinotecan concentrations. The overall ratio of SN-38 AUC to irinotecan AUC has been reported to be approximately 4%.[142] Irinotecan plasma concentrations are maximal immediately after the end of the drug infusion, whereas SN-38 plasma concentrations peak 2.2 ± 0.1 h (range 1.6–2.8 h) later.[128] Despite significant inter-patient variability, irinotecan plasma concentrations and AUC increase proportionally with increasing dose. However, analyses of the relationships between irinotecan and SN-38 pharmacokinetics have been somewhat conflicting. The results of some investigations have suggested that both SN-38 plasma concentrations and AUC plateau with increasing irinotecan dose, possibly due to saturation of the carboxylesterase

converting enzymes that are responsible for converting irinotecan to SN-38, whereas other results have demonstrated proportionality between SN-38 concentrations and irinotecan dose, albeit with inter-patient variability that might be interpreted as 'plateauing'.[124–127,130] In any case, these inconsistencies, as well as significant inter-individual variability, may result from many factors, including variability in the formation of SN-38 from irinotecan, variable rates of elimination by glucuronic acid conjugation and other modes of drug disposition, and significant differences in the clearance of irinotecan prior to metabolism.

Most investigators have characterized the concentrations of both irinotecan and SN-38 in plasma using either two- or three-compartment pharmacokinetic models.[122–128,130,131,138,143] In comparison with topotecan and other CPT analogues, SN-38 persists for long periods in plasma, with a terminal half-life of approximately 14.7 h for total drug and 8.7 h for the active lactone (Table 12.3).[124–128] The AUC of the irinotecan lactone represents approximately 38.2% of the total irinotecan AUC, and this value has been reported to be even greater (53.2%) for the SN-38 lactone.[124–128] Similar to topotecan, the V_{ss} of irinotecan is large, suggesting significant tissue binding; V_{ss} has been estimated to be approximately 263 ± 100 l/m² and 145 ± 4 l/m² for the lactone and total drug, respectively.[124–128] The pharmacokinetic behaviour of irinotecan in children appears to be similar.[144,145]

Protein binding

Plasma protein binding of irinotecan and SN-38, as determined from studies in which the agents were added to human plasma, is 30–43% and 92–96%, respectively.[146–148] Serum albumin was the major protein to which irinotecan (25–32%) and SN-38 (88–94%) are bound. Human serum albumin also affects the kinetics of lactone ring opening. The lactone form of SN-38 is preferentially stabilized by human

Table 12.3   Pharmacokinetic parameters for irinotecan and SN-38[124-126,128]

	Terminal half-life (h)	Clearance (l/h/m²)	V_{ss} (l/m²)	Urinary excretion (%)	Ratio of AUC lactone to AUC total (%)
Irinotecan lactone	7.0 ± 2.4	46.0 ± 7.3	76.3 ± 77.0	–	38.2 ± 5.2
Irinotecan total	10.5 ± 9.3	17.5 ± 3.2	145 ± 4	22.1 ± 13.0	–
SN-38 lactone	8.7 ± 4.0	–	–		53.2 ± 9.8
SN-38 total	14.7 ± 10.2	–	–	0.26 ± 0.19	

Data are mean values ± standard deviation from referenced studies of irinotecan.

serum albumin, and therefore albumin shifts the equilibrium between the lactone and carboxylate towards the formation of the lactone, in contrast with topotecan and CPT. In the absence and presence of human serum albumin, the half-lives for hydrolysis of the lactone forms were 25.6 min and 33.8 min, respectively, for irinotecan, and 20.9 and 35.9 min, respectively, for SN-38.[143] The importance of these findings is illustrated by the results of cytotoxicity studies involving MCF-7 and HL-60 cell lines, in which the IC_{50} of SN-38 increased 176-fold and 267-fold, respectively, in the presence of 50 mg/ml of human serum albumin.[105,143,144] These results also suggest that human serum albumin concentrations in plasma may be another important clinical variable with regard to drug toxicity and disease outcome.

Metabolism

CPT-11 is converted to SN-38 by carboxylesterases, ubiquitous enzymes located in the serum, liver, small intestine, and other tissues.[149–153] Another pathway of irinotecan metabolism is by cytochrome P450 3A-mediated oxidation of the terminal piperdine group on C-10, which results in the formation of several compounds (e.g. APC) that are much less active than SN-38.[154,155] The structures of these metabolites have recently been elucidated.[156,157]

SN-38 also undergoes glucuronidation to an inactive β-glucuronide derivative, which is mediated by uridine-diphosphate glucuronosyltransferase 1A1 (UGT 1A1).[158–160] The SN-38 glucuronide can potentially be converted back to SN-38 by β-glucuronidase activity mediated by intestinal microflora.[157,158] The actions of faecal β-glucuronidase may explain the absence of SN-38 glucuronide in the stool of some patients, and provide a rationale to concurrently treat patients with selective antibiotics to decrease the propensity for severe diarrhoea.[161,162]

Preliminary data suggest that genetic pleomorphisms in the conjugating enzymes may affect glucuronidation of SN-38 in patients.[163] Although pharmacogenomic factors have been proposed to account for the significant inter-individual variability in the metabolism of irinotecan and SN-38, the clearance of irinotecan and its metabolites did not differ significantly with gender or race in one prospective phase I study.[164,165]

The variability of the pharmacokinetics of CPT-11 and SN-38 is probably due to extensive inter-patient differences in conversion of CPT-11 to SN-38, metabolism of CPT-11 to APC, and glucuronidation of SN-38. Ratios of the AUCs of SN-38, SN-38 glucuronide, and APC to parent compound were observed to vary more

than 10-fold in patients enrolled in phase I and II trials.[166] In addition, a 13-fold range in the rate of SN-38 glucuronide formation by human hepatic microsomes has been noted.[167]

Elimination

The elimination of irinotecan occurs principally by urinary excretion, biliary excretion, and conversion to SN-38. Approximately 22% of the total dose of irinotecan is excreted unchanged in the urine, whereas less than 1% is excreted as SN-38.[124–128] Glucuronidation and biliary excretion appear to be the principal mechanisms of elimination for SN-38.[154–156,168]

Drug interactions

Irinotecan has been evaluated in combination with other chemotherapy agents. Agents that have shown synergism and lack of cross-resistance, as well as those selected due to the antitumour spectrum of irinotecan, have been selected. To date, pharmacokinetic interactions have been noted between irinotecan and both cisplatin and 5-fluorouracil. In a combination study of irinotecan and cisplatin using a fixed dose of cisplatin (60 mg/m^2), the pharmacokinetics of irinotecan were reported to be altered by cisplatin.[169] Specifically, the irinotecan C_{max} did not increase in a dose-proportional manner with increasing doses of irinotecan. In addition, there was a 2.19-fold increase in the C_{max} of SN-38 as the dose of irinotecan was increased 1.13-fold, along with a disproportionate increase in the AUC of SN-38. This drug interaction was confirmed in a larger population study of irinotecan and cisplatin.[170] Increasing the irinotecan dose from 80 to 90 mg/m^2 resulted in almost a doubling of the C_{max} and AUC of SN-38. The precise mechanism for this apparent interaction has not been determined.

The encouraging phase II results with irinotecan as a single agent in patients with colorectal carcinoma who have previously been treated with 5-fluorourail have resulted in a series of phase I evaluations of irinotecan in combination with 5-fluorouracil on several administration schedules. In one Japanese study, when treatment with irinotecan 100–150 mg/m^2 was followed by a 7 day continuous intravenous infusion of 5-fluorouracil 400 mg/m^2, both toxicity and antitumour activity were much less than expected.[171] In addition, irinotecan concentrations in plasma were much higher than those achieved in previous studies, and SN-38 concentrations were much less, which led to the hypothesis that 5-fluorouracil or a metabolite may inhibit the converting activity of carboxylesterases. In contrast, the pharmacokinetics of 5-fluorouracil were not affected by irinotecan. However, these results were not conclusive because irinotecan and SN-38 pharmacokinetics were not directly compared in the same patients with and without 5-fluorouracil. Soon after this report, a well-designed and controlled phase I study of 5-fluorouracil, leucovorin, and irinotecan did not demonstrate pharmacokinetic interactions when the same individual patients were treated with various sequence iterations of these agents.[172] Interestingly, irinotecan administered prior to 5-fluorouracil has resulted in additive cytotoxicity *in vitro*, whereas simultaneous treatment has produced antagonism.[173,174]

Irinotecan pharmacokinetics did not seem to be altered by etoposide in a phase I and pharmacokinetic evaluation of the drug combination.[175] The increase in the principal pharmacodynamic determinant (if any), SN-38 AUC, was proportional to dose, although the half-lives of elimination of both irinotecan and SN-38 were somewhat larger than in comparable patients receiving the single agent alone.

In preclinical studies, pretreatment of rats with valproic acid, a potent inhibitor of the conjugating enzyme, resulted in 99% inhibition in the formation of SN-38 glucuronide, whereas inducing the enzyme with phenobarbitol resulted in a 1.7-fold increase in the AUC of SN-38 glucuronide.[176] In addition, preclinical studies indicate that treatment with cyclosporin A before irinotecan increases the AUCs of irinotecan, SN-38, and SN-38 glucuronide, possibly by reducing excretion of the drug and metabolites into bile.[177]

Pharmacodynamics

The pharmacodynamic relationships for irinotecan have not been clearly elucidated. A summary of phar-macodynamic relationships evaluated during early phase I studies is given in Table 12.4. With regard to toxicity, acute diarrhoea is most probably due to the anticholinesterase activity of the parent compound, whereas myelosuppression is related to the inhibitory effects of the SN-38 lactone on topo I in haematopoietic cells. Several investigators have demonstrated that SN-38 AUC correlates with myelosuppression, whereas others have found relationships between CPT-11 AUC and myelosuppression.[127,128,171] Similarly, findings have been inconsistent with regard to relationships between SN-38 AUC and diarrhoea.

The decreased ability to detoxify SN-38 by glucuronidation may be associated with an increased propensity to develop severe diarrhoea. A biliary index, which reflects the relative ratio of SN-38 to SN-38 glucuronide in the bile and intestines, has been correlated with the development of severe diarrhoea.[164] The biliary index is calculated as the product of the irinotecan AUC and the ratio of the SN-38 to SN-38 glucuronide AUC. In one report, nine patients with grade 3 and 4 diarrhoea had significantly higher biliary indices than 12 patients with grades 0–2 diarrhoea.[164] Such observations have also suggested that the therapeutic index of irinotecan might be increased by agents that could increase SN-38 glucuronidation.[160,173] Interestingly, the ability to conjugate bilirubin, which is also dependent on UGT 1A1 activity, has been demonstrated to correlate with the serum concentration of conjugated bilirubin and is inversely related to myelosuppression.[178]

9-Amino-20(S)-CPT and 9-nitro-20(S)-CPT

9-Amino-20(S)-CPT (9-AC), a CPT analogue with poor aqueous solubility possessing an amino group sub-

Table 12.4 Pharmacodynamics of irinotecan in adult patients with solid tumours

Reference	Correlation of diarrhoea with:		Correlation of neutropenia with:	
	AUC (irinotecan)	AUC (SN-38)	AUC (irinotecan)	AUC (SN-38)
Single dose				
127	Not reported	Not reported	Not reported	Not reported
134	Yes (up to grade 2)	Yes (up to grade 2)	Yes	Yes
132	No	No	No	No
Weekly				
128	No	No	No	No
131	Yes	Yes	Yes	Yes
130	Not reported	Not reported	Not reported	Trend
5 day continuous infusion				
129	Yes	No	No	Yes
135	Yes	No	No	No

stitution at the 9 position of the A ring (Fig.12.1), was initially developed by the National Cancer Institute because of its impressive activity in preclinical studies. When administered as a subcutaneous suspension twice weekly, 9-AC induced disease-free remissions in athymic mice bearing advanced-stage human colon HT-29 tumour xenografts.[39] In addition, 9-AC administered either subcutaneously or intramuscularly on the same schedule was effective against human tumour xenografts of malignant melanoma, infiltrating ductal carcinoma of the breast, non-small-cell lung cancer, and hepatic metastases of colorectal carcinoma.[179–181] The agent was also active against tumours with multidrug resistance. Pharmacokinetic studies in mice showed that subcutaneous treatment with the suspension formulation simulated infusional schedules and demonstrated optimal activity when concentrations of the lactone were maintained at or above 10 nM repeatedly for approximately 48 h with brief periods of recovery between treatment.[182] Additional studies revealed that antitumour activity was enhanced when the duration of drug exposure above a threshold lactone concentration is prolonged and when the interval between treatments is short.[178,183,184]

Initially, phase I studies of 9-AC, formulated in dimethylacetamide, polyethylene glycol 400, and phosphoric acid (DMA–PEG–PO$_4$) and administered as a continuous infusion for 72 h repeated every 2–3 weeks, demonstrated that neutropenia was the principal dose-limiting toxicity.[180,185] Thrombocytopenia and anaemia were also prominent in patients treated at higher dose levels, precluding significant dose escalation of 9-AC using haematopoietic colony-stimulating factors. Following these initial phase I studies, as well as broad phase II studies evaluating this cumbersome administration schedule, a colloidal dispersion formulation of 9-AC was developed in order to enhance solubility and allow the use of shorter administration schedules.[186,187]

The colloidal dispersion formulation of 9-AC was initially evaluated on 24- and 72-h continuous infusion schedules.[182,183] More recently, bolus infusion daily for 5 days and a protracted (up to 21 days) continuous infusion schedule have been evaluated.[188,189] Preliminary results of phase I and pharmacokinetic studies of 9-AC administered orally as a colloidal dispersion formulation have demonstrated poor bioavailability and saturable absorption. However, a PEG oral formulation has been reported to have suitable bioavailability without evidence of saturable absorption.[186,187] Bioavailability of 9-AC administered orally in PEG has averaged 48.6 ± 17.6% and the active lactone has

accounted for <10% of total drug at the terminal disposition phase.[190,191] Nonetheless, substantial interindividual variability in pharmacokinetics was observed.

Pharmacokinetic studies with both 9-AC formulations have demonstrated significant inter-patient variability; plasma concentration data have been well characterized by two-compartment pharmacokinetic models.[180–183] Mean pharmacokinetic parameter values for 9-AC lactone in the DMA–PEG–PO$_4$ formulation included a clearance and terminal half-life of 24.5 ± 7.3 l/h/m^2 and 11.1 ± 4.5 h for 9-AC lactone.[7] The value of V_{ss} for the 9-AC lactone averaged 195 ± 114 l/m^2. The 9-AC lactone was estimated to account for 8.7% of total 9-AC circulating in the plasma. In addition, urinary excretion averaged 32.1 ± 8.3% of the total administered drug, and the drug was also detected in ascitic fluid. The pharmacokinetic behaviour of 9-AC in the colloidal dispersion formulation was similar.[182,183] The clearance of the lactone averaged 18 l/h/m^2 (range 10–55.6 l/h/m^2) and the terminal half-life averaged 10.7 h (range 2.2–34.7 h).[182]

9-Nitro-20(S)-CPT (9-NC) (Fig. 12.1), a waterinsoluble topo I inhibitor with a nitro group in the 9 position and broad antitumour activity in preclinical models, is also undergoing clinical evaluation. In human tumour xenografts, the antitumour activity of 9-NC is superior to the activity of several water-soluble compounds, and daily intragastric administration yielded results which were similar to those produced by continuous infusion and clearly superior to intravenous administration as a bolus infusion.[39,40] Enteric absorption in mice was relatively high, with 60% of the drug in the lactone form. Pharmacological studies have demonstrated that 9-NC is partially metabolized *in vivo* to 9-AC.[60,61] In a phase I and pharmacokinetic study in patients with advanced solid malignancies, 9-NC was administered orally with escalating doses from 1.0 to 2.25 mg/m^2/day for 5 consecutive days every week. Neutropenia was the principal toxicity, but thrombocytopenia, diarrhoea, chemical cystitis, nausea, and vomiting were also common. The maximum tolerated dose was determined to be 1.5 mg/m^2/ day. Major responses were observed in patients with pancreatic, breast, ovarian, and haematological malignancies. In this study, gastrointestinal absorption was moderately rapid, with peak lactone concentrations reported at a median of 1 h (range 0.5–6 h), whereas peak total drug concentrations occurred at a median of 4 h (range 2–6 h). A second peak, which may have been due to enterohepatic recirculation, was observed 6–8 h after drug administration. The mean percentage of the AUC of the lactone form versus the AUC of total drug was $14.7\% \pm 14.3$.

Other topoisomerase I targeting CPT analogues in clinical development

The recognition of topo I as a novel subcellular target, along with the efficacy demonstrated for topotecan and irinotecan in several common malignancies, has resulted in broad efforts to identify other topo I targeting agents with broader antitumour spectra and greater therapeutic indices. These efforts can be classified into three principal categories: (i) water-soluble CPT derivatives; (ii) lipophilic CPT derivatives; (iii) topo I derivatives that are not structurally related to CPT.

Among the water-soluble CPT derivatives, GI147211 (GG211; Fig. 12.1) and DX8951f have received the most attention with regard to clinical developmental efforts. GI147211 is the first of a series of 7-substituted 10,11-ethylenedioxy-20(S)-CPT analogues to undergo clinical development based on its water solubility and on its potency and broad spectrum of antitumour activity and favourable toxicity profile compared with both topotecan and CPT in preclinical studies.[192–194] To date, the agent has principally undergone phase I and II evaluations as a 30 min infusion daily for 5 days every 3 weeks, and a 72 h continuous infusion schedule has also been evaluated.[195,196] Neutropenia precluded dose escalation of GI147211 on the 30 min infusion daily for 5 days schedule, and recommended phase II doses were 1.5 mg/m^2/day and 1.0 mg/m^2/day for minimally pretreated and heavily pretreated patients, respectively.[191] Drug disposition in blood was described by a three-compartment model, with renal elimination accounting for only 11% of drug disposition. Mean values for pertinent pharmacokinetic parameters for the lactone (total drug) included a systemic clearance of 71 ± 29 (21 ± 9.6) l/h/m^2, a terminal half-life of elimination of 7.5 ± 2.8 (9.6 ± 48) h, and a V_{ss} of 432 ± 311 (149 ± 77) l/m^2.[191] In this study, no relationships were observed between the pharmacological exposure of the drug and effects on blood cells. The hydrolysis kinetics of GI147211 revealed not only a shift of the drug to the inactive carboxylate form in human serum albumin, but also stabilization of the lactone in erythrocytes, perhaps accounting for the observed lactone-to-carboxylate AUC ratio of 0.27.

DX-8951f is a synthetic hexacyclic CPT analogue that is a more potent topo I inhibitor than SN-38, topotecan, or CPT *in vitro*.[193] *In vivo*, DX-8951f showed similar or better efficacy than CPT-11 in a number of human tumour xenografts.[197] In addition, DX-8951f does not appear to be a substrate for the P-gp multidrug transporter.[193] Although the feasibility of DX-8951f on a diverse range of schedules is being evaluated in phase I studies, the schedule consisting of DX-8951f administered for 30 min daily for 5 days every 3 weeks is the most likely candidate for further clinical development because of its schedule-dependent characteristics in preclinical studies (i.e. superiority of protracted exposure *in vitro* and frequent dosing schedules *in vivo*) and its tolerability in preliminary clinical studies.[198] To date, the pharmacokinetics appears linear and does not change over 5 days of daily dosing.[194] Mean pharmacokinetic parameters that have been preliminarily reported for total drug include a total body clearance rate of 1.28 ± 0.39 l/h/m^2, a half-life of elimination of 8.27 ± 2.92 h, and a V_{ss} of 12.28 ± 3.3 l/m^2.

Advances in pharmaceutical formulation technologies have made it feasible to formulate, administer, and evaluate a variety of water-insoluble CPT analogues. Some of the most interesting water-insoluble CPT analogues are those that have a 10,11-methylenedioxyCPT backbone.[16] In addition, several chemical modifications of CPT, including one that is derived by the attachment of polyethylene glycol groups to the 20(S) position of CPT through an ester linkage, produce water-soluble prodrugs that undergo de-esterification in plasma.[199] The use of liposomes is an alternative way of administering both water-soluble and insoluble CPT analogues.[200,201] Liposomes with an internal acidic pH can be specifically devised to maintain a higher proportion of the CPT analogue in the active lactone form. In addition, several topo I inhibitors that are not CPT analogues are currently under evaluation, including indol (intoplicine), quinoline (TAS-103), anthraquinone antibiotics (saintopin), and indolocarbazole derivatives (NB-506. ED749).[202–204] Of these agents, intoplicine, TAS-103 and saintopin are dual inhibitors of topo I and topo II.

References

1. Wall ME, Wani MC, Cook CE, Palmer KH, McPhail AT, Sim GA (1966) The isolation and structure of camptothecin, a novel alkaloidal leukemia and tumor inhibitor from *Camptotheca acuminata*. *J Am Chem Soc*, 88, 3888.
2. Horwitz SB, Chang CSCK, Grollman AP (1971) Studies on camptothecin: I. Effects on nucleic acid and protein synthesis. *Mol Pharmacol*, 33, 2834–6.

3. Kessel D (1972) Selective interruption of high molecular weight RNA synthesis in HeLa cells by camptothecin. *Nature New Biol*, 237, 144–6.

4. Horwitz SB, Horwitz MS (1973) Effects of camptothecin on the breakage and repair of DNA during the cell cycle. *Cancer Res*, 33, 2834–6.

5. Abelson HT, Penman S (1974) Selective interruption of RNA metabolism by chemotherapeutic agents. *Handb Exp Pharmacol*, 38, 571–81.

6. Gottlieb JA, Guarino AM, Call JB, Oliverio VT, Block JB (1970) Preliminary pharmacologic and clinical evaluation of camptothecin sodium. *Cancer Chemother Rep*, 54, 461–70.

7. Creaven PR, Allen LM, Muggia FM (1972) Plasma camptothecin (NSC-100880) levels during a 5-day course of treatment: relation to dose and toxicity. *Cancer Chemother Rep*, 56, 573–8.

8. Muggia FM, Creaven PJ, Hansen HH, Cohen MH, Selawry OS (1972) Phase I clinical trial of weekly and daily treatment with camptothecin (NSC-100880): correlation with preclinical studies. *Cancer Chemother Rep*, 56, 515–21.

9. Moertel CG, Schutt AJ, Reitemeir RJ, Hahn RG (1972) Phase II study of camptothecin (NSC-100880) in the treatment of advanced gastrointenstinal cancer. *Cancer Chemother Rep*, 56, 95–101.

10. Gottlieb JA, Luce JK (1972) Treatment of malignant melanoma with camptothecin (NSC-100880). *Cancer Chemother Rep*, 56, 103–5.

11. Creaven PR, Allen LM (1973) Renal clearance of camptothecin (NSC-100880): effect of urine volume. *Cancer Chemother Rep*, 56, 95–101.

12. Slichenmyer WJ, Rowinsky EK, Donehower RC, Kaufmann SH (1993) The current status of camptothecin analogues as antitumor agents. *J Natl Cancer Inst*, 85, 271–91.

13. Bedeschi A, Candiani I, Geroni C, Capolongo L (1997) Water-soluble camptothecin derivatives. *Drugs Future*, 22, 1259–66.

14. Hertzberg RP, Caranga JM, Hecht SM (1989) On the mechanism of topoisomerase I inhibition by camptothecin: Evidence for binding to an enzyme-DNA complex. *Biochemistry*, 28, 4629–38.

15. Hertzberg RP, Caranfa MJ, Holden KG, *et al.* (1989) Modification of the hydroxy lactone ring of camptothecin: inhibition of mammalian topoisomerase I and biological activity. *J Med Chem*, 32, 715–20.

16. Jaxel C, Kohn KW, Wani MC, Wall ME, Pommier Y (1989) Structure–activity study of the actions of camptothecin derivatives on mammalian topoisomerase I: evidence for a specific receptor site and a relation to antitumor activity. *Cancer Res*, 49, 1465–9.

17. Rowinsky EK (1998) Topotecan in combination with cisplatin in patients with previously untreated non-small cell lung cancer. A phase I study. *10th NCI-EORTC Symposium on New Drug Development, Amsterdam. Ann Oncol*, 9 (suppl. 2), 70.

18. Kingsbury WD, Boehm JC, Jakas DR, *et al.* (1991) Synthesis of water-soluble (aminoalkyl)camptothecin analogues: inhibition of topoisomerase I and antitumor activity. *J Med Chem*, 34, 98–107.

19. Pommier Y, Kohlhagen G, Kohn KW, Leteurtre F, Wani MC, Wall ME (1995) Interaction of an alkylating camptothecin derivative with a DNA base at topoisomerase I-DNA cleavage sites. *Proc Natl Acad Sci USA*, 92, 8861–5.

20. Baker SD, Wadkins RM, Stewart CF, Beck WT, Danks MK (1995) Cell cycle analysis of amount and distribution of nuclear DNA topoisomerase I as determined by fluorescence digital imaging microscopy. *Cytometry*, 19, 134–45.

21. Wang JC (1996) DNA topoisomerases. *Annu Rev Biochem*, 65, 635–92.

22. Stewart L, Redinbo MR, Qiu X, Hol WG, Champoux JJ (1998) A model for the mechanism of human topoisomerase I. *Science*, 279, 1534–41.

23. D'Arpa P, Machlin PS, Ratrie HD, Rothfield NF, Cleveland DW, Earnshaw WC (1988) cDNA cloning of human DNA topoisomerase I: catalytic activity of a 67.7-kDa carboxyl-terminal fragment. *Proc Natl Acad Sci USA*, 85, 2543–7.

24. Champoux JJ (1998) Domains of human topoisomerase I and associated functions. *Prog Nucleic Acid Res Mol Biol*, 60, 111–32.

25. Alsner J, Svejstrup JQ, Kjeldsen E, Sorensen BS, Westergaard O (1992) Identification of an N-terminal domain of eukaryotic DNA topoisomerase I dispensable for catalytic activity but essential for *in vivo* function. *J Biol Chem*, 267, 12408–11.

26. Bharti AK, Olson MO, Kufe DW, Rubin EH (1996) Identification of a nucleolin binding site in human topoisomerase I. *J Biol Chem*, 271, 1993–7.

27. Lynn RM, Bjornsti MA, Caron PR, Wang JC (1989) Peptide sequencing and site-directed mutagenesis identify tyrosine-727 as the active site tyrosine of *Saccharomyces cerevisiae* DNA topoisomerase I. *Proc Natl Acad Sci USA*, 86, 3559–63.

28. Eng WK, Pandit SD, Sternglanz R (1989) Mapping of the active site tyrosine of eukaryotic DNA topoisomerase I. *J Biol Chem*, 264, 13373–6.

29. Svejstrup JQ, Christiansen K, Gromova II, Andersen AH, Westergaard O (1991) New technique for uncoupling the cleavage and religation reactions of eukaryotic topoisomerase I. The mode of action of camptothecin at a specific recognition site. *J Mol Biol*, 222, 669–78.

30. Hsiang YH, Hertzberg R, Hecht S, Liu LF (1985) Camptothecin induces protein-linked DNA breaks via mammalian DNA topoisomerase I. *J Biol Chem*, 260, 14873–8.

31. Porter SE, Champoux JJ (1989) The basis for camptothecin enhancement of DNA breakage by eukaryotic topoisomerase I. *Nucleic Acids Res*, 17, 8521–32.

32. Hsiang YH, Liu LF (1988) Identification of mammalian DNA topoisomerase I as an intracellular target of the anticancer drug camptothecin. *Cancer Res*, 48, 1722–6.

33. Subramanian D, Kraut E, Staubus A, Young DC, Muller MT (1995) Analysis of topoisomerase I/DNA complexes in patients administered topotecan. *Cancer Res*, 55, 2097–103.

34. Hochster H, Liebes L, Speyer J, *et al.* (1997) Effect of prolonged topotecan infusion on topoisomerase I levels: A phase I and pharmacodynamic study. *Clin Cancer Res*, 3, 1245–52.

35. Liebes L, Potmesil M, Kim T, *et al.* (1998) Pharmacodynamics of topoisomerase I inhibition: western blot

determination of topoisomerase I and cleavable complex in patients with upper gastrointestinal malignancies treated with topotecan. *Clin Cancer Res*, **4**, 545–57.

36. Covey JM, Jaxel C, Kohn KW, Pommier Y (1989) Protein-linked DNA strand breaks induced in mammalian cells by camptothecin, an inhibitor of topoisomerase I. *Cancer Res*, **49**, 5016–22.

37. Hsiang YH, Lihou MG, Liu LF (1989) Arrest of replication forks by drug-stabilized topoisomerase I-DNA cleavable complexes as a mechanism of cell killing by camptothecin. *Cancer Res*, **49**, 5077–82.

38. D'Arpa P, Beardmore C, Liu LF (1990) Involvement of nucleic acid synthesis in cell killing mechanisms of topoisomerase poisons. *Cancer Res*, **50**, 6919–24.

39. Giovanella BC, Stehlin JS, Wall ME, *et al.* (1989) DNA topoisomerase I-targeted chemotherapy of human colon cancer in xenografts. *Science*, **246**, 1046–8.

40. Giovanella BC, Hinz HR, Kozielski AJ, Stehlin JS Jr, Silber R, Potmesil M (1991) Complete growth inhibition of human cancer xenografts in nude mice by treatment with 20-(S)-camptothecin. *Cancer Res*, **51**, 3052–5.

41. Goldwasser F, Bae I, Valenti M, Torres K, Pommier Y (1995) Topoisomerase I-related parameters and camptothecin activity in the colon carcinoma cell lines from the National Cancer Institute anticancer screen. *Cancer Res*, **55**, 2116–21.

42. Dubrez L, Goldwasser F, Genne P, Pommier Y, Solary E (1995) The role of cell cycle regulation and apoptosis triggering in determining the sensitivity of leukemic cells to topoisomerase I and II inhibitors. *Leukemia*, **9**, 1013–24.

43. Bendixen C, Thomsen B, Alsner J, Westergaard O (1990) Camptothecin-stabilized topoisomerase I–DNA adducts cause premature termination of transcription. *Biochemistry*, **29**, 5613–19.

44. Goldwasser F, Shimizu T, Jackman J, *et al.* (1996) Correlations between S and G2 arrest and the cytotoxicity of camptothecin in human colon carcinoma cells. *Cancer Res*, **56**, 4430–7.

45. Whitacre CM, Berger NA (1997) Factors affecting topotecan-induced programmed cell death: adhesion protects cells from apoptosis and impairs cleavage of poly(ADP-ribose) polymerase. *Cancer Res*, **57**, 2157–63.

46. Pommier Y, Leteurtre F, Fesen MR, *et al.* (1994) Cellular determinants of sensitivity and resistance to DNA topoisomerase inhibitors. *Cancer Invest*, **12**, 530–42.

47. Rivory LP, Robert J (1995) Molecular, cellular, and clinical aspects of the pharmacology of 20(S)camptothecin and its derivatives. *Pharmacol Ther*, **68**, 269–96.

48. Chen AY, Yu C, Potmesil M, Wall ME, Wani MC, Liu LF (1991) Camptothecin overcomes MDR1-mediated resistance in human KB carcinoma cells. *Cancer Res*, **51**, 6039–44.

49. Hendricks CB, Rowinsky EK, Grochow LB, Donehower R, Kaufmann SH (1992) Effect of P-glycoprotein on the accumulation and cytotoxicity of topotecan (SK&F 104864), a new camptothecin analogue. *Cancer Res*, **52**, 2268–78.

50. Jansen WJ, Hulscher TM (1998) CPT-11 sensitivity in relation to the expression of P170-glycoprotein and multidrug resistance-associated protein. *Br J Cancer*, **77**, 359–65.

51. Yang CJ, Horton JK, Cowan KH, Schneider E (1995) Cross-resistance to camptothecin analogues in a mitoxantrone-resistant human breast carcinoma cell line is not due to DNA topoisomerase I alterations. *Cancer Res*, **55**, 4004–9.

52. Ma J, Maliepaard M, Nooter K, *et al.* (1998) Reduced cellular accumulation of topotecan: a novel mechanism of resistance in a human ovarian cancer cell line. *Br J Cancer*, **77**, 1645–52.

53. Maliepaard M, van Gastelen MA, Tohgo A, *et al.* (2001) Circumvention of breast cancer resistance protein (BCRP)-mediated resistance to camptothecins *in vitro* using non-substrate drugs or the BCRP inhibitor GF120918. *Clin Cancer Res*, **7**, 935–41.

54. Maliepaard M, Scheffer GL, Faneyte IF, *et al.* (2001) Subcellular localization and distribution of the breast cancer resistance protein transporter in normal human tissue. *Cancer Res*, **61**, 3458–64.

55. Schellens JH, Maliepaard M, Scheper RJ, *et al.* (2000) Transport of topoisomerase I inhibitors by the breast cancer resistance protein. Potential clinical implications. *Ann NY Acad Sci*, **922**, 188–94.

56. Kawato Y, Aonuma M, Hirota Y, Kuga H, Sato K (1991) Intracellular roles of SN-38, a metabolite of the camptothecin derivative CPT-11, in the antitumor effect of CPT-11. *Cancer Res*, **51**, 4187–91.

57. Tanizawa A, Fujimori A, Fujimori Y, Pommier Y (1994) Comparison of topoisomerase I inhibition, DNA damage, and cytotoxicity of camptothecin derivatives presently in clinical trials. *J Natl Cancer Inst*, **86**, 836–42.

58. Kanzawa F, Sugimoto Y, Minato K, *et al.* (1990) Establishment of a camptothecin analogue (CPT-11)-resistant cell line of human non-small cell lung cancer: characterization and mechanism of resistance. *Cancer Res*, **50**, 5919–24.

59. Niimi S, Nakagawa K, Sugimoto Y, *et al.* (1992) Mechanism of cross-resistance to a camptothecin analogue (CPT-11) in a human ovarian cancer cell line selected by cisplatin. *Cancer Res*, **52**, 328–33.

60. Danks MK, Morton CL, Pawlik CA, Potter PM (1998) Overexpression of a rabbit liver carboxylesterase sensitizes human tumor cells to CPT-11. *Cancer Res*, **58**, 20–2.

61. Morton CL, Wadkins RW, Danks MK, Potter PM (1999) The anticancer prodrug CPT-11 is a potent inhibitor of acetylcholinesterase but is rapidly catalyzed to SN-38 by butyrylcholinesterase. *Cancer Res*, **59**, 1458–63.

62. Takahashi R, Fujiwara Y, Yamakido M, Katoh O, Watanabe H, Mackenzie PI (1998) The role of glucuronidation in 7-ethyl-10-hydroxycamptothecin resistance *in vitro*. *Jpn J Cancer Res*, **88**, 1211–17.

63. Hinz HR, Harris NJ, Natelson EA, Giovanella BC (1994) Pharmacokinetics of the *in vivo* and *in vitro* conversion of 9-nitro-20(S)-camptothecin to 9-amino-20(S)-camptothecin in humans, dogs, and mice. *Cancer Res*, **54**, 3096–100.

64. Pantazis P, Harris N, Mendoza J, Giovanella B (1994) Conversion of 9-nitro-camptothecin to 9-amino-camptothecin by human blood cells *in vitro*. *Eur J Haematol*, 53, 246–8.

65. Benedetti P, Fiorani P, Capuani L, Wang JC (1993) Camptothecin resistance from a single mutation changing glycine 363 of human DNA topoisomerase I to cysteine. *Cancer Res*, 53, 4343–8.

66. Knab AM, Fertala J, Bjornsti MA (1993) Mechanisms of camptothecin resistance in yeast DNA topoisomerase I mutants. *J Biol Chem*, 268, 22322–30.

67. Tanizawa A, Beitrand R, Kohlhagen G, Tabuchi A, Jenkins J, Pommier Y (1993) Cloning of Chinese hamster DNA topoisomerase I cDNA and identification of a single point mutation responsible for camptothecin resistance. *J Biol Chem*, 268, 25463–8.

68. Rubin E, Pantazis P, Bharti A, Toppmeyer D, Giovanella B, Kufe D (1994) Identification of a mutant human topoisomerase I with intact catalytic activity and resistance to 9-nitro-camptothecin. *J Biol Chem*, 269, 2433–9.

69. Wang LF, Ting CY, Lo CK, *et al.* (1997) Identification of mutations at DNA topoisomerase I responsible for camptothecin resistance. *Cancer Res*, 57, 1516–22.

70. Li XG, Haluska P Jr, Hsiang YH, *et al.* (1997) Involvement of amino acids 361 to 364 of human topoisomerase I in camptothecin resistance and enzyme catalysis. *Biochem Pharmacol*, 53, 1019–27.

71. Redinbo MR, Stewart L, Kuhn P, Champoux JJ, Hol WGJ (1998) Crystal structures of human topoisomerase I in covalent and noncovalent complexes with DNA. *Science*, 279, 1504–13.

72. Buckwalter CA, Lin AH, Tanizawa A, Pommier YG, Cheng YC, Kaufmann SH (1996) RNA synthesis inhibitors alter the subnuclear distribution of DNA topoisomerase I. *Cancer Res*, 56, 1674–81.

73. Danks MK, Garrett KE, Marion RC, Whipple DO (1996) Subcellular redistribution of DNA topoisomerase I in anaplastic astrocytoma cells treated with topotecan. *Cancer Res*, 56, 1664–73.

74. Wadkins RM, Danks MK, Horowitz L, Baker SD (1998) Characterization of topotecan-mediated redistribution of DNA topoisomerase I by digital imaging microscopy. *Exp Cell Res*, 241, 332–9.

75. Baker SD, Wall ME, Wani MC, Wadkins RM (1998) Correlation of structural composition of camptothecin (CPT) analogs and their ability to affect subcellular distribution of topoisomerse I (topo I). *Proc Am Assoc Cancer Res*, 39, 421.

76. Sorensen M, Sehested M, Christensen IJ, Larsen JK, Jensen PB (1998) Low-level resistance to camptothecin in a human small-cell lung cancer cell line without reduction in DNA topoisomerase I or drug-induced cleavable complex formation. *Br J Cancer*, 77, 2152–61.

77. Caserini C, Pratesi G, Tortoreto M, *et al.* (1997) Apoptosis as a determinant of tumor sensitivity to topotecan in human ovarian tumors: preclinical *in vitro*/invivo studies. *Clin Cancer Res*, 3, 955–61.

78. Sane AT, Bertrand R (1998) Distinct steps in DNA fragmentation pathway during camptothecin-induced apoptosis involved caspase-, benzyloxycarbonyl- and

N-tosyl-L-phenylalanylchloromethyl ketone-sensitive activities. *Cancer Res*, 58, 3066–72.

79. Rowinsky EK, Adjei A, Donehower RC, *et al.* (1994) Phase I and pharmacodynamic study of the topoisomerase I-inhibitor topotecan in patients with refractory acute leukemia. *J Clin Oncol*, 12, 2193–203.

80. Rowinsky EK, Kaufmann SH, Baker SD, *et al.* (1996) A phase I and pharmacological study of topotecan infused over 30 minutes for five days in patients with refractory acute leukemia. *Clin Cancer Res*, 2, 1921–30.

81. Kantarjian HM, Beran M, Ellis A, *et al.* (1993) Phase I study of topotecan, a new topoisomerase I inhibitor, in patients with refractory or relapsed acute leukemia. *Blood*, 81, 1146–51.

82. Takimoto CH, Arbuck SG (1997) Clinical status and optimal use of topotecan. *Oncology*, 11, 1635–46.

83. Takimoto CH, Kieffer LV, Kieffer ME, Arbuck SG, Wright J. (1999) DNA topoisomerase I poisons. *Cancer Chemother Biol Response Modif*, 18: 81–124.

84. Arbuck SG, Takimoto CH (1998) An overview of topoisomerase I-targeting agents. *Semin Hematol*, 35, (suppl 4), 3–12.

85. Hochster H, Liebes L, Speyer J, *et al.* (1994) Phase I trial of low-dose continuous topotecan infusion in patients with cancer: an active and well-tolerated regimen. *J Clin Oncol*, 12, 553–9.

86. Underberg WJM, Goossen RMJ, Smith BR, Beijnen JH (1990) Equilibrium kinetics of the new experimental antitumour compound SK&F 104684-A in aqueous solution. *J Pharmacol Biomed Anal*, 8, 8–12.

87. Fassberg J, Stella VJ (1992) A kinetic and mechanistic study of the hydrolysis of camptothecin and some analogues. *J Pharm Sci*, 81, 676–84.

88. Beijnen JH, Smith BR, Keijer WJ, *et al.* (1990) High-performance liquid chromatographic analysis of the new antitumour drug SK&F 104864-A (NSC 609699) in plasma. *J Pharm Biomed Anal*, 8, 789–94.

89. Grochow LB, Rowinsky EK, Johnson R, *et al.* (1992) Pharmacokinetics and pharmacodynamics of topotecan in patients with advanced cancer. *Drug Metab Dispos*, 20, 706–13.

90. Wall JG, Burris HA, Hoff DDV, *et al.* (1992) A phase I clinical and pharmacokinetic study of the topoisomerase I inhibitor topotecan (SK&F 104864) given as an intravenous bolus every 21 days. *Anticancer Drugs*, 3, 337–45.

91. Saltz L, Sirott M, Young C, *et al.* (1993) Phase I clinical and pharmacology study of topotecan given daily for 5 consecutive days to patients with advanced solid tumors, with attempt at dose intensification using recombinant granulocyte colony-stimulating factor. *J Natl Cancer Inst*, 85, 1499–1507.

92. Verweij J, Lund B, Beijnen J, *et al.* (1993) Phase I and pharmacokinetic study of topotecan, a new topoisomerase I inhibitor. *Ann Oncol*, 4, 673–8.

93. Rowinsky EK, Grochow LB, Sartorius SE, *et al.* (1996) Phase I and pharmacologic study of high doses of the topoisomerase I inhibitor topotecan with granulocyte colony-stimulating factor in patients with solid tumors. *J Clin Oncol*, 14, 1224–35.

94. Rowinsky EK, Kaufmann SH, Baker SD, *et al.* (1997) A phase I and pharmacologic study of topotecan infused

over 30 minutes for 5 days in patients with refractory acute leukemia. *Clin Cancer Res*, **12**, 2193–203.

95. Blaney SM, Balis FM, Cole DE, *et al.* (1993) Pediatric phase I trial and pharmacokinetic study of topotecan administered as a 24-hour continuous infusion. *Cancer Res*, **53**, 1032–6.

96. Stewart CF, Baker SD, Heideman RL, Jones D, Crom WR, Pratt CB (1994) Clinical pharmacodynamics of continuous infusion topotecan in children: systemic exposure predicts hematologic toxicity. *J Clin Oncol*, **12**, 1946–1511.

97. Pratt CB, Stewart C, Santana VM, *et al.* (1994) Phase I study of topotecan for pediatric patients with malignant solid tumors. *J Clin Oncol*, **12**, 539–43.

98. Tubergen DG, Stewart CF, Pratt CB, *et al.* (1996) Phase I trial and pharmacokinetic (PK) and pharmacodynamic (PD) study of topotecan using a five-day course in children with refractory solid tumors: a pediatric oncology group study. *J Ped Hematol Oncol*, **18**, 352–61.

99. Furman WL, Baker SD, Pratt CB, Rivera GK, Evans WE, Stewart CF (1996) Escalating systemic exposure of continuous infusion topotecan in children with recurrent acute leukemia. *J Clin Oncol*, **14**, 1504–11.

100. Kuhn J, Rizzo J, Eckardt J, *et al.* (1995) Phase I bioavailability study of oral topotecan. *Proc Am Soc Clin Oncol*, **14**, 474.

101. Schellens JHM, Creemers GJ, Beijnen JH, *et al.* (1996) Bioavailability and pharmacokinetics of oral topotecan: a new topoisomerase I inhibitor. *Br J Cancer*, **73**, 1268–71.

102. Creemers GJ, Gerrits CJ, Eckardt JR, *et al.* (1997) Phase I and pharmacologic study of oral topotecan administered twice daily for 21 days to adult patients with solid tumors. *J Clin Oncol*, **15**, 1087–93.

103. Gerrits CJH, Burris H, Schellens JHM, *et al.* (1998) Oral topotecan given once or twice daily for ten days: a phase I and pharmacology study in adult patients with solid tumors. *Clin Cancer Res*, **4**, 1153–8.

104. Gore M, Rustin G, Calvert H, *et al.* (1998) A multicenter randomized phase III study of topotecan administered intravenously or orally for advanced epithelial ovarian cancer. *Proc Am Soc Clin Oncol*, **17**, 349a.

105. Plaxe SC, Christen RD, O'Quigley J (1998) Phase I and pharmacokinetic study of intraperitoneal topotecan. *Invest New Drugs*, **16**, 147–53.

106. Hofstra LS, deVries EGE, van der Zee AGJ, Beijnen JH, Aalders JG, Willemse PHB (1998) Phase I-II and pharmacokinetic study of intraperitoneal topotecan. *Proc Am Soc Clin Oncol*, **17**, 244a.

107. O'Reilly S, Rowinsky E, Slichenmyer EW, *et al.* (1996) Phase I and pharmacologic study of topotecan in patients with impaired hepatic function. *J Natl Cancer Inst*, **88**, 817–24.

108. Burke TG, Mi Z (1994) The structural basis of camptothecin interactions with human serum albumin: impact on drug stability. *J Med Chem*, **37**, 40–6.

109. Mi Z, Malak H, Burke TG (1995) Reduced albumin promotes the stability and activity of topotecan in human blood. *Biochemistry*, **34**, 13722–8.

110. Blaney SM, Cole DE, Balis FM, Godwin K, Poplack DG (1993) Plasma and cerebrospinal fluid pharmacokinetic study of topotecan in nonhuman primates. *Cancer Res*, **53**, 725–7.

111. Sung C, Blaney SM, Cole DE, Balis FM, Dedrick RL (1994) A pharmacokinetic model of topotecan clearance from plasma and cerebrospinal fluid. *Cancer Res*, **54**, 5118–22.

112. Baker SD, Heideman RL, Crom WR, Kuttesch JF, Gajjar A, Stewart CF (1996) Cerebrospinal fluid pharmacokinetics and penetration of continuous infusion topotecan in children with central nervous system tumors. *Cancer Chemother Pharmacol*, **37**, 195–202.

113. Rosing H, Herben VM, van Gortel-van Zomeren DM, *et al.* (1997) Isolation and structural confirmation of N-desmethyl topotecan, a metabolite of topotecan. *Cancer Chemother Pharmacol*, **39**, 498–504.

114. Zamboni WC, Houghton PJ, Johnson RK, *et al.* (1998) Probenecid alters topotecan systemic and renal disposition by inhibiting renal tubular secretion. *J Pharmacol Exp Ther*, **284**, 89–94.

115. O'Reilly S, Rowinsky EK, Slichenmyer EW, *et al.* (1996) Phase I and pharmacologic studies of topotecan in patients with impaired renal function. *J Clin Oncol*, **14**, 3062–73.

116. Rowinsky EK, Kaufmann SH, Baker SD, *et al.* (1996) Sequences of topotecan and cisplatin: phase I, pharmacologic, and *in vitro* studies to examine sequence dependence. *J Clin Oncol*, **14**, 3074–84.

117. deJonge MJA, Sparreboom A, Planting AST, *et al.* (1998) Sequence-dependent effects of oral topotecan with intravenous cisplatin in a phase I and pharmacologic study in patients with advanced solid tumors. *Proc Am Soc Clin Oncol*, **17**, 204a.

118. Zamboni WC, Gajjar AJ, Heideman RL, *et al.* (1998) Phenytoin alters the disposition of topotecan and N-desmethyl topotecan in a patient with medulloblastoma. *Clin Cancer Res*, **4**, 783–9.

119. Kawato Y, Sekiguchi M, Akahane K, *et al.* (1993) Inhibitory activity of camptothecin derivatives against acetylcholinesterase in dogs and their binding activity to acetylcholine receptors in rats. *J Pharm Pharmacol*, **45**, 444–8.

120. van Warmerdam LJ, Verweij J, Schellens JH, *et al.* (1995) Pharmacokinetics and pharmacodynamics of topotecan administered daily for 5 days every 3 weeks. *Cancer Chemother Pharmacol*, **35**, 237–45.

121. Haas NB, LaCreta FP, Walczak J, *et al.* (1994) Phase I/pharmacokinetic study of topotecan by 24-hour continuous infusion weekly. *Cancer Res*, **54**, 1220–6.

122. van Warmerdam LJ, ten Bokkel Huinink WW, Rodenhuis S, *et al.* (1995) Phase I clinical and pharmacokinetic study of topotecan administered by a 24-hour continuous infusion. *J Clin Oncol*, **13**, 1768–76.

123. van Warmerdam LJ, Verweij J, Rosing H, Schellens JH, Maes RA, Beijnen JH (1994) Limited sampling models for topotecan pharmacokinetics. *Ann Oncol*, **5**, 259–64.

124. Minami H, Beijnen JH, Verweij J, Ratain MJ (1996) Limited sampling model for area under the concentration time curve for total topotecan. *Clin Cancer Res*, **2**, 43–6.

125. Kaneda N, Nagata H, Furuta T, Yokokura T (1990) Metabolism and pharmacokinetics of the camptothecin analogue CPT-11 in the mouse. *Cancer Res*, **50**, 1715–20.

126. Fukuoka M, Negoro S, Niitani H, *et al.* (1990) A phase I study of weekly administration of CPT-11 in lung cancer. *Gan To Kagaku Ryoho*, **17**, 993–7 (in Japanese).

127. Taguchi T, Wakui A, Hasegawa K, *et al.* (1990) Phase I clinical study of CPT-11. Research group of CPT-11. *Gan To Kagaku Ryoho*, **17**, 115–20.

128. Negoro S, Fukuoka M, Masuda N, *et al.* (1991) Phase I study of weekly intravenous infusions of CPT-11, a new derivative of camptothecin, in the treatment of advanced non-small-cell lung cancer. *J Natl Cancer Inst*, **83**, 1164–8.

129. Ohe Y, Sasaki Y, Shinkai T, *et al.* (1992) Phase I study and pharmacokinetics of CPT-11 with 5-day continuous infusion. *J Natl Cancer Inst*, **84**, 972–4.

130. Rothenberg ML, Kuhn JG, Burris HAd, *et al.* (1993) Phase I and pharmacokinetic trial of weekly CPT-11. *J Clin Oncol*, **11**, 2194–204.

131. de Forni M, Bugat R, Chabot GG, *et al.* (1994) Phase I and pharmacokinetic study of the camptothecin derivative irinotecan, administered on a weekly schedule in cancer patients. *Cancer Res*, **54**, 4347–54.

132. Rowinsky EK, Grochow LB, Ettinger DS, *et al.* (1994) Phase I and pharmacological study of the novel topoisomerase I inhibitor 7-ethyl-10-[4-(1-piperidino)-1-piperidino]carbonyloxycamptothecin (CPT-11) administered as a ninety-minute infusion every 3 weeks. *Cancer Res*, **54**, 427–36.

133. Abigerges D, Armand JP, Chabot GG, *et al.* (1994) Irinotecan (CPT-11) high-dose escalation using intensive high-dose loperamide to control diarrhea. *J Natl Cancer Inst*, **86**, 446–9.

134. Abigerges D, Chabot GG, Armand JP, Herait P, Gouyette A, Gandia D (1995) Phase I and pharmacologic studies of the camptothecin analog irinotecan administered every 3 weeks in cancer patients. *J Clin Oncol*, **13**, 210–21.

135. Catimel G, Chabot GG, Guastalla JP, *et al.* (1995) Phase I and pharmacokinetic study of irinotecan (CPT-11) administered daily for three consecutive days every three weeks in patients with advanced solid tumors. *Ann Oncol*, **6**, 133–40.

136. Fukuoka M, Niitani H, Suzuki A, *et al.* (1992) A phase II study of CPT-11, a new derivative of camptothecin, for previously untreated non-small-cell lung cancer. *J Clin Oncol*, **10**, 16–20.

137. Masuda N, Fukuoka M, Kusunoki Y, *et al.* (1992) CPT-11: a new derivative of camptothecin for the treatment of refractory or relapsed small-cell lung cancer. *J Clin Oncol*, **10**, 1225–9.

138. Gandia D, Abigerges D, Armand JP, *et al.* (1993) CPT-11-induced cholinergic effects in cancer patients. *J Clin Oncol*, **11**, 196–7.

139. Saliba F, Hagipantelli R, Misset J-L, *et al.* (1998) Pathophysiology and therapy of irinotecan-induced delayed-onset diarrhea in patients with advanced colorectal cancer: a prospective assessment. *J Clin Oncol*, **16**, 2745–51.

140. Rivory LP, Robert J (1994) Reversed-phase high-performance liquid chromatographic method for the simultaneous quantitation of the carboxylate and lactone forms of the camptothecin derivative irinotecan, CPT-11, and its metabolite SN-38 in plasma. *J Chromatogr B Biomed Appl*, **661**, 133–41.

141. Rivory LP, Chatelut E, Canal P, Mathieu-Boue A, Robert J (1994) Kinetics of the *in vivo* interconversion of the carboxylate and lactone forms of irinotecan (CPT-11) and of its metabolite SN-38 in patients. *Cancer Res*, **54**, 6330–3.

142. Sasaki Y, Hakusui H, Mizuno S, *et al.* (1995) A pharmacokinetic and pharmacodynamic analysis of CPT-11 and its active metabolite SN-38. *Jpn J Cancer Res*, **86**, 101–10.

143. Chabot GG, Abigerges D, Catimel G, *et al.* (1995) Population pharmacokinetics and pharmacodynamics of irinotecan (CPT-11) and active metabolite SN-38 during phase I trials. *Ann Oncol*, **6**, 141–51.

144. Stewart CF, Ma M, Furman WL, *et al.* (1998) Pharmacokinetics of irinotecan and its active metabolite SN-38 in children with recurrent solid tumors after protracted low dose iv irinotecan. *Proc Am Soc Clin Oncol*, **17**, 186.

145. Vassal G, Santos A, Deroussent A, *et al.* (1998) Clinical pharmacology of irinotecan (CPT-11) in children. *Proc Am Soc Clin Oncol*, **17**, 187.

146. *Investigator Brochure: Irinotecan Hydrochloride Trihydrate*. Upjohn Company, Kalamazoo, MI, June 1992.

147. Burke, T.G., Munshi, C.B., Mi, Z., Jiang, Y. (1995) The important role of albumin in determining the relative human blood stabilities of the camptothecin anticancer drugs. *J Pharm Sci*, **84**, 518–19.

148. Burke T, Mi Z, Roy D, Munshi C (1995) The pivotal role of albumin in determining the relative blood stabilities of camptothecin analogs currently in clinical trials. *Proc Am Soc Clin Oncol*, **14**, 463.

149. Tsuji T, Kaneda N, Kado K, Yokokura T, Yoshimoto T, Tsuru D (1991) CPT-11 converting enzyme from rat serum: purification and some properties. *J Pharmacobiodyn*, **14**, 341–9.

150. Rivory LP, Bowles MR, Robert J, Pond SM (1996) Conversion of irinotecan (CPT-11) to its active metabolite, 7-ethyl-10-hydroxycamptothecin (SN-38), by human liver carboxylesterase. *Biochem Pharmacol*, **52**, 1103–11.

151. Zamboni WC, Houghton PJ, Thompson J, *et al.* (1998) Altered irinotecan and SN-38 disposition after intravenous and oral administration of irinotecan in mice bearing human neuroblastoma xenografts. *Clin Cancer Res*, **4**, 455–62.

152. Atsumi R, Okazaki O, Hakusui H (1995) Metabolism of irinotecan to SN-38 in a tissue-isolated tumor model. *Biol Pharm Bull*, **18**, 1024–6.

153. Potter PM, Pawlik CA, Morton CL, Naeve CW, Danks MK (1998) Isolation and partial characterization of a cDNA encoding a rabit liver carboxylesterase that activates the prodrug irinotecan (CPT-11). *Cancer Res*, **58**, 2646–51.

154. Lokiec F, Sorbier BMd, Sanderink GJ (1996) Irinotecan (CPT-11) metabolites in human bile and urine. *Clin Cancer Res*, **2**, 1943–9.

155. Haaz MC, Rivory L, Riche C, Vernillet L, Robert J (1998) Metabolism of irinotecan (CPT-11) by human hepatic microsomes: participation of cytochrome

P-450 3A and drug interactions. *Cancer Res*, 58, 468–72.

156. Rivory LP, Riou JF, Haaz MC, *et al.* (1996) Identification and properties of a major plasma metabolite of irinotecan (CPT-11) isolated from the plasma of patients. *Cancer Res*, 56, 3689–94.

157. Dodds HM, Haaz MC, Riou JF, Robert J, Rivory LP (1998) Identification of a new metabolite of CPT-11 (irinotecan): pharmacological properties and activation to SN-38. *J Pharmacol Exp Ther*, 286, 578–83.

158. Rivory LP, Robert J (1995) Identification and kinetics of a beta-glucuronide metabolite of SN-38 in human plasma after administration of the camptothecin derivative irinotecan. *Cancer Chemother Pharmacol*, 36, 176–9.

159. Haaz MC, Rivory L, Jantet S, Ratanasavanh D, Robert J (1997) Glucuronidation of SN-38, the active metabolite of irinotecan, by human hepatic microsomes. *Pharmacol Toxicol*, 80, 91–6.

160. Iyer L, King CD, Whitington PF, *et al.* (1998) Genetic predisposition to the metabolism of irinotecan (CPT-11). Role of uridine diphosphate glucuronosyltransferase isoform 1A1 in the glucuronidation of its active metabolite (SN-38) in human liver microsomes. *J Clin Invest*, 101, 847–54.

161. Takasuna K, Kasai Y, Kitano Y, *et al.* (1995) Protective effects of kampo medicines and baicalin against intestinal toxicity of a new anticancer camptothecin derivative, irinotecan hydrochloride (CPT-11), in rats. *Jpn J Cancer Res*, 86, 978–84.

162. Takasuna K, Hagiwara T, Hirohashi M, *et al.* (1996) Involvement of beta-glucuronidase in intestinal microflora in the intestinal toxicity of the antitumor camptothecin derivative irinotecan hydrochloride (CPT-11) in rats. *Cancer Res*, 56, 3752–7.

163. Saka H, Ando Y, Sugiura S, Asai G (1998) UGT1A1*2B28 pleomorphism may affect glucuronidation of SN-38 in CPT-11 chemotherpay. *Proc Am Soc Clin Oncol*, 17, 195.

164. Gupta E, Mick R, Ramirez J, *et al.* (1997) Pharmacokinetic and pharmacodynamic evaluation of the topoisomerase inhibitor irinotecan in cancer patients. *J Clin Oncol*, 15, 1502–10.

165. Ratain MJ, Mick R, Gupta E, Lestingi TM, Schilsky RL, Vokes EE (1996) Prospective evaluation of the effect of race and gender on irinotecan (CPT-11) pharmacokinetics (PK) and intestinal toxicity. *Proc Am Soc Clin Oncol*, 15, 472.

166. Rivory LP, Haaz M-C, Canal P, Lokiec F, Armand J-P, Robert J (1997) Pharmacokinetic interrelationships of irinotecan (CPT-11) and its three major plasma metabolites in patients enrolled in phase I/II trials. *Clin Cancer Res*, 3, 1261–6.

167. Iyer L, Roy SK, Ratain MJ (1996) *In vitro* glucuronidation of SN-38, the active metabolite of irinotecan (CPT-11) in human liver microsomes. *Proc Am Soc Clin Oncol*, 15, 497.

168. Gupta E, Lestingi TM, Mick R, Ramirez J, Vokes EE, Ratain MJ (1994) Metabolic fate of irinotecan in humans: correlation of glucuronidation with diarrhea. *Cancer Res*, 54, 3723–5.

169. Masuda N, Fukuoka M, Kudoh S, *et al.* (1993) Phase I and pharmacologic study of irinotecan in combination with cisplatin for advanced lung cancer. *Br J Cancer*, 68, 777–82.

170. Kudoh S, Fukuoka M, Masuda N, *et al.* (1995) Relationship between the pharmacokinetics of irinotecan and diarrhea during combination chemotherapy with cisplatin. *Jpn J Cancer Res*, 86, 406–13.

171. Sasaki Y, Ohtsu A, Shimada Y, Ono K, Saijo N (1994) Simultaneous administration of CPT-11 and fluorouracil: alteration of the pharmacokinetics of CPT-11 and SN-38 in patients with advanced colorectal cancer. *J Natl Cancer Inst*, 86, 1096–8.

172. Saltz LB, Kanowitz J, Kemeny NE, *et al.* (1996) Phase I clinical and pharmacokinetic study of irinotecan, fluorouracil, and leucovorin in patients with advanced solid tumors. *J Clin Oncol*, 14, 2959–67.

173. Harstrick A, Vanhoefer U, Muller C, *et al.* (1997) Combination of CPT-11 and 5FU in colorectal cancer: preclinical rationale and initial phase I results. *Proc Am Assoc Cancer Res*, 38, 318.

174. Grivicich I, Mans DRA, Rocha ABd, Costa HSD, Schwartsmann G (1997) The cytotoxicity of irinotecan (CPT-11)-5-fluorouracil (5-FU) combinations in human colon carcinoma cell lines is related to the sequence dependent introduction of DNA-lesions. *Proc Am Assoc Cancer Res*, 38, 318.

175. Masuda N, Fukuoka M, Kudoh S, *et al.* (1994) Phase I and pharmacologic study of irinotecan and etoposide with recombinant human granulocyte colony-stimulating factor support for advanced lung cancer. *J Clin Oncol*, 12, 1833–41.

176. Gupta E, Wang X, Ramirez J, Ratain MJ (1997) Modulation of glucuronidation of SN-38, the active metabolite of irinotecan, by valproic acid and phenobarbital. *Cancer Chemother Pharmacol*, 39, 440–4.

177. Gupta E, Safa AR, Wang X, Ratain MJ (1996) Pharmacokinetic modulation of irinotecan and metabolites by cyclosporin A. *Cancer Res*, 56, 1309–14.

178. Wasserman E, Myara A, Lokiec F, *et al.* (1998) Bilirubin and SN-38 metabolism: Pharmacodynamics of CPT-11 toxicity. *Proc Am Soc Clin Oncol*, 17, 185.

179. Potmesil M, Giovanella BC, Liu LF, *et al.* (1991) Preclinical studies of DNA topoisomerase I-targeted 9-amino and 10, 11-methylenedioxycamptothecin. In Potmesil M, Kohn KW (eds) *DNA Topoisomerases in Cancer*. New York: Oxford University Press, 299–311.

180. Pantazis P, Hinz HR, Mendoza JT, *et al.* (1992) Complete inhibition of growth followed by death of human malignant melanoma cells *in vitro* and regression of human melanoma xenografts in immunodeficient mice induced by camptothecins. *Cancer Res*, 52, 3980–7.

181. Potmesil M, Giovanella BC, Wall ME, *et al.* (1993) Preclinical and clinical development of DNA topoisomerase I inhibitors in the United States. In Andoh T (ed) *The International Symposium on DNA Topoisomerases in Chemotherapy*. New York: CRC, 301–11.

182. Supko JG, Plowman J, Dykes DJ, Zaharko DS (1992) Relationship between the schedule-dependence of 9-amino-20(S)-camptothecin (AC; NSC 603071) antitumor activity in mice and its plasma pharmacokinetics. *Proc Am Assoc Cancer Res*, 33, 432.

183. Supko JG, Malspeis L (1993) Pharmacokinetics of the 9-amino and 10,11-methylenedioxy derivatives of camptothecin in mice. *Cancer Res*, **53**, 3062–9.

184. Dahut W, Harold N, Takimoto C, *et al.* (1996) Phase I and pharmacologic study of 9-aminocamptothecin given by 72-hour infusion in adult cancer patients. *J Clin Oncol*, **14**, 1236–44.

185. Rubin E, Wood V, Bharti A, *et al.* (1995) A phase I and pharmacokinetic study of a new camptothecin derivative, 9-aminocamptothecin. *Clin Cancer Res*, **1**, 269–76.

186. Siu LL, Oza AM, Eisenhauer EA, *et al.* (1998) Phase I and pharmacologic study of 9-aminocamptothecin colloidal dispersion formulation given as a 24-hour continuous infusion weekly times four every 5 weeks. *J Clin Oncol*, **16**, 1122–30.

187. Eder JP, Supko JG, Lynch T, *et al.* (1998) Phase I trial of the colloidal dispersion formulation of 9-amino-20(S)-camptothecin administered as a 72-hour continuous intravenous infusion. *Clin Cancer Res*, **4**, 317–24.

188. Beijnen JH, Herben VMM, ten Bokkel Huinink WW, *et al.* (1998) A phase I and pharmacokinetic study of a daily times 5 intravenous bolus schedule of 9-aminocamptothecin in patients with advanced solid tumors. *Proc Am Soc Clin Oncol*, **17**, 197.

189. Hochster H, Liebes L, Speyer J, *et al.* (1997) Phase I and pharmacodynamic study of prolonged infusion 9-aminocamptothecin in two formulations. *Proc Am Soc Clin Oncol*, **16**, 201.

190. Mani S, Iyer L, Janisch L, *et al.* (1997) Phase I clinical and pharmacokinetic study of oral 9-aminocamptothecin (NSC-603071). *Proc Am Soc Clin Oncol*, **16**, 201.

191. Sparreboom A, Jonge MJAd, Punt CJA, *et al.* (1998) Pharmacokinetics and bioavailability of oral 9-aminocamptothecin given capsules in adult patients with solid tumors. *Clin Cancer Res*, **4**, 1915–19.

192. Verschraegen CF, Natelson EA, Giovanella BC, *et al.* (1998) A phase I clinical and pharmacological study of oral 9-nitrocamptothecin, a novel water-insoluble topoisomerase I inhibitor. *Anticancer Drugs*, **9**, 36–44.

193. Emerson DL, Besterman JM, Brown HR, *et al.* (1995) *In vivo* antitumor activity of two new seven-substituted water-soluble camptothecin analogues. *Cancer Res*, **55**, 603–9.

194. Besterman JM (1996) Topoisomerase I inhibition by the camptothecin analog GI147211C. From the laboratory to the clinic. *Ann NY Acad Sci*, **803**, 202–9.

195. Eckhardt SG, Baker SD, Eckardt JR, *et al.* (1998) Phase I and pharmacokinetic study of GI147211, a water-soluble camptothecin analogue, administered for five consecutive days every three weeks. *Clin Cancer Res*, **4**, 595–604.

196. Gerrits CJ, Creemers GJ, Schellens JH, *et al.* (1996) Phase I and pharmacological study of the new topoisomerase I inhibitor GI147211, using a daily × 5 intravenous administration. *Br J Cancer*, **73**, 744–50.

197. Kumazawa E, Jimbo T, Ochi Y, Tohgo A (1998) Potent and broad antitumor effects of DX-8951f, a water-soluble camptothecin derivative, against various human tumors xenografted in nude mice. *Cancer Chemother Pharmacol*, **42**, 210–20.

198. Johnson T, Geyer C, Jager D, *et al.* (1998) A phase I and pharmacokinetic study of DX-8951f, a novel hexacyclic camptothecin analog, on a 30 minute infusion daily for 5 days every 3 week schedule. *Proc. 10th NCI-EORTC Symp. on New Drugs in Cancer Therapy*, 64.

199. Greenwald RB, Pendri A, Conover C, Gilbert C, Yang R, Xia J (1996) Drug delivery systems. 2. Camptothecin 20-O-poly(ethylene glycol) ester transport forms. *J Med Chem*, **39**, 1938–40.

200. Lynam E, Landfair DJ, Luzzio MJ, Wiles ME (1998) Camptothecin analogue efficacy *in vitro*. Effect of liposomal encapsulation of GI147211 (Lurotecan) on *in vitro* cytotoxcity for multiple tumor types. *Proc Am Assoc Cancer Res*, **39**, 421.

201. Madden TD, Burke TG, Redelmeir TE, Bally MB (1998) Encapsulation of topotecan in lipid-based carrier systems. Evaluation of drug stability and plasma elimination in a murine model, and comparison of antitumor efficacy against murine L1210 and B16 tumors. *Proc Am Soc Clin Oncol*, **17**, 196.

202. Eckardt JR, Burris HA 3rd, Kuhn JG, *et al.* (1994) Activity of intoplicine (RP60475), a new DNA topoisomerase I and II inhibitor, against human tumor colony-forming units *in vitro*. *J Natl Cancer Inst*, **86**, 30–3.

203. Yoshinari T, Matsumoto M, Arakawa H, *et al.* (1995) Novel antitumor indolocarbazole compound 6-N-formyl-amino-12,13-dihydro-1,11-dihydroxy-13-(beta-D-glucopyranosyl)-5H-indolo[2,3-a]pyrrolo[3,4-c]carbazole-5,7(6H)-dione (NB-506): induction of topoisomerase I-mediated DNA cleavage and mechanisms of cell line-selective cytotoxicity. *Cancer Res*, **55**, 1310–15.

204. Donehower RC, Elza-Brown K, O'Reily S, Israel B, Grochow L (1998) A phase I dose escalation, safety, tolerability, and pharmacokinetic study of TAS-103 in patients with refractory solid tumors. *Proc Am Soc Clin Oncol*, **17**, 209.

13 | *Platinum agents*

Steven W. Johnson, James P. Stevenson and Peter J. O'Dwyer

Introduction

Platinum complexes represent a unique and important class of antitumour drugs. Although *cis*-diamminedichloroplatinum(II) (cisplatin) was initially synthesized in 1845, it was not realized that platinum compounds exhibited antitumour activity until the work of Barnett Rosenberg published in 1969.[1] These studies led to the clinical development of *cis*-diamminedichloroplatinum(II) (cisplatin) for the treatment of various solid tumours. It was soon discovered that nephrotoxicity and the development of tumour cell resistance limited the overall success of cisplatin-based

Summary

	Cisplatin	Carboplatin	Oxaliplatin
Brand names	Platinol	Paraplatin	Eloxatin
Molecular weight (Da)	300.0	371.25	397.3
Mechanism of action	DNA damage	DNA damage	DNA damage
Cell-cycle specificity	None	None	None
Route of administration	Intravenous	Intravenous or intraperitoneal	Intravenous
Metabolism	Aquation	Aquation	Aquation
Elimination	Renal	Renal	Renal
Plasma Pt half-lives			
$t_{1/2\,\alpha}$ (min)	14–49	12–98	26
$t_{1/2\,\beta}$ (h)	1–5	1.3–1.7	
$t_{1/2\,\gamma}$ (h)	24–127	8.2–40	38.7
Ultrafilterable Pt half-lives			
$t_{1/2\,\alpha}$ (min)	10–30	7.6–87	21
$t_{1/2\,\beta}$ (h)	0.7–0.8	1.7–5.9	24.2
Protein binding (4 h) (%)	>90	24	85
Urinary excretion (24 h) (%)	23–50	54–82	>50
Toxicities	Nephrotoxicity, neurotoxicity	Myelosuppression	Neurotoxicity
Unique features	Leucocyte DNA adduct formation correlates with response/toxicity	AUC correlates with glomerular filtration rate	Activity in cisplatin and carboplatin resistant cells

chemotherapy. Therefore, over the last three decades, many investigators have embarked on the development of cisplatin analogues in an attempt to improve the efficacy and to ameliorate the toxicity profile observed with cisplatin. It was also believed that novel platinum analogues could be designed to circumvent pathways responsible for cisplatin resistance. Only one other platinum drug, carboplatin, currently has Food & Drug Administration (FDA) approval in the United States for the treatment of cancer. Another platinum compound that has shown promising activity in the treatment of colorectal cancer is oxaliplatin, which received marketing approval in France in 1996. In this chapter, the pharmacokinetic and pharmacodynamic properties of cisplatin, carboplatin, and oxaliplatin will be discussed. Reviews of other platinum compounds currently undergoing preclinical and clinical investigation can be found elsewhere.[2,3]

Clinical use

Cisplatin, carboplatin, and oxaliplatin have all been shown to exhibit activity in a wide variety of solid tumours (Table 13.1). The observed toxicities and efficacies associated with these three platinum(II) complexes are largely due to the structure of their leaving groups and carrier ligands, respectively. In aqueous environments with a low chloride content, the dichloro ligands of cisplatin and the cyclobutanedicarboxylate ligand of carboplatin become aquated to yield the same active species [*cis*-diamminediaquoplatinum(II)], although the rate of carboplatin aquation is slower. As a result, most diseases respond similarly to either cisplatin or carboplatin and the two drugs exhibit similar cross-resistance profiles in drug-resistant tumour cells. The major difference between these two drugs is in their toxicity profiles, which have influenced their overall clinical use.

In contrast, oxaliplatin contains a 1,2-diaminocyclohexane (DACH) carrier ligand. This feature is responsible for the lack of cross-resistance observed in cisplatin and carboplatin-refractory tumour cells. Preclinical studies suggest that weak nucleophiles, such as bicarbonate and dihydrogen phosphate, can displace the oxalate group from oxaliplatin.[4] The resulting species is rapidly converted into monoaqua-1,2-DACH-monochloroplatinum(II) or 1,2-DACH-dichloroplatinum(II).[5] These reactive compounds are analogous to those of cisplatin and carboplatin. Many clinical trials have been conducted to determine which platinum drug is most effective in the treatment of particular types of cancer. Attempts have also been made to optimize other factors, such as dose, scheduling, and combination with other anticancer drugs, to yield safe and efficacious regimens.

Testicular cancer

The most significant contribution of platinum drugs to the treatment of solid tumours has occurred in testicular cancer. Prior to the use of cisplatin-based regimens, the survival of most patients with advanced germ-cell tumours was less than 2 years. In an early phase I trial, single-agent cisplatin was reported to be very active against testicular germ-cell tumours, yielding response rates of 70% and complete remission rates of 50%.[6] In recent years, the use of cisplatin in combination with etoposide and bleomycin has revolutionized treatment, producing cure rates of 85–90%.[7] At standard doses, carboplatin is less effective than cisplatin in this disease; however, evidence suggests that high-dose chemotherapy regimens incorporating carboplatin may salvage some patients with resistant disease.

Table 13.1 Clinical use of platinum drugs

Tumour	Platinum drug used in combination chemotherapy	Outcome
Testicular	Cisplatin or carboplatin	High cure rate (>80%)
Anal	Cisplatin or carboplatin	High cure rate (>50%)
Ovarian	Cisplatin or carboplatin	Low cure rate (<25%)
Small-cell lung	Cisplatin	Low cure rate (20%)
Bladder	Cisplatin	Low cure rate (?%)
Non-small-cell lung	Cisplatin or carboplatin	Prolonged survival
Colon	Oxaliplatin	Prolonged survival
Head and neck	Cisplatin or carboplatin	Tumour shrinkage
Other (gastric, cervical, endometrial)	Cisplatin or carboplatin	Tumour shrinkage

Ovarian cancer

In the treatment of advanced-stage ovarian cancer, cisplatin-based chemotherapy is more effective than single alkylating agent therapy or non-platinum combination regimens. Carboplatin may be substituted for cisplatin with equivalent efficacy; it is much easier to administer and it is less toxic at clinically relevant doses.[8] The current standard of care in the United States is the combination of *carboplatin and paclitaxel*. This is based on a study by the Gynaecologic Oncology Group (GOG) showing that the combination of cisplatin and paclitaxel was superior to the combination of cisplatin and cyclophosphamide in advanced stage ovarian cancer.[9] Advances in haematopoietic support to alleviate myelosuppression have extended the application of high-dose carboplatin chemotherapy in the treatment of ovarian cancer.[10]

Bladder cancer

Cisplatin has been shown to have significant activity in the treatment of bladder cancer, with approximately 35% of patients responding in phase II clinical trials.[11] However, metastatic bladder cancer is most effectively treated with combination chemotherapy. The widely used combination of methotrexate, vinblastine, doxorubicin, and cisplatin (M-VAC) has been reported to yield response rates of 39–72%.[12] Cisplatin in combination with gemcitabine is also highly active in this disease. The response rates of patients treated with single-agent carboplatin are relatively low (14%);[13] however, *carboplatin in combination with paclitaxel* appears to yield high response rates. Ongoing randomized trials will determine the best platinum-based regimen for bladder cancer.

Head and neck cancer

Cisplatin-based chemotherapy has been used successfully to complement surgery and radiation therapy for the treatment of advanced head and neck cancer. In a recent study, high-dose single-agent cisplatin yielded a response rate of 59% in patients with locally advanced head and neck cancer.[14] Combinations of cisplatin and 5-fluorouracil or cisplatin with bleomycin and methotrexate are among the most active regimens currently used, yielding response rates of 60–90%.[15–17] Recently, two studies showed that the combination of cisplatin and paclitaxel also yields high response rates in previously untreated patients.[18–20] Hopefully, high dose response rates will translate into a hitherto elusive survival advantage.

Lung cancer

Non-small-cell lung cancer (NSCLC) is generally refractory to most chemotherapy; however, cisplatin-based regimens have been part of standard therapy for metastatic NSCLC.[21] Typically, response rates of 15–30% are observed, although median survival is less than 1 year. Recently, improvements have been made by combining cisplatin with paclitaxel or carboplatin with paclitaxel. Response rates of 31–47% and 12–62%, respectively, have been observed with these regimens.[21] In addition, the combination of carboplatin and *gemcitabine* has produced favourable response rates (30–54%).[21] Cisplatin and carboplatin used as single agents are also active against *small-cell lung* cancer, yielding response rates of approximately 30%. Cisplatin-based combination chemotherapy also results in significant responses (70–80%).[22]

Colorectal cancer

Fluoropyrimidines have been used as standard treatment for colorectal cancer for decades. Until recently, the use of platinum drugs for this disease was unsuccessful. Several trials exploring the activity of single-agent cisplatin or carboplatin resulted in poor responses (<10%). However, oxaliplatin has been shown to have activity as a single agent in previously untreated and fluoropyrimidine-refractory colorectal cancer (response rates of 12–24% and 10–11%, respectively).[23] Oxaliplatin combined with 5-fluorouracil–leucovorin has produced response rates of 32–70% in previously untreated patients.[24] Ongoing research is likely to define an important role for oxaliplatin in the treatment of colorectal cancer.

Formulation

Cisplatin (Platinol) for injection is available from Bristol-Myers Oncology Division (Princeton, NJ) as a lyophilized powder in 10 mg and 50 mg vials. It is reconstituted by adding sterile water to obtain a final concentration of 1 mg/ml. This solution is stable at room temperature for 20 h. Carboplatin (Paraplatin) for injection is available from Bristol-Myers Oncology Division (Princeton, NJ) as a lyophilized powder in 50 mg, 150 mg, and 450 mg vials. It is reconstituted by adding Sterile Water for Injection USP, Dextrose 5% in Water USP, or Sodium Chloride Injection USP to obtain a final concentration of 10 mg/ml. This solution is stable at room temperature for 8 h. Oxaliplatin is available from Sanofi Pharmaceuticals (Collegeville, PA) as a lyophilized powder in 50 and 100 mg vials. It is reconstituted by adding Sterile Water for Injection USP to obtain a final concentration of 2 mg/ml. This solution is stable at room temperature for 1 week.

Mechanism of action

Several observations have led investigators to believe that DNA is the primary cytotoxic target of the platinum drugs. First, during his experiments studying the effects of electricity on the growth of bacteria, Rosenberg discovered that *cis*-diamminedichloroplatinum(II) induced the filamentous growth of bacteria while inhibiting cell division.[25] This observation, in conjunction with other studies,[26,27] indicated that cisplatin inhibits DNA synthesis, while RNA and protein synthesis still occurs. Secondly, cisplatin has been shown to form a variety of DNA lesions including intra- and inter-strand cross-links. The formation of cross-links by other DNA reactive drugs has been implicated in their cytotoxic effects. Finally, studies of fibroblasts isolated from patients with xeroderma pigmentosum, known to contain defects in nucleotide excision repair, have been shown to exhibit hypersensitivity to cisplatin and other DNA-damaging agents.[28,29]

The differential cytotoxic effects observed with platinum drugs are influenced by the structure and relative amount of DNA adducts formed. Platinum drugs react with the N-7 position of guanine and adenine residues to form a variety of monofunctional and bifunctional adducts.[30] The predominant bidentate lesions that are formed with DNA *in vitro* or in cultured cells are the d(GpG)Pt, d(ApG)Pt, and d(GpNpG)Pt intra-strand cross-links.[31,32] In a study of cisplatin-treated Chinese hamster ovary cells, these lesions were determined to account for approximately 60%, 15%, and 20% of the total platinum DNA adducts, respectively.[33] Cisplatin also forms inter-strand cross-links between guanine residues located on opposite strands that account for >5% of the total DNA bound platinum. These adducts may contribute to the drug's cytotoxicity as they impede certain cellular processes, such as replication and transcription, that require the separation of both DNA strands.

The adducts that are formed by the reaction of carboplatin with DNA in cultured cells are essentially the same as those of cisplatin; however, higher concentrations of carboplatin are required (20–40-fold for cells) to obtain equivalent total platinum–DNA adduct levels because of its slower rate of aquation.[34] The relative amounts of each lesion are different, with the d(GpNpG)Pt intra-strand adduct being the most prevalent (~40%) followed by the d(GpG)Pt (~30%) and d(ApG)Pt (~15%) intra-strand adducts. [33] As with cisplatin, a relatively small number of monoadducts and inter-strand cross-links are observed. The relative amounts and frequencies of the DNA adducts formed in cultured cells by oxaliplatin has also been examined.[35] Higher concentrations of oxaliplatin are required to obtain total platinum–DNA adduct levels similar to that of cisplatin. Oxaliplatin forms predominantly d(GpG)Pt and d(ApG)Pt intra-strand cross-links at similar ratios to those of cisplatin.

Different cytotoxicity profiles are often observed between cisplatin and carboplatin compared with oxaliplatin *in vitro*.[36] Based on crystallographic data, computer modelling of the d(GpG)Pt adduct formed by oxaliplatin indicated that the DACH group projects into the major groove of DNA, producing a bulkier adduct than that formed with cisplatin.[37] Thus damage-recognition proteins, such as the mismatch repair complex, may be prevented from recognizing oxaliplatin adducts because of steric hindrance caused by the DACH ring.[5] These results emphasize the importance of the carrier ligand in determining the overall structure of the DNA lesion, which may influence DNA damage recognition and the intracellular signalling events that follow. Such pathways may ultimately be important in determining the fate of a cell.

Mechanisms of resistance

The major limitation to the successful treatment of solid tumours with platinum-based chemotherapy is the emergence of drug-resistant tumour cells. Platinum drug resistance may be intrinsic or acquired and can occur through a variety of mechanisms (Table 13.2). These mechanisms can be classified into two major groups: those that limit the formation of cytotoxic platinum–DNA adducts, and those that prevent cell death from occurring following platinum–DNA adduct formation. The first group of mechanisms includes decreased drug accumulation and increased drug inactivation by cellular protein and non-protein thiols.

Table 13.2 Mechanisms of resistance to platinum drugs

Mechanism	Phenotype	Molecular basis
Reduced Pt–DNA adduct formation:	Decreased drug uptake	Unknown
	Inactivation	Glutathione, metallothioneins
Repair Pt–DNA adducts:	Nucleotide excision repair	ERCC1–XPF complex
Tolerate Pt–DNA adducts:	Replicative bypass of adducts	Mismatch repair proteins
	Defective programmed cell death	Unknown

The second group of mechanisms includes increased platinum–DNA adduct repair and increased platinum–DNA damage tolerance.[38]

Decreased platinum accumulation is a common phenotype observed in cell lines selected for cisplatin resistance *in vitro* and the accumulation difference between the sensitive and resistant counterpart may reach as high as 14-fold.[39–42] The precise mechanism(s) of cisplatin uptake is unknown, but the process is believed to occur through a combination of passive diffusion and carrier-mediated transport processes.[43] However, differences in platinum drug accumulation do not always correlate strongly with drug sensitivity in unrelated cell lines, suggesting that it may not be a clinically relevant resistance mechanism.[44]

In addition to reduced drug accumulation, a variety of intracellular factors may affect the activity of cisplatin and also preclude it from binding to DNA. Sulfhydryl-rich proteins and glutathione have been implicated in the inactivation of cisplatin and other alkylating agents by drug-resistant cells. Glutathione (GSH) is a ubiquitous tripeptide that is involved in the detoxification of a variety of exogenous and endogenous molecules. Two groups have reported evidence for the formation of a GSH–Pt complex in cells exposed to cisplatin.[45,46] Several investigators have observed increased glutathione levels in cell lines selected for cisplatin resistance *in vitro*.[47–50] GSH has also been found to be associated with cisplatin sensitivity in some unrelated cell lines.[50] Alternatively, platinum drugs may be covalently bound to metallothionein (MT). The MTs constitute a family of sulfhydryl-rich proteins of low molecular weight that participate in heavy metal detoxification. Manipulating MT levels by overexpression or knockout has been shown to influence cisplatin sensitivity.[51,52]

If decreased drug accumulation and/or inactivation pathways fail to prevent the formation of cytotoxic platinum–DNA adducts, cells must either repair or tolerate the damage in order to survive. The capacity to *repair DNA damage* rapidly and efficiently may play a role in determining the sensitivity of a tumour cell to platinum drugs and other DNA-damaging agents. For example, there is recent evidence to suggest that cell lines derived from tumours that are unusually sensitive to cisplatin, such as testicular non-seminomatous germ-cell tumours, are deficient in their ability to repair platinum–DNA adducts.[53] Similarly, the relative unresponsiveness of non-small-cell lung cancer compared with small-cell lung cancer has been associated with an elevated DNA repair capacity.[54] Increased repair of platinum–DNA lesions in cisplatin-resistant cell lines compared with their sensitive counterparts has been shown to occur in several human cancer cell lines including ovarian,[55,56] breast,[57] and glioma,[58] as well as in murine leukaemia cell lines.[59] Evidence for increased repair of cisplatin inter-strand cross-links in specific gene and non-gene regions in cisplatin-resistant cell lines has also been demonstrated.[56,60]

Platinum–DNA damage tolerance is a phenotype that has been observed in both cisplatin-resistant cells derived from chemotherapy-refractory patients and cells selected for primary cisplatin resistance *in vitro*. The contribution of this mechanism to resistance is significant, and it has been shown to correlate strongly with cisplatin resistance as well as with resistance to other drugs in two ovarian cancer model systems.[44,56] Like other cisplatin resistance mechanisms, this phenotype may result from alterations in a variety of cellular pathways. Assuming that DNA is the cytotoxic target of cisplatin, there are at least two ways a cell can exhibit increased platinum–DNA damage tolerance. Enhanced replicative bypass enables cellular DNA replication machinery to synthesize DNA past a lesion. Subsequent repair of the lesion could then be completed at the G_2 checkpoint prior to mitosis. This process was previously demonstrated to occur in two cisplatin-resistant human ovarian cancer cell lines.[61] It has also been shown that DNA polymerase can efficiently bypass a (dGpG)Pt intra-strand adduct *in vitro*.[62]

Another possible explanation for the platinum–DNA damage tolerance phenotype is that cisplatin-resistant cells may require higher drug concentrations in order to activate programmed cell death (apoptosis). Since apoptosis is a highly regulated process, it is conceivable that disruption of one or more components of the pathway could elicit the multidrug resistance phenotype observed in clinically refractory tumour cells. Failure of cisplatin-resistant murine leukaemia cells to undergo apoptosis when exposed to normally toxic concentrations of cisplatin has recently been demonstrated.[63] Alternatively, over-expression of a gene which suppresses apoptosis could also result in decreased drug sensitivity. For example, over-expression of members of the *bcl-2* gene family, *bcl-2* and *bcl-x$_l$*, has been shown to protect cells from apoptotic cell death when exposed to cisplatin and other chemotherapeutic agents.[64,65] Overall, identifying the components of platinum-drug-induced cell-death pathways will be necessary for the molecular basis for the tolerance phenotype to be understood.

Chemistry

Cisplatin, carboplatin, and oxaliplatin are platinum(II) complexes with molecular weights 300 Da, 371.25 Da, and 397.3 Da, respectively (Fig. 13.1). Cisplatin contains two chlorine atoms and two amino groups arranged in a *cis* configuration. Carboplatin contains two amino groups and a 1,1-dicyclobutanedicarboxylate group. Oxaliplatin consists of a 1,2-dicyclohexane and an oxalato group. As mentioned above, the differences in the structures of the leaving groups and carrier ligands impact on both the toxicity and efficacy of these agents.

Analytical methodology

During the initial period of preclinical and clinical development, the measurement of platinum for phar-

macokinetic studies involved using radionuclides (platinum-193m or platinum-195m) or flameless atomic absorption spectrometry (FAAS). For FAAS, plasma and urine samples can be diluted in 0.2% nitric acid–0.1% Triton X-100 prior to injection onto the spectrometer. The detection limit using this method is approximately 5 mg platinum per litre of sample, which makes this technique suitable for standard pharmacokinetic measurements. Inductively coupled plasma mass spectrometry (ICP–MS) has been used when a higher level of sensitivity is required. This technique has been reported to be 4000 times more sensitive than FAAS[66] and has been used for measuring long-term pharmacokinetics in patients treated with cisplatin, carboplatin, and oxaliplatin.[67,68]

High-performance liquid chromatography (HPLC) in conjunction with UV detection, electrochemical detection, or mass spectrometry is also valuable for the analysis of platinum drug metabolites. For example, in ultrafiltrate and urine samples of patients treated with carboplatin, it is often necessary to determine the amount of carboplatin and the relative amount of platinum that exists as decarboxylated free platinum and platinum bound to small molecules. A variety of techniques have been employed for the determination of platinum–DNA adduct levels in patient white blood cells (WBCs), including FAAS[69] and enzyme-linked immmunosorbent assay (ELISA).[70,71]

Pharmacokinetics

In general, the pharmacokinetic differences observed between platinum drugs can be attributed to the structure of their leaving groups. Platinum complexes containing leaving groups that are less easily displaced exhibit reduced plasma protein binding, longer plasma half-lives, and higher rates of renal clearance. These

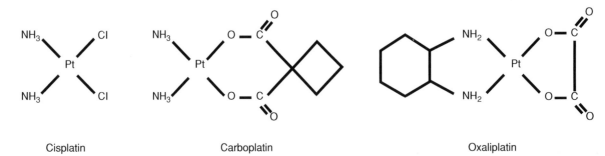

Cisplatin   Carboplatin   Oxaliplatin

Figure 13.1.   Chemical structures of cisplatin, carboplatin, and oxaplatin.

features are evident in the pharmacokinetic properties of cisplatin, carboplatin, and oxaliplatin, which are summarized in Tables 13.3–13.5. Other aspects of platinum drug pharmacokinetics have been thoroughly reviewed elsewhere.[72–75]

Cisplatin

In the first few hours after infusion, cisplatin rapidly diffuses into tissues and becomes covalently bound to plasma protein. More than 90% of platinum is bound to plasma protein at 4 h post-infusion.[76] The protein-bound platinum is inactive, exhibiting no cytotoxicity in *in vitro assays*.[77] In *in vitro* studies, cisplatin decomposes rapidly, binding to plasma proteins with a half-life of 1.5–3.6 h.[77,78]

The disappearance of cisplatin from plasma following a bolus or intravenous infusion occurs in a biphasic or triphasic fashion. The half-life of the initial phase is rapid (14–49 min), whereas the half-life of the second phase has been reported to be between 0.7 and 5 h (Table 13.3). Both of these half-lives represent elimination of free drug from the circulation by either excretion or diffusion into tissues. The terminal phase, which consists of the removal of platinum bound to plasma protein, has been reported to have a half-life of 24–127 h.[79] The variability associated with these values may be due to the selection of time points for sampling and the use of different assays to measure platinum at the later time points. The disappearance of ultrafilterable platinum is rapid and occurs in a biphasic fashion. Half-lives of 10–30 min and 0.7–0.8 h have been reported for the initial and terminal phases, respectively.[80,81]

Efficient removal of cisplatin is dependent on adequate renal function, which accounts for the majority of its elimination. The percentage of platinum excreted in the urine has been reported to be between 23% and 40% at 24 h post-infusion.[77,81] Only a small percentage of the total platinum is excreted in the bile.[82]

Carboplatin

The differences in pharmacokinetics observed between cisplatin and carboplatin depend primarily on the slower rate of conversion of carboplatin to a reactive species. Thus the stability of carboplatin as well as its mechanism of clearance has been attributed to the low nephrotoxicity observed with its use. Like cisplatin, carboplatin diffuses rapidly into tissues following infusion; however, it is considerably more stable in plasma. A half-life of 30 h was reported for its binding to plasma at 37°C in *in vitro* studies,[83] and only 24% was reported to be bound to plasma at 4 h post-infusion *in vivo*.[83] At 24 h post-infusion, 87% of the remaining platinum is bound to plasma protein.

Pharmacokinetic studies of carboplatin include both the analysis of plasma, which contains protein-bound and unbound platinum, and ultrafilterable platinum, which consists of the parent drug and carboplatin metabolites. The ultrafilterable species are responsible for both the antitumour activity and the toxicity associated with the drug. The disappearance of platinum from plasma following short intravenous infusions of carboplatin has been reported to occur in a biphasic or triphasic manner. The initial half-lives for total platinum, which vary considerably among several studies, are listed in Table 13.4. The half-lives for total platinum range from 12 to 98 min during the first phase ($t_{1/2\,\alpha}$) and from 1.3 to 1.7 h during the second phase ($t_{1/2\,\beta}$). Half-lives reported for the terminal phase range from 8.2 to 40 h. The disappearance of ultrafilterable

Table 13.3 Pharmacokinetics of cisplatin (adapted from selected references)*

	Ref. 76	Ref. 77	Ref. 80	Ref. 100	Ref. 79	Ref. 81
Plasma Pt						
$t_{1/2\,\alpha}$ (min)	25–49	23	20		14.4	
$t_{1/2\,\beta}$ (h)			1	0.7	4.6	
$t_{1/2\,\gamma}$ (h)	58–73	67	>24		127	
Ultrafilterable Pt						
$t_{1/2\,\alpha}$ (min)			20–30		9.7	30
$t_{1/2\,\beta}$ (h)					0.7	0.8
Protein binding (4 h) (%)	>90					
Urinary excretion (24 h) (%)	27–45 (5 days)	23		49.5	28	40

*Data were obtained from patients given bolus injections or short-term infusions.

Table 13.4 Pharmacokinetics of carboplatin (adapted from selected references)

Reference	Ref. 83	Ref. 101	Ref. 102	Ref. 103	Ref. 104
Plasma Pt					
$t_{1/2\,\alpha}$ (min)	98	26–49		66	12–24
$t_{1/2\,\beta}$ (h)					1.3–1.7
$t_{1/2\,\gamma}$ (h)		8.2–20		15	22–40
Ultrafilterable Pt					
$t_{1/2\,\alpha}$ (min)	87	7.6–21.4	10	31	30
$t_{1/2\,\beta}$ (h)	5.9	1.7–3.9	2.2	2.7	2.2
Protein binding (%)	24 (4 h)		18 (0.5 h)		40–50 (6–24 h)
Urinary excretion (24 h) (%)	65	54	66		57–82

platinum is biphasic with $t_{1/2\,\alpha}$ and $t_{1/2\,\beta}$ values ranging from 7.6 to 87 min and 1.7 to 5.9 h, respectively.

Carboplatin is excreted predominantly by the kidneys. During the first 24 h, the cumulative urinary excretion of platinum is 54–82%. Of this, 32–80% has been reported to exist as unmodified carboplatin. The large variation in these values is probably due to the degradation of carboplatin in urine samples during collection and storage, and so it is likely that the majority of the platinum exists as the parent drug. The renal clearance of carboplatin is closely correlated with the glomerular filtration rate (GFR).[83] This observation enabled Calvert et al.[84] to design a carboplatin dosing formula based on an individual patient's GFR.

Oxaliplatin

Following oxaliplatin infusion, platinum accumulates into three compartments: plasma-bound platinum, ultrafilterable platinum, and platinum associated with erythrocytes. Approximately 85% of the total platinum is bound to plasma at 2–5 h post-infusion.[68] The disappearance of total platinum and ultrafiltrates is biphasic. The half-lives for the initial and terminal phases are 26 min and 38.7 h, respectively, for total platinum, and 21 min and 24.2 h, respectively, for ultrafilterable platinum (Table 13.5).[75] A prolonged retention of platinum is observed in red blood cells, and this may be responsible for oxaliplatin toxicity. Unlike cisplatin, which accumulates as both protein-bound and free platinum, total plasma platinum does not accumulate to any significant level following multiple courses of oxaliplatin treatment.[68] This may explain why neurotoxicity associated with oxaliplatin therapy is reversible. Oxaliplatin is eliminated predominantly by the kidneys, with more than 50% being excreted in the urine at 48 h.

Table 13.5 Pharmacokinetics of oxaliplatin (adapted from selected references)

	Ref. 75	Ref. 68
Plasma Pt		
$t_{1/2\,\alpha}$ (min)	26	
$t_{1/2\,\beta}$ (h)	38.7	
Ultrafilterable Pt		
$t_{1/2\,\alpha}$ (min)	21	
$t_{1/2\,\beta}$ (h)	24.2	
Protein binding (2–5 h) (%)		85
Urinary excretion (48 h) (%)	>50	

Toxicity

A number of toxicities are associated with the intravenous administration of platinum drugs. The differences in pharmacokinetics and pharmacodynamics for the three platinum compounds discussed above are largely responsible for their unique toxicity profiles.

Cisplatin

The major dose-limiting toxicity of cisplatin is nephrotoxicity, which nearly led to its abandonment in the 1970s. Cvitkovic and coworkers[85,86] introduced the use of aggressive hydration accompanied by mannitol diuresis prior to cisplatin therapy, which resulted in an acceptable incidence of moderate and reversible nephrotoxicity. The other side effects of cisplatin include nephrotoxicity, myelosuppression, ototoxicity, neuropathy, nausea, and vomiting. Administering antiemetics alleviates the latter two. Ototoxicity and neuropathy are cumulative and only partially reversible. This toxicity may result from the long-term retention of platinum in tissues following repeated dosing. A linear relationship was observed between post-mortem platinum levels in neurological tissue and the cumulative dose of cisplatin administered.[87] Other infrequent toxicities associated with cisplatin therapy include visual impairment, seizures, arrhythmias, acute ischaemic vascular effects, glucose intolerance, and pancreatitis.

Carboplatin

The dose-limiting toxicity of carboplatin is myelosuppression, particularly thrombocytopenia.[88] Leucopenia and anaemia also occur but are less severe. Following a single dose of carboplatin, the lowest *platelet counts* are observed 17–21 days later and recovery usually occurs by day 28. Other toxicities include alopecia, nausea, and vomiting. Nephrotoxicity and neurotoxicity are uncommon; however, these toxicities may become more severe in high-dose carboplatin studies in which myelosuppression is controlled by autologous bone marrow transplantation.

Oxaliplatin

The dose-limiting toxicity of oxaliplatin is sensory neuropathy, particularly paraesthesia and dysaesthesia in the extremities, triggered or enhanced by exposure to cold. The severity depends on the cumulative oxaliplatin dose and it is mostly or completely reversible. Other toxicities associated with oxaliplatin treatment include haematological toxicity, nausea, vomiting, and diarrhoea. Unlike cisplatin, little nephrotoxicity is observed.

Pharmacodynamics

Platinum pharmacodynamics has involved predicting both toxicity and tumour response to platinum-based chemotherapy. To achieve these goals, investigators have used pharmacokinetic parameters and cellular determinants such as platinum–DNA adduct levels and relative gene expression in leucocytes and tumour samples. As with other anticancer agents, the observed inter-patient variability in toxicity and perhaps response is attributable to inter-patient pharmacokinetic differences. For example, Calvert *et al.*[84] showed that the dose of carboplatin required to achieve the same ultrafilterable platinum AUC in a group of patients varied two- to threefold. This difference was accounted for by inter-patient variability in renal clearance or

GFR. As mentioned above, the result of this study was the development of a carboplatin dosing formula which has improved the therapeutic index of carboplatin. A subsequent study by Jodrell *et al.*[89] showed that carboplatin AUC was a predictor of tumour response, thrombocytopenia, and leucopenia. The likelihood of tumour response increased with increasing AUC up to a level of 5–7 mg·min/ml, above which the response rates did not increase significantly.

Unlike carboplatin, cisplatin clearance does not correlate strongly with renal clearance and so patient dosing is still based on body surface area. As a result, the AUCs measured for cisplatin vary widely.[80,90] However, several clinical studies have established relationships between cisplatin dose (dose intensity and cumulative dose) and tumour response and toxicity.[91–94] Differences in the dose–response and dose–toxicity relationships may be explained by inter-patient differences in dose–AUC relationship or by other pharmacodynamic factors.

Peripheral leucocytes offer a convenient and easily obtainable tissue for monitoring platinum–DNA adduct formation. In fact, Fichtinger-Schepman *et al.*[95] demonstrated that the amount of platinum in tumour tissue correlates closely with the amount in healthy tissues, suggesting that WBCs are a reliable surrogate tissue for determining whether platinum–DNA adduct levels correlate with patient response to platinum-based chemotherapy. Several investigators have shown that the formation of platinum–DNA adducts in WBCs is predictive of response. For example, Reed *et al.*[96] measured the formation of intra-strand cross-links in WBC DNA from ovarian cancer patients treated with platinum-based chemotherapy using an ELISA assay. Peak adduct levels were associated with the response of the patients to chemotherapy. Patients whose WBCs contained an undetectable amount of platinum–DNA adducts showed no response to therapy. This group also demonstrated a correlation between adduct formation in WBCs and the occurrence of a complete response in patients with poor prognosis testicular cancer.[97] In a paediatric study, Peng *et al.*[98] used ELISA to measure platinum–DNA adducts in the WBCs of 24 children with solid tumours following cisplatin or carboplatin therapy. Platinum–DNA adduct levels did not correlate with AUC, suggesting that both pharmacokinetic and cellular factors are responsible for platinum–DNA adduct formation.

Using FAAS, Schellens *et al.*[99] found a significant correlation between ultrafilterable cisplatin AUC and the area under the platinum–DNA adduct–time curve

(AUA) in the WBCs of patients treated with cisplatin. AUC and AUA were also significantly higher in responding patients than in non-responding patients. They concluded that dosing patients with cisplatin by AUC or AUA might lead to improved response rates. Overall, these studies indicate that, in addition to tumour cell resistance, clinical resistance to platinum-based chemotherapy may be the result of host factors that influence the bioavailability of drug.

Future directions

In the past three decades, platinum drugs have made a significant impact in cancer chemotherapy. At the present time, most solid tumours are treated with combination regimens that contain a platinum drug. Also, new analogues that have the potential of being less toxic and offering a different spectrum of activity than existing platinum drugs are undergoing phase I clinical trials. It is hoped that the development of new drugs and new combinations will increase the therapeutic index of these novel transition metal complexes. Understanding the molecular basis for resistance to platinum drugs and the pharmacodynamics of platinum-based chemotherapy may also lead to the development of effective resistance modulators.

References

1. Rosenberg B, Van Camp L, Trosko JE, Mansour VH (1969) Platinum compounds: a new class of potent antitumour agents. *Nature*, **222**, 385–6.
2. O'Dwyer PJ, Johnson SW, Hamilton TC (1997) In De Vita VTJ (ed) *Cancer: Principles and Practice of Oncology* (5th edn). Philadelphia, PA: JB Lippincott, 418–32.
3. Kelland LR (1997) In Teicher BA (ed) *Cancer Therapeutics: Experimental and Clinical Agents*. Totowa, NJ: Humana Press, 93–112.
4. Mauldin SK, Plescia M, Richard FA, Wyrick SD, Voyksner RD, Chaney SG (1988) Displacement of the bidentate malonate ligand from (d,l-trans-1,2-diaminocyclohexane)malonatoplatinum(II) by physiologically important compounds *in vitro*. *Biochem Pharmacol*, **37**, 3321–33.
5. Raymond E, Faivre S, Woynarowski JM, Chaney SG (1998) Oxaliplatin: mechanism of action and antineoplastic activity. *Semin Oncol*, **25** (Suppl 5), 4–12.
6. Higby DJ, Wallace HJ, Albert DJ, Holland JF (1974) Diaminodichloroplatinum: a phase I study showing responses in testicular and other tumors. *Cancer*, **33**, 1219–25.
7. Loehrer PJ, Einhorn LH, Elson PJ, *et al.* (1992) A randomized comparison of cisplatin alone or in combination with methotrexate, vinblastine, and doxorubicin in patients with metastatic urothelial carcinoma: a cooperative group study. *J Clin Oncol* **10**, 1066–73.
8. Qazi F, McGuire WP (1995) The treatment of epithelial ovarian cancer. *CA Cancer J Clin*, **45**, 88–101.
9. McGuire WP, Hoskins WJ, Brady MF, *et al.* (1996) Cyclophosphamide and cisplatin compared with paclitaxel and cisplatin in patients with stage III and stage IV ovarian cancer. *N Engl J Med*, **334**, 1–6.
10. Schilder RJ, Shea TC (1998) Multiple cycles of high-dose chemotherapy for ovarian cancer. *Semin Oncol*, **25**, 349–55.
11. Roth BJ (1996) Chemotherapy for advanced bladder cancer. *Semin Oncol*, **23**, 633–44.
12. Waxman J, Wasan H (1994) Platinum-based chemotherapy for bladder cancer. *Semin Oncol*, **21** (suppl 12), 54–60.
13. Mottet-Auselo N, Bons-Rosset F, Costa P, Louis JF, Navratil H (1993) Carboplatin and urothelial tumors. *Oncology*, **50**, 28–36.
14. Planting AS, de Mulder PH, de Graeff A, Verweij J (1997) Phase II study of weekly high-dose cisplatin for six cycles in patients with locally advanced squamous cell carcinoma of the head and neck. *Eur J Cancer*, **33**, 61–5.
15. Vogl SE, Schoenfeld DA, Kaplan BH, Lerner HJ, Engstrom PF, Horton J (1985) A randomized prospective comparison of methotrexate with a combination of methotrexate, bleomycin, and cisplatin in head and neck cancer. *Cancer*, **56**, 432–42.
16. Ervin TJ, Clark JR, Weichselbaum RR, *et al.* (1987) An analysis of induction and adjuvant chemotherapy in the multidisciplinary treatment of squamous-cell carcinoma of the head and neck. *J Clin Oncol*, **5**, 10–20.
17. Chang TM (1988) Induction chemotherapy for advanced head and neck cancers: a literature review. *Head Neck Surg*, **10**, 150–9.
18. Schilling T, Heinrich B, Kau R, *et al.* (1997) Paclitaxel administered over 3 h followed by cisplatin in patients with advanced head and neck squamous cell carcinoma: a clinical phase I study. *Oncology*, **54**, 89–95.
19. Hitt R, Hornedo J, Colomer R, *et al.* (1997) Study of escalating doses of paclitaxel plus cisplatin in patients with inoperable head and neck cancer. *Semin Oncol*, **24** (Suppl 2), 58–64.
20. Kelsen D, Ginsberg R, Bains M, *et al.* (1997) A phase II trial of paclitaxel and cisplatin in patients with locally advanced metastatic esophageal cancer: a preliminary report. *Semin Oncol*, **24** (Suppl 19), S77–81.
21. Sweeney CJ, Sandler AB (1998) Treatment of advanced (stages III and IV) non-small-cell lung cancer. *Curr Probl Cancer*, **22**, 85–132.
22. Sandler AB (1997) Current management of small cell lung cancer. *Semin Oncol*, **24**, 463–76.
23. Becouarn Y, Rougier P (1998) Clinical efficacy of oxaliplatin monotherapy: phase II trials in advanced colorectal cancer. *Semin Oncol*, **25** (Suppl 5), 23–31.
24. Bleiberg H, de Gramont A (1998) Oxaliplatin plus 5-fluorouracil: clinical experience in patients with

advanced colorectal cancer. *Semin Oncol*, **25** (Suppl 5), 32–9.

25. Rosenberg B, Van Camp L, Krigas T (1965) Inhibition of cell division in Escherichia coli by electrolysis products from a platinum electrode. *Nature*, **205**, 698–9.

26. Harder HC, Rosenberg B (1970) Inhibitory effects of anti-tumor platinum compounds on DNA, RNA and protein syntheses in mammalian cells *in vitro*. *Int J Cancer*, **6**, 207–16.

27. Howle JA, Gale GR (1970) Cis-dichlorodiammineplatinum(II) Persistent and selective inhibition of deoxyribonucleic acid synthesis *in vivo*. *Biochem Pharmacol*, **19**, 2757–62.

28. Fraval HN, Rawlings CJ, Roberts JJ (1978) Increased sensitivity of UV-repair-deficient human cells to DNA bound platinum products which unlike thymine dimers are not recognized by an endonuclease extracted from *Micrococcus luteus*. *Mutat Res*, **51**, 121–32.

29. Poll EHA, Abrahams PJ, Arwert F, Eriksson AW (1984) Host-cell reactivation of *cis*-diamminedichloroplatinum(II)-treated SV40 DNA in normal human, Fanconi anaemia and xeroderma pigmentosum fibroblasts. *Mutat Res*, **132**, 181–7.

30. Eastman A (1987) The formation, isolation and characterization of DNA adducts produced by anticancer platinum complexes. *Pharmacol Ther*, **34**, 155–66.

31. Plooy ACM, Fichtinger-Schepman AMJ, Schutte HH, van Dijk M, Lohman PHM (1985) The quantitative detection of various Pt–DNA-adducts in Chinese hamster ovary cells treated with cisplatin: application of immunochemical techniques. *Carcinogenesis*, **6**, 561–6.

32. Fichtinger-Schepman AMJ, van der Veer JL, den Hartog JHJ, Lohman PHM, Reedijk J (1985) Adducts of the antitumor drug *cis*-diamminedichloroplatinum(II) with DNA: formation, identification, and quantitation. *Biochemistry*, **24**, 707–13.

33. Blommaert FA, van Kijk-Knijnenburg HCM, Dijt FJ, *et al.* (1995) Formation of DNA adducts by the anticancer drug carboplatin: different nucleotide sequence preferences *in vitro* and in cells. *Biochemistry*, **34**, 8474–80.

34. Knox RJ, Friedlos F, Lydall DA, Roberts JJ (1986) Mechanism of cytotoxicity of anticancer platinum drugs: evidence that *cis*-diamminedichloroplatinum(II) and *cis*-diammine-(1,1-cyclobutanedicarboxylato)platinum(II) differ only in the kinetics of their interaction with DNA. *Cancer Res*, **46**, 1972–9.

35. Saris CP, van de Vaart PJM, Rietbroek RC, Blommaert FA (1996) *In vitro* formation of DNA adducts by cisplatin, lobaplatin and oxaliplatin in calf thymus DNA in solution and in cultured human cells. *Carcinogenesis*, **17**, 2763–9.

36. Rixe O, Ortuzar W, Alvarez M, *et al.* (1996) Oxaliplatin, tetraplatin, cisplatin, and carboplatin: spectrum of activity in drug-resistant cell lines and in the cell lines of the National Cancer Institute's Anticancer Drug Screen panel. *Biochem Pharmacol*, **52**, 1855–65.

37. Scheeff ED, Briggs J, Howell S (1999) Molecular modeling of the intrastrand guarine-guarine DNA adducts produced by cisplatin and oxaliplatin. *Mol Pharmacol*, **56**, 633–43.

38. Johnson SW, Ferry KV, Hamilton TC (1998) Recent insights into platinum drug resistance in cancer. *Drug Resist Updates*, **1**, 243–54.

39. Waud WR (1987) Differential uptake of *cis*-diamminedichloroplatinum(II) by sensitive and resistant murine L1210 leukemia cells. *Cancer Res*, **47**, 6549–55.

40. Richon VM, Schulte N, Eastman A (1987) Multiple mechanisms of resistance to *cis*-diamminedichloroplatinum(II) in murine leukaemia L1210 cells. *Cancer Res*, **47**, 2056–61.

41. Teicher BA, Holden SA, Kelley MJ, *et al.* (1987) Characterization of a human sqamous carcinoma cell line resistant to *cis*-diamminedichloroplatinum(II). *Cancer Res*, **47**, 388–93.

42. Johnson SW, Shen D, Pastan I, Gottesman MM, Hamilton TC (1996) Cross-resistance, cisplatin accumulation, and platinum–DNA adduct formation and removal in cisplatin-sensitive and resistant human hepatoma cell lines. *Exp Cell Res*, **226**, 133–9.

43. Gately DP, Howell SB (1993) Cellular accumulation of the anticancer agent cisplatin: a review. *Br J Cancer*, **67**, 1171–6.

44. Johnson SW, Laub PB, Beesley JS, Ozols RF, Hamilton TC (1997) Increased platinum–DNA damage tolerance is associated with cisplatin resistance and cross-resistance to various chemotherapeutic agents in unrelated human ovarian cancer cell lines. *Cancer Res*, **57**, 850–6.

45. Ishikawa T, Ali-Osman F (1993) Glutathione-associated *cis*-diamminedichloroplatinum(II) metabolism and ATP-dependent efflux from leukemia cells. Molecular characterization of glutathione-platinum complex and its biological significance. *J Biol Chem*, **268**, 20116–25.

46. Mistry P, Loh SY, Kelland LR, Harrap KR (1993) Effect of buthionine sulfoximine on PtII and PtIV drug accumulation and the formation of glutathione conjugates in human ovarian-carcinoma cell lines. *Int J Cancer*, **55**, 848–56.

47. Godwin AK, Meister A, O'Dwyer PJ, Huang CS, Hamilton TC, Anderson ME (1992) High resistance to cisplatin in human ovarian cancer cell lines is associated with marked increase of glutathione synthesis. *Proc Natl Acad Sci USA*, **89**, 3070–4.

48. Hosking LK, Whelan RD, Shellard SA, Bedford P, Hill BT (1990) An evaluation of the role of glutathione and its associated enzymes in the expression of differential sensitivities of antitumour agents shown by a range of human tumour cell lines. *Biochem Pharmacol*, **40**, 1833–42.

49. Britten RA, Green JA, Broughton C, Browning PG, White R, Warenius HM (1991) The relationship between nuclear glutathione levels and resistance to melphalan in human ovarian tumour cells. *Biochem Pharmacol*, **41**, 647–9.

50. Mistry P, Kelland LR, Abel G, Sidhar S, Harrap KR (1991) The relationships between glutathione, glutathione-*S*-transferase and cytotoxicity of platinum drugs and melphalan in eight human ovarian carcinoma cell lines. *Br J Cancer*, **64**, 215–20.

51. Kelley SL, Basu A, Teicher BA, Hacker MP, Hamer DH, Lazo JS (1988) Overexpression of metallothionein confers resistance to anticancer drugs. *Science*, **241**, 1813–15.

52. Kondo Y, Woo ES, Michalska AE, Choo KH, JS L (1995) Metallothionein null cells have increased sensitivity to anticancer drugs. *Cancer Res*, 55, 2021–3.

53. Köberle B, Grimaldi KA, Sunters A, Hartley JA, Kelland LR, Masters JR (1997) DNA repair capacity and cisplatin sensitivity of human testis tumour cells. *Int J Cancer*, 70, 551–5.

54. Zeng Rong N, Paterson J, Alpert L, Tsao MS, Viallet J, Alaoui Jamali MA (1995) Elevated DNA repair capacity is associated with intrinsic resistance of lung cancer to chemotherapy. *Cancer Res*, 55, 4760–4.

55. Johnson SW, Perez RP, Godwin AK, et al. (1994) Role of platinum–DNA adduct formation and removal in cisplatin resistance in human ovarian cancer cell lines. *Biochem Pharmacol*, 47, 689–97.

56. Johnson SW, Swiggard PA, Handel LM, et al. (1994) Relationship between platinum–DNA adduct formation and removal and cisplatin cytotoxicity in cisplatin-sensitive and -resistant human ovarian cancer cells. *Cancer Res*, 54, 5911–16.

57. Yen L, Woo A, Christopoulopoulos G, et al. (1995) Enhanced host cell reactivation capacity and expression of DNA repair genes in human breast cancer cells resistant to bi-functional alkylating agents. *Mutat Res*, 337, 179–89.

58. Ali Osman F, Berger MS, Rairkar A, Stein DE (1994) Enhanced repair of a cisplatin-damaged reporter chloramphenicol-O-acetyltransferase gene and altered activities of DNA polymerases alpha and beta, and DNA ligase in cells of a human malignant glioma following *in vivo* cisplatin therapy. *J Cell Biochem* 54, 11–9.

59. Eastman A, Schulte N (1988) Enhanced DNA repair as a mechanism of resistance to *cis*-diamminedichloroplatinum(II) *Biochemistry*, 27, 4730–4.

60. Zhen W, Link CJJ, O'Connor PM, et al. (1992) Increased gene-specific repair of cisplatin interstrand cross-links in cisplatin-resistant human ovarian cancer cell lines. *Mol Cell Biol*, 12, 3689–98.

61. Mamenta EL, Poma EE, Kaufmann WK, Delmastro DA, Grady HL, Chaney SG (1994) Enhanced replicative bypass of platinum–DNA adducts in cisplatin-resistant human ovarian carcinoma cell lines. *Cancer Res*, 54, 3500–5.

62. Hoffmann JS, Pillaire MJ, Maga G, Podust V, Hübscher U, Villani G (1995) DNA polymerase beta bypasses *in vitro* a single d(GpG)-cisplatin adduct placed on codon 13 of the HRAS gene. *Proc Natl Acad Sci USA*, 92, 5356–60.

63. Segal Bendirdjian E, Jacquemin Sablon A (1995) Cisplatin resistance in a murine leukemia cell line is associated with a defective apoptotic process. *Exp Cell Res*, 218, 201–12.

64. Miyashita T, Reed JC (1993) Bcl-2 oncoprotein blocks chemotherapy-induced apoptosis in a human leukemia cell line. *Blood*, 81, 151–7.

65. Minn AJ, Rudin CM, Boise LH, Thompson CB (1995) Expression of bcl-xL can confer a multidrug resistance phenotype. *Blood*, 86, 1903–10.

66. Minami T, Ichii M, Okazaki Y (1995) Comparison of three different methods for measurement of tissue platinum level. *Biol Trace Elem Res*, 48, 37–44.

67. Tothill P, Klys HS, Matheson LM, McKay K, Smyth JF (1992) The long-term retention of platinum in human tissues following the administration of cisplatin or carboplatin for cancer chemotherapy. *Eur J Cancer*, 28, 1358–61.

68. Gamelin E, Le Bouil A, Boisdron-Celle M, et al. (1997) Cumulative pharmacokinetic study of oxaliplatin, administered every three weeks, combined with 5-fluorouracil in colorectal cancer patients. *Clin Cancer Res*, 3, 891–9.

69. Ma J, Verweij J, Planting AST, et al. (1995) Current sample handling methods for measurement of platinum–DNA adducts in leucocytes in man lead to discrepant results in DNA adduct levels and DNA repair. *Br J Cancer*, 71, 512–7.

70. Poirier MC, Lippard SJ, Zwelling LA, et al. (1982) Antibodies elicited against *cis*-diamminedichloroplatinum(II)-modified DNA are specific for *cis*-diamminedichloroplatinum(II)-DNA adducts formed *in vivo* and *in vitro*. *Proc Natl Acad Sci USA*, 79, 6443–7.

71. Tilby MJ, Johnson C, Knox RJ, Cordell J, Roberts JJ, Dean CJ (1991) Sensitive detection of DNA modifications induced by cisplatin and carboplatin *in vitro* and *in vivo* using a monoclonal antibody. *Cancer Res*, 51, 123–9.

72. Zwelling LA, Kohn KW (1982) In Chabner B (ed) *Pharmacologic Principles of Cancer Treatment*. Philadelphia, PA: W.B. Saunders, 309–339.

73. van der Vijgh WJF (1991) Clinical pharmacokinetics of carboplatin. *Clin Pharmacokinet*, 21, 242–61.

74. Duffull SB, Robinson BA (1997) Clinical pharmacokinetics and dose optimisation of carboplatin. *Clin Pharmacokinet*, 33, 161–83.

75. Extra JM, Marty M, Brienza S, Misset JL (1998) Pharmacokinetics and safety profile of oxaliplatin. *Semin Oncol*, 25 (Suppl 5), 13–22.

76. De Conti RC, Toftness BR, Lange RC, Creasey WA (1973) Clinical and pharmacological studies with *cis*-diamminedichloroplatinum(II). *Cancer Res*, 33, 1310–15.

77. Gormley PE, Bull JM, LeRoy AF, Cysyk R (1979) Kinetics of *cis*-dichlorodiammineplatinum. Clin *Pharmacol Ther*, 25, 351–7.

78. Repta AJ, Long DF (1980) In Prestayko AW, Crooke ST, Carter SK (ed) *Cisplatin. Current Status and New Developments*. New York: Academic Press, 285–304.

79. Vermorken JB, Van der Vijgh WJF, Klein I, Hart AA, Gall HE, Pinedo HM (1984) Pharmacokinetics of free and total platinum species after short-term infusion of cisplatin. *Cancer Treat Rep*, 68, 505–13.

80. Himmelstein KJ, Patton TF, Belt RJ, Taylor S, Repta AJ, Sternson LA (1981) Clinical kinetics on intact cisplatin and some related species. *Clin Pharmacol Ther*, 29, 658–64.

81. Belt RJ, Himmelstein KJ, Patton TF (1979) Pharmacokinetics of non-protein-bound platinum species following administration of *cis*-dichlorodiammineplatinum(II). *Cancer Treat Rep*, 63, 1515–21.

82. Casper ES, Kelsen DP, Alcock NW, Young CW (1979) Platinum concentrations in bile and plasma following rapid and 6-hour infusions of *cis*-dichlorodiammineplatinum(II) *Cancer Treat Rep*, 63, 2023–5.

83. Harland SJ, Newell DR, Siddik ZH, Chadwick R, Calvert AH, Harrap KR (1984) Pharmacokinetics of *cis*-diammine-1,1-cyclobutane dicarboxylate platinum(II). in patients with normal and impaired renal function. *Cancer Res*, **44**, 1693–7.

84. Calvert AH, Newell DR, Gumbrell LA, *et al.* (1989) Carboplatin dosage: prospective evaluation of a simple formula based on renal function. *J Clin Oncol*, **7**, 1748–56.

85. Cvitkovic E, Spaulding J, Bethune C, Martin J, Whitmore W (1977) Improvement of *cis*-dichloro-diammineplatinum (NSC 119875): therapeutic index in an animal model. *Cancer*, **39**, 1357–61.

86. Hayes DM, Cvitkovic E, Goldberg RB, Scheiner E, Helson L, Krakoff IH (1977) High dose *cis*-platinum diammine dichloride: amelioration of renal toxicity by mannitol diuresis. *Cancer*, **39**, 1372–81.

87. Gregg RW, Molepo JM, Monpetit VJ, *et al.* (1992) Cisplatin neurotoxicity: the relationship between dosage, time, and platinum concentration in neurologic tissues, and morphologic evidence of toxicity. *J Clin Oncol*, **10**, 795–803.

88. Calvert AH, Harland SJ, Newell DR, *et al.* (1982) Early clinical studies with *cis*-diammine-1,1-cyclobutane dicarboxylate platinum II. *Cancer Chemother Pharmacol*, **9**, 140–7.

89. Jodrell DI, Egorin MJ, Canetta RM, *et al.* (1992) Relationships between carboplatin exposure and tumor response and toxicity in patients with ovarian cancer. *J Clin Oncol*, **10**, 520–8.

90. Reece PHA, Stafford I, Russell J, Khan M, Fill PG (1987) Creatinine clearance as a predictor of ultra-filterable platinum disposition in cancer patients treated with cisplatin: relationship between peak ultrafilterable platinum plasma levels and nephrotoxicity. *J Clin Oncol*, **5**, 304–9.

91. Ozols RF, Idhe DC, Linehan M, Jacob J, Ostchega Y, Young RC (1988) A randomized trial of standard chemotherapy v a high-dose chemotherapy regimen in the treatment of poor prognosis nonseminomatous germ-cell tumors. *J Clin Oncol*, **6**, 1031–40.

92. Kaye SB, Lewis CR, Paul J, *et al.* (1992) Randomised study of two doses of cisplatin with cyclophosphamide in epithelial ovarian cancer. Lancet, **340**, 329–33.

93. Levin L, Simon R, Hryniuk W (1993) Importance of multiagent chemotherapy regimens in ovarian carcinoma: dose intensity analysis. *J Natl Cancer Inst*, **85**, 1732–42.

94. Bruckner HW, Wallach R, Cohen CJ, *et al.* (1981) High-dose platinum for the treatment of refractory ovarian cancer. *Gynecol Oncol*, **12**, 64–7.

95. Fichtinger-Schepman AMJ, van der Velde-Visser SD, van Dijk-Knijnenburg HCM, van Oosterom AT, Baan RA, Berends F (1990) Kinetics of the formation and removal of cisplatin–DNA adducts in blood cells and tumor tissue of cancer patients receiving chemotherapy: comparison with *in vitro* adduct formation. *Cancer Res*, **50**, 7887–94.

96. Reed E, Ozols RF, Tarone R, Yuspa SH, Poirier MC (1987) Platinum–DNA adducts in leukocyte DNA correlate with disease response in ovarian cancer patients receiving platinum-based chemotherapy. *Proc Natl Acad Sci USA*, **84**, 5024–8.

97. Reed E, Ozols RF, Tarone R, Yuspa SH, Poirier MC (1988) The measurement of cisplatin-DNA adduct levels in testicular cancer patients. *Carcinogenesis*, **9**, 1909–11.

98. Peng B, Tilby MJ, English MW, *et al.* (1997) Platinum–DNA adduct formation in leucocytes of children in relation to pharmacokinetics after cisplatin and carboplatin therapy. *Br J Cancer*, **76**, 1466–73.

99. Schellens JHM, Ma J, Planting AST, *et al.* (1996) Relationship between the exposure to cisplatin, DNA-adduct formation in leucocytes and tumour response in patients with solid tumours. *Br J Cancer*, **73**, 1569–75.

100. Patton TF, Himmelstein KH, Belt R, Bannister SJ, Sternson LA, Repta AJ (1978) Plasma levels and urinary excretion of filterable platinum species following bolus injection and iv infusion of cis-dichlorodiamineplatinum-(II) in man. *Cancer Treat Rep*, **62**, 1359–62.

101. Van Echo DA, Egorin MJ, Whitaere MY, Olman EA, Aisner J (1984) Phase I clinical and pharmacologic trial of carboplatin daily for 5 days. *Cancer Treat Rep*, **68**, 1103–14.

102. Iler JM, Trump DL, Tutsch LD, Earhart RH, Davis TE, Tormey DC (1986) Phase I clinical trial and pharmacokinetics of carboplatin (NSC 241240) by single monthly 30-minute infusion. *Cancer*, **57**, 222–5.

103. Lee EJ, Egorin MJ, Van Echo DA, Cohen AE, Tait N, Schiffer CA (1988) Phase I and pharmacokinetic trial of carboplatin in refractory adult leukemia. *J Natl Cancer Inst*, **80**, 131–5.

104. Oguri S, Sakakibara T, Mase H, Shimizu T, Ishikawa K, Kimura K, Smyth RD (1988) Clinical pharmacokinetics of carboplatin. *J Clin Pharmacol*, **28**, 208–15.

14 | *Novel tyrosine kinase inhibitors: focus on imatinib and gefitinib*

Wandena S. Lakhai, Jos H. Beijnen, and Jan H. M. Schellens

Introduction

Signal transduction is the chemistry that allows communication at the cellular level. Cells sense signals from both the outside environment and other cells, and in response they regulate all aspects of cell function. Receptors are pivotal in signal transduction pathways. Binding of ligands to receptors leads to a conformational change in the receptor that initiates signalling. The final response of the cell can be metabolism, cell division, death, survival, differentiation, or movement.

Receptor tyrosine kinases

Receptor tyrosine kinases are transmembrane proteins that can be divided into those that contain a tyrosine

Summary

	Imatinib	Gefitinib
Brand names	Glivec	Iressa
Other names	STI571	ZD1839
Molecular weight (Da)	589.7	446.9
Mechanism of action	Binding to part of the ATP binding pocket and stabilizing the inactive non-ATP binding form	Competes for the ATP binding site in the cytoplasmic tail of EGFR tyrosine kinase
Cell-cycle specificity	None	None
Route of administration	Oral	Oral
Protein binding (%)	95	90
Metabolism	CYP 3A4; major metabolite *N*-desmethyl imatinib	CYP 3A4; major metabolite *O*-desmethyl gefitinib
Elimination	Faeces (68%), urine (13%)	Faeces (86%), urine (< 4%)
Half-life (h)	18	28
Toxicities	Haematological, nausea, vomiting, dyspepsia and/or upper abdominal pain, oedema	Diarrhoea, rash, acne, dry skin, nausea, vomiting
Unique features		No significant myelosuppression

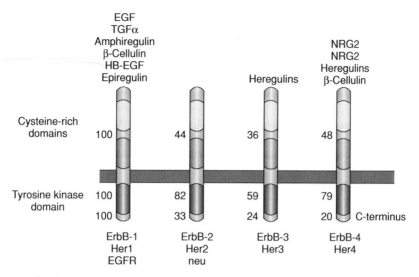

Figure 14.1. The HER family and ligands.

kinase activity as an integral part of the receptor molecule, and those that are inactive in this respect but can recruit a kinase as a result of ligand binding.

Receptors with integral kinase activity

Receptors with integral kinase activity have an extracellular ligand binding domain, a transmembrane region, and a multifunctional cytoplasmic tail. The tail has an ATP binding site plus tyrosine kinase activity capable of phosphorylating itself (autophosphorylation) as well as other proteins.[1]

The EGFR (HER) family of tyrosine kinase receptors is a good example of these types of receptors. The four members of the EGFR family are EGFR (HER1 or erbB1), HER2/neu (erbB2), HER3 (erbB3), and HER4 (erbB4) (Fig. 14.1).

Except for the kinase-deficient HER3, there is an approximate 80% homology in the tyrosine kinase domains.[2] The extracellular ligand binding domain is less conserved. Binding of ligands to the extracellular domain results in receptor dimerization and activation of the receptor's tyrosine kinase activity by autophosphorylation.[3] Subsequently, the phosphorylated tyrosines serve as binding sites for a number of cytoplasmic signal-transducing molecules. Activation of these pathways downstream of the EGFR leads to cell proliferation, migration, differentiation, adhesion, protection from apoptosis, and gene transcription.[4]

The specificity of the signalling response from activated EGFR is highly dependent on the identity of the ligand and the cellular levels of the co-receptors. EGFR can homodimerize with another EGFR monomer or heterodimerize with HER2/neu (erbB2), HER3 (erbB3), or HER4 (erbB4) (Fig. 14.2).[5]

For example, when EGFR heterodimerize with HER3 or HER4, the phosphatidylinositol-3 kinase and the downstream protein kinase Akt are activated.[6] After activation, Akt transduces signals that regulate a variety of biological processes including apoptosis and cellular proliferation.[5] The identity of the ligand is also important for the specificity of the signalling output. The EGFR (erbB1, HER1) can bind the ligand's epidermal growth factor (EGF), transforming growth factor-α (TGF-α) and amphiregulin polypeptides, whereas HER2/neu (erbB2) has no obvious ligands. A summary of the HER family of receptors and their ligands is shown in Figure 14.1.

Some ligands are dimeric; therefore the ligand is able to bind two receptors simultaneously. Other ligands

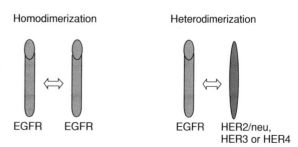

Figure 14.2. Homodimerization and heterodimerization of EGFR.

are monomeric but have two receptor binding sites that allow them to induce receptor dimerization. Both the ligands and the co-receptors stimulate the receptor dimerization that is needed to activate the receptor.

Receptors that recruit tyrosine kinases

A number of receptors do not have intrinsic enzymatic activity but stimulate associated tyrosine kinases. The cytokine and interferon receptors associate constitutively with members of the Janus kinase (Jak) family of tyrosine kinases.[7] The kinases appear to be inactive in the absence of ligand but, as happens in receptors with intrinsic tyrosine kinase activity, signalling is initiated by ligand-stimulated heterodimerization of the receptors. Dimerization of the receptors brings the Jak kinases into proximity with each other or with other tyrosine kinases, and transphosphorylation leads to their activation. Downstream signalling is dependent on the active Jak kinases and other substrates.

Linking tyrosine kinase receptors with cancer and progression

Tyrosine kinases are altered in many cancers. Excessive EGFR signalling in tumours is usually the result of EGFR over-expression and/or the excessive production and availability of receptor ligands. For example, several human cancers, including those of the upper aerodigestive tract, lung, colon, pancreas, breast, ovary, bladder, and kidney, as well as gliomas, display EGFR mRNA and/or protein over-expression. This over-expression is sometimes the result of EGFR gene amplification and is often associated with increased expression of the receptor ligands transforming TGF-α or amphiregulin.[5] Other possible mechanisms of aberrant EGFR signalling include heterodimerization with other erbB receptors such as erbB2 (HER2), transactivation by heterologous signalling networks, loss of regulatory mechanisms of receptor signalling,[8] and activating mutations. For example, the most common mutant of the EGFR is the EGFRvIII, which lacks an external ligand binding domain and has a constitutively activated tyrosine kinase.[9] The result of excessive signalling is tumour progression, including the promotion of proliferation, angiogenesis, invasion/metastasis, and inhibition of apoptosis.[10,11] The expression of EGFR in tumours has been correlated with disease progression, poor survival, poor response to therapy,[12] and the development of resistance to cytotoxic agents.[13]

Oncogenes with kinase activity

Of considerable interest is the description of a number of oncogenes with constitutive kinase activity. These molecules are derived from genes including c-ABL, c-FMS, FLT3, c-KIT, and PDGFRβ which are normally involved in the regulation of hematopoiesis.[14] The kinase activity of the oncogene is constitutively activated by mutations that remove inhibitory domains of the molecule or induce the kinase domain to adopt an activated configuration. As a result of such constitutive activation a number of signalling cascades, such as the Jak pathways and the phosphatidylinositol-3 kinase pathway, are activated that enhance tumour progression.

Tyrosine kinases as a target for cancer therapy

An ideal molecular target in tumours would be one that is differentially expressed or differentially functional in tumour versus non-tumour tissues. In addition, molecular epidemiology has identified that such a target is a dominant predictor of poor disease outcome. Some tyrosine kinases are such targets. The activation of tyrosine kinases is tightly regulated in normal cells, but in tumour cells the signal transduction pathways are disrupted in such a way that excessive signalling results in tumour progression.

EGFR inhibitors

Several *in vitro* and *in vivo* studies have shown that interruption of signalling with various EGFR inhibitors that recognize the extracellular or intracellular domain of the receptor (Fig. 14.1) results in inhibition of tumour cell proliferation and/or viability.[11] These observations, together with the association of EGFR over-expression with poor patient prognosis, the ability to identify EGFR-expressing human tumours in diagnostic tissues, and the lack of a critical physiological role of EGFR in healthy persons, have all suggested this signalling network as an ideal target for novel cancer therapeutic strategies.[2]

The first antireceptor strategy has been the use of monoclonal antibodies that recognize the receptor's extracellular domain. These monoclonal antibodies compete for ligand binding and induce EGFR dimerization and downregulation from the cell surface. In some cases, antibody-induced receptor internalization may be followed by routing to a lysosomal compartment.

The ability to induce receptor downregulation and to block its catalytic function has been shown with the 528 mouse IgG2a, the 225 mouse IgG1, and the 225 humanized monoclonal antibody.[15] In tumour cells with EGFR over-expression, the result was inhibition of EGFR signalling leading to cell-cycle arrest and cell death. In a phase I trial with the EGFR mouse monoclonal antibody 225Mab it was also shown that the antibody localized specifically in squamous cell cancers of the lung that had not been screened for EGFR expression before the study.[16]

This study proves that the differential expression of EGFR in tumour versus non-tumour tissue can provide a therapeutic window for cancers with a high level of receptor expression (e.g. in the treatment of head and neck cancer) because these tumour types are characterized by a high level of EGFR over-expression (80–100%).[8] The first monoclonal antibody approved for cancer therapy was trastuzumab.[17] Trastuzumab binds to and blocks HER2/neu (erbB2). Over-expression of HER2/neu occurs in approximately 25% of breast cancers and is associated with a poor prognosis. Currently, trastuzumab is approved for the treatment of metastatic breast cancer, alone or in combination with paclitaxel.[18] Trastuzumab is also studied alone and in combination with other anticancer agents in HER2-expressing cancers, such as prostate and non-small cell lung cancer (NSCLC). In both tumour types, HER2 reaches its highest expression in poorly differentiated tumours and is associated with poor survival.[19,20]

There are also monoclonal antibodies (MDX-447) that compete with ligands for binding to EGFR and recruit Fc-receptor-expressing immune effector cells, such as natural killer cells. These immune effector cells can mediate tumour cell lysis (antibody-dependent cellular toxicity).[21] These monoclonal antibodies show that both kinase blockade and immune mechanisms may contribute to the antitumour activity.

The second antireceptor approach was based on the observation that mutations in the ATP binding pocket of the EGFR cytoplasmic tail affect its tyrosine kinase function, suggesting that the receptor's tyrosine kinase is essential for EGFR-mediated tumour progression. This approach resulted in random screening from natural or synthetic compound libraries of small molecules (molecular weight ~300–500 Da) that compete for the ATP binding site in the EGFR cytoplasmic tail.[22,23] These small molecules inhibit ATP binding to the tyrosine kinase domain of the receptor, thereby inhibiting tyrosine kinase activity and autophosphorylation, and subsequently blocking signal transduction from the EGFR.

Several small-molecule inhibitors of the EGFR receptor are currently in clinical development and some of them have already been studied in phase II and III trials. Several studies have shown that higher concentrations of these inhibitors are required for continuous blockage of EGFR phosphorylation in intact cells (*in vivo*) than to inhibit purified EGFR *in vitro*. This is because of the high intracellular concentration of ATP.[24] The approximately 80% homology between EGFR and HER2 kinases has also initiated the development of bifunctional inhibitors, such as EKB-569, CI-1033 and GW572016, which inhibit both receptor kinases directly.[25]

Of the small-molecule inhibitors, imatinib (Glivec) and gefitinib (Iressa) have recently been accepted for registration. Because of this, these two agents will be discussed in greater detail in this chapter.

Imatinib (Glivec, STI571)

Imatinib exemplifies the successful development of a rationally designed molecularly targeted therapy for the treatment of a specific cancer. It received authorization from the U.S. Food and Drug Administration (FDA) in May 2001 and from the European Commission in November 2001. The product is presented as hard gelatin capsules available in doses of 50 or 100 mg. The active substance is the mesylate salt form of imatinib, a phenylaminopyrimidine derivate and is the 4-[(4-methyl-1-piperazinyl)methyl]-N-[4-methyl-3-] [4-(3-pyridinyl)-2-pyrimidinyl] amino]-phenyl]-benzamide methanesulphonic acid salt (Fig. 14.3).[26]

Therapeutic indications

Imatinib is indicated for the treatment of patients with newly diagnosed Philadelphia chromosome positive (Ph+) chronic myeloid leukaemia (CML) for whom

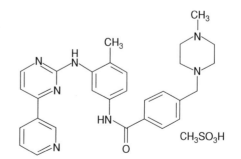

Figure 14.3. Chemical structure of imatinib.

stem-cell transplantation is not considered as first-line treatment.[27] Formerly, interferon-α (IFN) alone or in combination with cytosine-arabinoside (Ara-C) was the first-line standard treatment for CML patients who were not candidates for stem-cell transplantation. A phase III study compared treatment with either single-agent imatinib or a combination of IFN and Ara-C in a total of 1106 newly diagnosed patients with CML. The estimated rate of patients free of progression at 12 months was significantly higher in the imatinib arm than in the IFN-Ara-C arm. The estimated rate of progression-free survival at 12 months was 97.2% in the imatinib arm and 80.3% in the control arm. Other studies showed that some patients stopped IFN treatment because of toxicity. There were also patients who did not respond to IFN at all and some of them also developed resistance. Because of these failures, imatinib is now considered as the new gold standard for treatment of CML.[28–30]

CML is a myeloproliferative disorder. It accounts for 15%–20% of all cases of leukaemia. Clinically, the disease progresses through distinct phases referred to as chronic, accelerated and blast phase. The chronic or stable phase of the disease is characterized by excess numbers of myeloid cells that differentiate normally. Within an average of 4–6 years, the disease transforms through an accelerated phase to a fatal acute leukaemia, also known as blast crisis.[31] The hallmark of CML is the Ph chromosome. This chromosome results from a reciprocal translocation t(9;22) in a hematopoietic stem cell and results in the transfer of the Abelson (*abl*) oncogene to an area of chromosome 22 termed the breakpoint cluster region (*bcr*) and creates a fused *bcr–abl* gene.[27,32] The final product of this genetic rearrangement is an abnormal 210 kDa cytoplasmic fusion protein. This oncoprotein is responsible for most phenotypic abnormalities of chronic phase CML. The *bcr–abl* protein is oncogenic because its *abl*-derived tyrosine kinase is constitutively activated and transduces signals to various pathways in an autonomous fashion.[33] This results in increased proliferation, protection from apoptosis, and possibly genetic instability, leading to disease progression.[34]

Imatinib is also indicated for the treatment of adult patients with Kit (CD117) positive unresectable and/or metastatic gastrointestinal stromal tumours (GISTs).[27] GISTs predominantly affect middle-aged and older patients with a median age of 50–60 years.[35] About 60%–70% of GISTs occur in the stomach, 20%–30% in the small intestine, and 10% or less in the oesophagus, colon, and rectum.[36] CD117, the c-Kit proto-oncogene protein, is a transmembrane receptor for a growth factor known as the stem-cell factor (SCF). It is encoded by the c-Kit proto-oncogene located on chromosome 4q11–21.[37,38] Binding of SCF ligand to the receptor leads to dimerization, activation of the tyrosine kinases in the cytoplasmic tail, and activation of further signalling cascades controlling cell proliferation, adhesion, and differentiation. In GISTs the *c-Kit* gene is mutated, resulting in gain of function with permanent activation of the receptor in the absence of binding of the SCF ligand.[39] This results in uncontrolled growth of the tumour. *In vitro* and *in vivo* studies showed that imatinib can inhibit various types

Table 14.1   Inhibitory effect of imatinib on various types of Kit

Reference	Type of Kit	Phosphorylation Kit	Cell proliferation	
			In vitro	*In vivo*
Buchdunger *et al.*[40]	Wild	+	NE	NE
Heinrich *et al.*[30]	Wild	+	NE	NE
	Kit[560Gly]	+	+	NE
Ma *et al.*[41]	Wild	+	NE	NE
	Kit[816Val]	−	NE	NE
	Kit[816F]	−	NE	NE
	Kit[816Y]	−	NE	NE
	Kit[560Gly] + Kit[816Val]	−	−	NE
Tuveson *et al.*[42]	Kit[558AsnPro]	+	+	NE
	Kit[642Glu]	+	+	NE
Chen *et al.*[43]	Wild	+	+	+
	Kit[del559–560]	+	+	+
	Kit[642Glu]	+	+	+
	Kit[820Tyr]	+	+	+

+, inhibited; −, not inhibited; NE, not examined

of activating mutant Kit found in GISTs.[30,40–43] The effect of imatinib on Kit autophosphorylation, *in vitro* cellular proliferation, and *in vivo* tumorgenicity was examined in transfectants expressing various types of mutant Kit. The results are shown in Table 14.1.

Recently, imatinib has also been indicated for the treatment of dermatofibrosarcoma protuberans which is a slow-growing infiltrating dermal neoplasm of intermediate malignancy. Tumour cells are characterized by either ring chromosomes or linear translocations. Both the rings and linear translocations contain a specific fusion of the collagen type I alpha 1 (COL1A1) gene with the platelet-derived growth factor B-chain (PDGFB) gene. In all dermatofibrosarcoma protuberans cases that underwent molecular investigations, the breakpoint localization in PDGFB was found to be constant, placing exon 2 under the control of the COL1A1 promotor. In contrast, the COL1A1 breakpoint was found to be variably located within exon 6–49. The result of the fusion product is that PDGFB acts as a mitogen by autocrine stimulation of the PDGFR. It is constantly activated by the COL1A1 promotor. The preferred treatment of dermatofibrosarcoma protuberans is wide surgical excision with pathologically negative margins. Imatinib can also inhibit PDGFR tyrosine kinase, and such targeted therapy is encouraging for the treatment of the few dermatofibrosarcoma protuberans cases that are not manageable by surgery.[44]

In summary, imatinib has a restricted activity against various types of mutant Kit, bcr–abl, and PDGFR. Imatinib is not able to inhibit a wide variety of other tyrosine kinases, including members of the Jak kinase receptors, HER2/neu, the vascular epithelial growth factor receptors (VEGFRs), and many others.[45] The characteristics that distinguish sensitive from resistant kinases are only partially understood. Based on a crystal structure of the catalytic domain of *abl* complexed with imatinib, initial drug binding requires that the kinase is in an inactive conformation in which the activation loop is unphosphorylated. Unlike the active conformation, the inactive conformation is diverse among protein kinases. One factor possibly contributing to the specificity of imatinib for *abl* was reported to be the preservation of an ion pair between lysine and glutamine residue side chains in the inactive conformation of *abl* that appears to contribute to drug–substrate interaction.[45] Threonine residue 315 (T315) was also suggested to be necessary for the interaction of imatinib with *abl*. In accordance with this, T315 in *abl* is conserved in imatinib substrates PDGFR and Kit but is

replaced by a methionine in the imatinib-insensitive Jak2.[45]

Overall, these results indicate that imatinib can be used to treat tumours that express bcr–abl, various Kit mutations, and PDGFR. Tumours that are characterized by Jak kinase receptor, HER2/neu, or VEGFR over-expression cannot be treated efficiently with imatinib.

Mechanism of action

Imatinib was originally thought to inhibit kinase activity by acting as a competitive inhibitor of the ATP binding pocket. However, recent structural resolution of the *abl* catalytic domain complexed with imatinib showed that the drug occupies only part of the ATP binding pocket and that it produces its inhibitory effects by binding to and stabilizing the inactive non-ATP binding form of bcr–abl. As a consequence of imatinib binding to bcr–abl, three related effects are produced: inhibition of bcr–abl autophosphorylation, inhibition of substrate phosphorylation, and inhibition of cell proliferation.[46,47] Thus the specific signal transduction pathway abnormally activated in the leukaemic transformation process is inactivated by imatinib while the normal pathways are unaffected. Wild-type *abl* is also inhibited by imatinib, but owing to redundancy in signal transduction pathways, this phenomenon does not appear clinically to alter normal processes.[48]

Clinical pharmacology

The clinical development programme of imatinib mainly focused on the different stages of CML, including Ph+ acute lymphoblastic leukaemia (ALL) or acute myeloid leukaemia (AML).

Shortly thereafter, clinical trials were initiated in GIST patients.[49] c-Kit is also expressed in a variety of other tumours, including AML, small-cell lung carcinoma, germ-cell tumours, melanoma, myeloma, and neuroblastoma.[49] Whether c-Kit contributes to the pathogenesis of these diseases is not clear. Clinical trials in these disorders will be required to determine the activity of imatinib in these diseases. PDGFR expression occurs in dermatofibrosarcoma protuberans, glioblastomas, and many other tumours. The precise contribution of PDGFR to the growth and survival of these tumours is not clear. Again, clinical trials of imatinib have been initiated and may define the contribution of this pathway.

Pharmacodynamics

The pharmacodynamics of imatinib were investigated in one dose-finding study carried out in adult (>18 years) and paediatric (<18 years) patients. The study included 84 adult patients with chronic-phase CML intolerant to IFN and 59 adult patients with either CML in blast crisis (*n* = 48) or ALL/AML (*n* = 11). The study also included a limited population of paediatric patients (*n* = 6).[24] In this study, the relative response expressed as the percentage reduction in white blood cells (WBCs) was used to measure the pharmacodynamic activity, because hyperleucocytosis is a prominent characteristic of CML and the normalization of WBCs is an important therapeutic goal.[50] Because the results from the paediatric patients formed a limited database, only the results obtained from the adult patients will be described here.

In patients with chronic-phase CML intolerant to IFN, complete haematological responses were seen even at a low dose level of imatinib (140 mg).[26] Once doses ≥300 mg were reached, significant clinical benefits were observed. Of the 84 patients, 77 were fully assessable. Of these 77 patients, 28 patients were treated at doses <300 mg and 49 patients at doses ≥300 mg. In the cohort treated with imatinib <300 mg, complete haematological responses were achieved in 39% (11/28). Of the patients treated with a dose ≥300 mg, 98% (48/49) achieved complete haematological responses. In this study, it was also shown that a major cytogenetic response was achieved in 41% of assessable patients in the chronic phase of CML and was complete in 18%.[26] A complete cytogenetic response indicates that there are no detectable Ph+ metaphases and that the leukaemia clone of the cells is eliminated.[31]

The 59 patients with CML in blast crisis or ALL/AML were divided into two cohorts. Patients with lymphoid blast crisis and ALL were grouped as the lymphoid phenotype, and the patients with myeloid blast crisis and AML were grouped as the myeloid phenotype. The patients were treated with dose levels ranging from 300 to 1000 mg/day. The overall rate of haematological response was 70% and 54% in the patients with a lymphoid and a myeloid phenotype, respectively. The duration of the response was shorter in lymphoid phenotypes. A major cytogenetic response was achieved in 14% of patients with a myeloid blast crisis and 30% of those with lymphoid blast crisis.[26]

This and other clinical trials[51,52] have confirmed that imatinib induces haematological and cytogenetic re-sponses in patients with leukaemia. Imatinib reduces the number of WBCs in patients with hyperleucocytosis.

Pharmacokinetics

The pharmacokinetics of imatinib have been evaluated in several studies.[26,51,53,54] These studies have investigated the pharmacokinetics over a dosage range of 25–1000 mg.

When imatinib was administered in capsule formulation, the mean absolute bioavailability was 98%. There was a high inter-patient variability in plasma imatinib AUC levels after oral dosing. When the patient swallowed the capsule with a high-fat meal, the rate of absorption was minimally reduced.[55] It was also shown that, at clinically relevant concentrations of imatinib, binding to plasma proteins was approximately 95%, mostly to albumin and a1-acid glycoprotein, with little binding to lipoproteins. Metabolism studies showed that the major radioactive compound in plasma was imatinib, followed by the N-desmethyl metabolite of imatinib CGP 74588. This is the major metabolite *in vitro* as well as *in vivo* and has comparable potency to the parent. Imatinib and the N-desmethyl metabolite together accounted for about 65% of the circulating radioactivity. The remaining radioactivity consisted of a number of minor metabolites. The human cytochrome P450 enzyme CYP 3A4 is mainly responsible for the biotransformation of imatinib. In addition, imatinib competitively inhibited CYP 2C9, CYP 2D6, and CYP 3A4/5. This was shown in *in vitro* studies using human liver microsomes.[26] Imatinib was excreted slowly; the bulk of the carbon-14 radioactivity dose was recovered within 7 days. Excretion was mainly in faeces (68% of dose) and to a minor extent in urine (13% of dose). Unchanged imatinib accounted for 25% of the dose (5% urine, 20% faeces), the remainder being inactive metabolites.[55]

Plasma pharmacokinetics were studied in healthy volunteers, CML populations, and in patients with GISTs. Healthy volunteers were randomly assigned to receive imatinib in the dose range 25–1000 mg. The half-life following oral administration of a single dose of imatinib was approximately 18 h. This suggests that once-daily dosing is appropriate. The increase in mean AUC with increasing dose was linear and dose proportional in the range 25–1000 mg imatinib after oral administration. There was no change in the kinetics of imatinib on repeated dosing.[55] CML populations were studied in a multiple-dose pharmacokinetic study. The pharmacokinetics were examined on day 1 (first dose) and day 28 (multiple dose, steady state). Imatinib was rapidly absorbed after oral administration with C_{max} being reached about 2–4 h post-dose. At steady state, plasma $AUC_{(0-24)}$ rose 1.5- to 3-fold after multiple dosing on a once-daily schedule. Mean $AUC_{(0-24)}$ rose linearly with dose from 25 to 1000 mg for both single and multiple doses. The metabolite CGP 74588 showed the same dose dependency as imatinib, but its half-life was longer (27–58 h). Furthermore, the influence of dosing by body weight or body surface area on plasma AUC showed no reduction in inter-patient variability in AUC, indicating no advantage in normalizing the dose of imatinib to match differences in body size. There was no effect of gender on the kinetics of imatinib.[26]

Plasma pharmacokinetics in GIST patients were also examined in a multicentre phase II trial.[26,56] Patients included in the trial were randomly assigned to receive imatinib 400 mg or 600 mg daily. Imatinib was rapidly absorbed after the first administration. The $AUC_{(0-24)}$ values indicate 1.2-fold higher drug exposure for the 600 mg dose than for 400 mg at steady state. There was considerable inter-patient variability of pharmaco-kinetics.

The pharmacokinetics of imatinib in GIST patients seemed to differ from that in CML patients. Peak plasma concentrations and systemic exposure observed in GIST patients were higher than those observed in CML patients at 400 and 600 mg. This may have been related to differences in liver function as GIST patients have liver metastases more frequently than CML patients. The presence of hepatic metastases is related to hepatic insufficiency and this, in turn, is expected to reduce the metabolism of imatinib in GIST patients.[26] A summary of imatinib pharmacokinetics is given in Table 14.2.

Table 14.2   Summary of imatinib pharmacokinetics

Dose range	25–1000 mg
Administration	Oral
Bioavailability	98%
Effect of food	Of no importance
Binding to plasma proteins	95%, mostly to albumin and α1-acid glycoprotein
Metabolizing enzyme	CYP 3A4
Major metabolite	N-desmethyl imatinib
Excretion	Faeces (68%) and urine (13%)
Plasma pharmacokinetics	C_{max} 2–4 h post-dose Half-life, 18 h Mean AUC rose linearly with dose from 25 to 1000 mg Inter-patient variability in mean $AUC_{(0-24)}$, coefficient of variation was 40%
Effect of hepatic dysfunction	No clinical studies conducted, but imatinib should be used cautiously in patients with hepatic impairment
Effect of renal dysfunction	No clinical studies conducted, but a decrease in total body clearance is not expected in patients with renal insufficiency

Data from EMEA.[26]

Table 14.3   Recommended doses of imatinib for treatment of CML patients

CML	Criteria in blood and bone marrow	Recommended dose of imatinib
Chronic phase	Blasts <15% *and* peripheral blood basophils <20% *and* platelets >100 × 10⁹/litre	400 mg/day
Accelerated phase	Blasts ≥15% but ≥30% *or* blasts + promyelocytes ≥30% *or* peripheral blood basophils ≥20% *or* platelets <100 × 10⁹/litre unrelated to therapy	600 mg/day
Blast crisis	Blasts ≥30%	600 mg/day

Recommended doses

Several clinical studies have been performed to determine the recommended doses of imatinib.[54,55] Table 14.3 summarizes the daily doses that are frequently used currently in CML patients. In clinical trials, treatment with imatinib was continued until disease progression.

Dosing for children should be on the basis of body surface area (mg/m^2). Doses of 260 mg/m^2 and 340 mg/m^2 daily are recommended for children with chronic-phase and advanced-phase CML, respectively. Dosing in children at 260 mg/m^2 and 340 mg/m^2 achieved the same exposure as doses of 400 mg and 60 mg, respectively, in adult patients. This dose recommendation is currently based on a small number of paediatric patients.[55]

The recommended dose of imatinib for patients with unresectable and/or metastatic malignant GISTs is 400 mg/day in one single dose. There are limited data available for the effect of dose increases from 400 to 600 mg in patients progressing at the lower dose. In clinical trials with GIST patients, treatment with imatinib was continued until disease progression.[55]

If non-haematological or haematological adverse events occur in CML and GIST patients, treatment with imatinib may be continued at a reduced daily dose. In adults the dose should be reduced from 400 to 300 mg or from 600 to 400 mg, and in children from 260 to 200 mg/m^2 day or from 340 to 260 mg/m^2 day.[55]

Toxicity

Non-haematological toxicity

Imatinib is well tolerated in patients with CML, but the majority experience adverse events at some point. The most commonly reported related adverse events are nausea, sometimes accompanied by vomiting, dyspepsia, and/or upper abdominal pain.[28,57] Imatinib can also induce gastrointestinal haemorrhage by damaging blood vessels during tumour regression, especially in GISTs. Another commonly reported toxicity is oedema. It can appear at various sites, but is most frequent in the periorbital region, limbs, and face. Some patients also have a variety of musculoskeletal symptoms including muscle cramps, arthralgia, and myalgia. Another miscellaneous drug-related adverse event is fluid retention. This may present clinically as pleural effusion, pulmonary oedema, ascites, and rapid weight gain with or without superficial oedema. Some patients also have serious skin rashes and urticaria. Liver toxicity mani-

festing as elevated transaminases, sometimes accompanied by elevated bilirubin and/or alkaline phosphatase, is also common in CML patients treated with imatinib. Renal toxicity is sometimes observed during imatinib therapy.[26,51]

The non-haematological toxicity profile of imatinib in GIST patients is mainly similar to that observed in CML patients. GIST patients experience an increased frequency of oedema and develop gastrointestinal bleeding more often than CML patients.[56]

Haematological toxicity

Cytopenias, particularly neutropenia and thrombocytopenia, have been a consistent finding in all studies of CML. Neutropenia and thrombocytopenia appear with a higher frequency at high doses (≥ 750 mg).[26,58] In patients with CML, the occurrence of cytopenias is also dependent on the stage of the disease. For example, the frequencies of grade 3 or 4 neutropenias (ANC $< 1.0 \times 10^9$/litre) and thrombocytopenias (platelet count $< 50 \times 10^9$/litre) are about four and six times higher, respectively, in blast crisis and accelerated phase CML than in newly diagnosed patients in chronic phase CML.[26,51] The duration of grade 3 or 4 neutropenia or thrombocytopenia is also longer in patients with advanced CML. The median durations of the neutropenic and thrombocytopenic episodes are 2–3 weeks and 3–4 weeks, respectively.[55]

The haematological toxicity in GIST patients is lower than in CML patients. Neutropenia and thrombocytopenia are less frequent, but anemia is more common. This can be related to the higher frequency of gastrointestinal bleeding in GIST patients.[26]

The non-haematological and haematological toxicities can usually be managed by dose reduction or interruption of treatment with imatinib.

Drug–drug interactions

Imatinib is mainly metabolized by the CYP 3A4 liver enzyme. Several drugs can alter the plasma concentration of imatinib. For example, ketoconazole, itraconazole, clarithromycin, and erythromycin inhibit CYP 3A4 activity.[55] This results in decreased metabolism and increased imatinib plasma concentrations. Compounds such as phenytoin, dexamethasone, carbamazepine, phenobarbital, rifampicin, and extract of *Hypericum perforatum* (St John's wort) are inducers of CYP 3A4 activity.[55] These compounds can increase the metabolism of imatinib and decrease its plasma exposure. This could potentially increase the risk of therapeutic failure. In a study where patients were pretreated with multiple doses of rifampicin 600 mg followed by a single 400 mg dose of imatinib, it was shown that C_{max} and AUC of imatinib decreased by at least 54% and 74%, respectively, of their values without rifampicin treatment.[55]

Imatinib can also alter exposure to other drugs due to inhibition of CYP 3A4. For example, imatinib increases the mean C_{max} and AUC of simvastatin, indicating an inhibition of the CYP 3A4 enzyme. Imatinib may also increase the plasma concentration of other CYP 3A4 metabolized drugs, such as triazolo-benzodiazepines and dihydropyridine calcium-channel blockers.[55] A summary is given in Tables 14.4 and 14.5.

Imatinib can also competitively inhibit CYP 2C9 and CYP 2D6. Therefore systemic exposure to substrates of CYP 2C9 and CYP 2D6 is potentially increased during co-administration with imatinib.

Mechanisms of resistance to imatinib

Resistance to imatinib includes *de novo* resistance and relapse after an initial response. Patients with relapse/resistance mechanisms can be separated in two cate-

Table 14.4   Drugs that alter imatinib plasma concentrations

Drug	Plasma concentration of imatinib
Ketoconazole	Increase
Itraconazole	Increase
Clarithromycin	Increase
Erythromycin	Increase
Phenytoin	Decrease
Dexamethasone	Decrease
Carbamazepine	Decrease
Phenobarbital	Decrease
Rifampicin	Decrease
H. perforatum extract	Decrease

Table 14.5   Imatinib alters plasma concentrations of some drugs

Drug	Plasma concentration of drug
Simvastatin	Increase
Triazolo-benzodiazepines	Increase
Dihydropyridine calcium-channel blockers	Increase

gories. The first category includes patients with persistent inhibition of the *bcr–abl* kinase, and the second category includes patients with reactivation of the *bcr–abl* kinase.[31] Patients with persistent inhibition of the *bcr–abl* kinase could have additional molecular abnormalities, such as new mutations, driving the growth and survival of the malignant leukaemia cells in addition to *bcr–abl*. In contrast, patients with persistent *bcr–abl* kinase activity or reactivation of the kinase could have resistance mechanisms that either prevent imatinib from reaching its target or render the target insensitive to imatinib. Mechanisms like drug efflux and protein binding could prevent imatinib from reaching its target in the *abl* kinase. Drug efflux regulated by P-glycoprotein (P-gp) was investigated in cell lines over-expressing the multidrug resistance (MDR1) gene that encodes for P-gp. It was shown that the K562/DOX cell line grew continuously in the presence of 1 mM imatinib, but died in 4–5 days if the P-gp pump modulators verapamil or PSC833 were added to the imatinib-treated culture.[59] It was also shown that retroviral-mediated transfection of the *bcr–abl*(+) AR230 cell line with the MDR1 gene decreased its sensitivity to imatinib. This could also be reversed by verapamil.[59] These results indicate that the intracellular accumulation of imatinib can be affected by the MDR phenomenon. In addition to mechanisms that prevent imatinib from reaching its target, the target itself could become insensitive by mutations in the *bcr–abl* kinase and amplification of the *bcr–abl* protein.[31]

The majority of patients who relapse after an initial response to imatinib have reactivation of the *bcr–abl* kinase.[60] No changes in drug levels have been observed in these patients and their leukaemic cells have decreased cellular sensitivity to imatinib.[60] This suggests that resistance is due to intrinsic cellular properties rather than drug metabolism or protein binding of imatinib. Several studies[61–63] have shown that the majority of these patients have developed point mutations in the *abl* kinase that render it less sensitive to imatinib. The point mutations could be at contact sites between imatinib and the *abl* kinase,[60,64] at residues adjacent to contact points, or in the kinase activation loop.[63,64]

A minority of patients who relapse after an initial response have *bcr–abl* amplification.[62] In these patients, *bcr–abl* remains a good target for therapy but different potent *abl* inhibitors are required. *bcr–abl* mutations and amplification have not commonly been seen in patients with *de novo* imatinib resistance. Studies to identify the mechanisms of resistance in these patients are ongoing.[31]

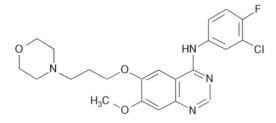

Figure 14.4. Chemical structure of gefitinib.

Gefitinib (Iressa, ZD1839)

Gefitinib is an orally active EGFR tyrosine kinase inhibitor currently available in Japan, the United States, and Australia. It was approved by the FDA in May 2003. The brown film-coated tablets contain 250 mg of gefitinib and are available for daily oral administration. Gefitinib is an anilinoquinazoline with the chemical name 4-quinazolinamine,N-(3-chloro-4-fluorophenyl)-7-methoxy-6-[3–4-morpholin)propoxy] (Fig. 14.4).[65]

Therapeutic indications

Gefitinib is currently indicated as second-line treatment of patients with advanced NSCLC after platinum pre-treatment. Phase I trials in patients with previously treated NSCLC showed objective responses.[66] After completion of the phase I studies, two phase II trials of gefitinib monotherapy were performed in patients with recurrent NSCLC.[67,68] These multicentre studies conducted in Japan, Europe, and Australia (IDEAL 1) and in North America (IDEAL 2). Patients enrolled in IDEAL 1 were required to have failed only one prior platinum-containing regimen,[67] whereas patients enrolled in IDEAL 2 were required to have failed two prior chemotherapy regimens including a platinum-containing regimen and docetaxel.[68] Patients were randomized between 250 and 500 mg/day of gefitinib and followed until disease progression. In IDEAL 1, the overall response rates were 18.4% and 19% with the 250 mg and 500 mg doses, respectively. One-year survival rates were 35% and 30% in the 250 mg and 500 mg groups, respectively. The overall response rates in IDEAL 2 were 11.8% and 8.8%, and the one-year survival rates were 29% and 24% with the 250 mg and 500 mg doses, respectively. Grade 3 and 4 toxicities were relatively uncommon.

Two phase III trials were undertaken in which chemotherapy plus gefitinib was compared with chemo-therapy alone in chemotherapy-naive patients with advanced NSCLC.[69,70] In the INTACT-1 trial cisplatin plus gemcitabine served as the chemotherapy regimen, and in the INTACT-2 trial the regimen was carboplatin plus paclitaxel. Unfortunately, neither INTACT-1 nor INTACT-2 revealed an improvement in overall survival. There was also no improvement in times to progression among patients receiving gefitinib. Toxicities were not significantly different among patients given gefitinib compared with the placebo group. An explanation for the failure of the INTACT trials could be the lack of a priori patient selection. Gefitinib targets the EGFR tyrosine kinase, and the expression of EGFR, but possibly also HER2 co-expression, can be crucial for determining the response to gefitinib. Currently there are no specific guidelines for selection of patients who may respond. When gefitinib is combined with other active drugs, such as carboplatin and paclitaxel, it does not have a positive impact on survival in chemo-therapy-naive NSCLC patients. Randomized studies are required to establish whether gefitinib as mono-therapy in second-line treatment of patients with NSCLC improves time to progression and/or survival. In addition, gefitinib is also being studied in trials including patients with prostate, breast, head and neck, ovarian, glioma, renal, bladder, and cervical cancers.[71] These studies have not yet resulted in registration for any of these indications.

Mechanism of action

Gefitinib is an inhibitor of the EGFR tyrosine kinase. Several epithelial tumours, particularly carcinomas of the upper aerodigestive tract including NSCLC, display EGFR over-expression.[72] Gefitinib competes for the ATP binding site in the cytoplasmic tail of the EGFR tyrosine kinase. The result is inhibition of auto-phosphorylation of the tyrosine kinase, thereby inhibiting the signal transduction pathways downstream of the EGFR and leading to inhibition of cellular proliferation, angiogenesis, tumour invasion, and metastases. Gefitinib also appears to induce apoptosis as well.[72]

Clinical pharmacology

The clinical pharmacology of gefitinib has been studied in several phase I, II, and III trials. Most of these studies included patients with NSCLC, but there are also trials in prostate, breast, and colorectal cancer patients. A summary of the results obtained in the phase I trials is given here.

Pharmacodynamics

The pharmacodynamics of gefitinib were studied in two phase I trials in which the effects of gefitinib on EGFR tyrosine kinase activity in cancer patients were evaluated.[73] Skin expresses EGFR tyrosine kinase and can serve as a surrogate tissue for detecting EGFR tyrosine kinase blockade in patients. In the first study, skin biopsies from 16 patients before and after 28 days of treatment with gefitinib were evaluated for molecular markers and downstream effects on proliferation known to be changed by EGFR tyrosine kinase inhibition.[74] The skin biopsies were processed for immunohistochemistry with antibodies for activated signal transduction molecules or proliferation. The mitogen-activated protein kinase (MAPK) is a signal transduction molecule downstream in the EGFR pathway. Labelling for MAPK was seen in pretreatment samples. After treatment with gefitinib the expression of MAPK declined. Treatment with gefitinib was also associated with a reduction in proliferation, assessed by staining for the nuclear antigen Ki-67 and with an increase in p27[kip-1], a marker for EGFR pathway inhibition and growth arrest.[73] No dose response was observed with respect to the degree of inactivation of downstream signal molecules or reduction in expression of proliferation markers.[75]

In the second study, skin biopsies from 65 cancer patients were evaluated before and after 28 days of therapy.[73] The results in this larger patient population were consistent and similar to results in the earlier study, showing that daily oral treatment with gefitinib inhibited EGFR tyrosine kinase activation and downstream signalling in skin biopsies.

Recently, the pharmacodynamic effects of gefitinib were evaluated immunohistochemically in tumour biopsy samples of gastric carcinomas obtained at baseline and after 28 days of treatment. In each tumour sample the percentage of tumour cells expressing EGFR, the activated phosphorylated form of EGFR (pEGFR), activated MAPK, and Ki-67 were determined. This study indicated that gefitinib achieved an almost complete inhibition of pEGFR and decreased activated MAPK in gastric tumours.[76]

Pharmacokinetics

The pharmacokinetics of gefitinib have been evaluated in phase I studies including healthy volunteers[77] and patients with advanced malignancies.[78–79]

In healthy volunteers, the peak plasma levels of gefitinib were observed 3–7 h after a single oral dose. AUC and C_{max} increased approximately linearly with once-daily doses ranging from 10 to 100 mg. The terminal elimination half-life ($t_{1/2\ \beta}$) was 28 h (range 12–51 h). Gefitinib was primarily cleared by the liver. The enzyme CYP 3A4 is mainly responsible for its metabolism.

Excretion was predominantly via faeces (86%), with renal elimination of drug and metabolites accounting for less than 4% of the administered dose.[77] Five

Table 14.6   Summary of gefitinib pharmacokinetics

Dose range	50–1000 mg
Administration	Oral
Bio-availability	60%
Effect of food	Of no importance
Binding to plasma proteins	90%, mostly to albumin and α1-acid glycoprotein
Metabolizing enzyme	CYP 3A4
Major metabolite	O-desmethyl gefitinib
Excretion	Faeces (86%) and urine (<4%)
Plasma pharmacokinetics	C_{max} 3–7 h post-dose Half-life, 28 h Mean AUC rose linearly with dose from 10 to 100 mg Inter-patient variability in mean AUC$_{(0-24)}$, 1.823–38.493 ng/h/ml
Effect of hepatic dysfunction	Patients with moderately and severely elevated biochemical liver abnormalities had gefitinib pharmacokinetics similar to individuals without liver abnormalities
Effect of renal dysfunction	No clinical studies conducted, but a decrease in total body clearance is not expected in patients with renal insufficiency

Data from Arteaga and Johnson.[72]

metabolites were identified in human plasma. The major metabolite identified in human plasma is *O*-desmethyl gefitinib. It is 14-fold less potent than gefitinib at inhibiting EGFR-stimulated cell growth and therefore it is unlikely that it contributes significantly to the clinical activity of gefitinib.[65]

In patients with advanced malignancies, C_{max} was also achieved within 3–7 h of oral dosing and $t_{1/2\,\beta}$ ranged from 24 to 58 h. Excretion was also predominantly via faeces[78] To date, several phase I studies have been completed in patients with advanced malignancies.[79] These studies also showed that gefitinib exhibits a dose-proportional increase in C_{max} and AUC over the investigated dose range of 50–1000 mg/day. C_{max} and AUC increase linearly with once-daily doses ranging from 10 to 100 mg. The phase I trials also revealed that the mean oral bioavailability was ±60%. Bioavailability was not significantly altered by food.[65] *In vitro* studies showed that binding of gefitinib to plasma proteins was 90%, mostly to serum albumin and α1-acid glycoprotein. This was independent of drug concentrations.[65] Gefitinib pharmacokinetics are summarized in Table 14.6.

Recommended doses

Several clinical trials have been performed to determine the recommended dose of gefitinib. These trials have studied gefitinib in a wide dose range and in patients with several cancers.[70,80,81] The recommended daily dose is one 250 mg tablet with or without food. Several studies showed that higher doses did not give a better response and caused increased toxicity. Patients who received 500 mg instead of 250 mg gefitinib showed a higher rate of most of the adverse events described in the next section.[65] In patients who receive gefitinib in combination with a potent CYP 3A4 inducer, a dose increase to 500 mg daily can be considered in the absence of severe drug reactions.[65]

Toxicity

Non-haematological toxicity

The most common non-haematological toxicities reported at the recommended 250 mg daily dose are diarrhoea, rash, acne, dry skin, nausea, and vomiting. Adverse events reported to a lesser extent are pruritus, anorexia, asthenia, weight loss, peripheral oedema, amblyopia, dyspnoea, conjunctivitis, vesiculobullous rash, and mouth ulceration.[65,81,82] There are also reports of eye pain and corneal erosion/ulceration, sometimes in association with

aberrant eyelash growth. There are also rare reports of pancreatitis and very rare reports of corneal membrane sloughing, ocular ischaemia/haemorrhage, and allergic reactions including urticaria.[65]

Cases of interstitial lung disease at an overall incidence of about 1% have been observed in patients receiving gefitinib. Approximately one-third of the cases have been fatal. Reports have described this adverse event as interstitial pneumonia, pneumonitis, and alveolitis. Interstitial lung disease has occurred in patients who have received prior chemotherapy (57% of reported cases), prior radiation therapy (31% of reported cases), and no previous therapy (12% of reported cases). In the event of acute onset or worsening of pulmonary symptoms (dyspnoea, cough, fever), gefitinib therapy should be interrupted.[65]

Haematological toxicity

No significant myelosuppression was observed in patients treated with gefitinib as monotherapy.[79]

Drug–drug interactions

Gefitinib is mainly metabolized by the CYP 3A4 liver enzyme. Studies with human liver microsomes have shown that gefitinib had no inhibitory effect on CYP 1A2, CYP 2C9, and CYP3A4. At high concentrations, gefitinib inhibited CYP 2C19 and CYP 2D6.[65]

Substances that are inducers of CYP 3A4 activity increase the metabolism of gefitinib and decrease its plasma concentration–time profile. For example, rifampicin (CYP 3A4 inducer) reduced the mean AUC of gefitinib by 85% in healthy male volunteers. Substances that are potent inhibitors of CYP 3A4 activity decrease gefitinib metabolism and increase its plasma concentration. When itraconazole (CYP 3A4 inhibitor) was concomitantly administered with gefitinib, the mean AUC of gefitinib was increased by 88% in healthy male volunteers.[65]

Furthermore, it was shown that drugs that cause significant sustained elevation in gastric pH, such as ranitidine or cimetidine, may reduce plasma concentrations of gefitinib and therefore potentially may reduce efficacy. A plausible explanation is that gefitinib is almost insoluble at pH > 7.[65] A summary is given in Table 14.7.

Mechanisms of resistance to gefitinib

Tumour cells can develop several mechanisms that may result in resistance to gefitinib. Patients who relapse

Table 14.7   Drugs that alter gefitinib plasma concentrations

Drugs	Plasma concentration of gefitinib
Rifampicin and other CYP 3A4 inducers	Decrease
Itraconazole and other CYP 3A4 inhibitors	Increase
Ranitidine and cimetidine	Decrease

after an initial response frequently have mutations in the EGFR gene. Amplification of the EGFR gene is detected in 40% of human gliomas, where a significant proportion exhibit EGFR gene rearrangements.[83] The mutation can take place in the ATP binding pocket, with the result that the target becomes insensitive to gefitinib. Mechanisms like drug efflux and protein binding could also prevent gefitinib from binding to its target.

A phase III study showed that additional oncogenic changes downstream of the EGFR (e.g. changes in the phosphatidylinositol-3 kinase–Akt pathway) can also result in resistance to gefitinib.[84] When Akt is phosphorylated, it inactivates the pro-apoptotic and cell-cycle regulatory molecules, thus enhancing tumour cell survival and proliferation. When EGFR is inhibited by gefitinib, Akt can still be active due to Akt gene amplification and over-expression, as well as loss of the PTEN phosphatase that can turn off Akt activity.[85] In this case, combined blockade of the EGFR tyrosine kinase and Akt should be considered as a therapeutic approach. Co-expression of HER2 may also be associated with resistance to gefitinib. However, this should be further investigated in clinical tumour material.

Future perspectives

In addition to imatinib and gefitinib, other small-molecule inhibitors of the EGFR tyrosine kinase are currently in clinical development or have been studied in phase I, II, or III trials. One example is OSI-774 (erlotinib) which works similarly to gefitinib. It also competes for the ATP binding site in the cytoplasmic tail of the EGFR.[86] OSI-774 halts excessive cellular growth by inhibiting the EGFR process within a cell. Clinical trials evaluating OSI-774 in a variety of cancers are currently under way.[87] Gefitinib and OSI-774 are examples of target-molecule-specific drugs. These drugs were developed to block only one target,

in this case the EGFR tyrosine kinase. There are also small molecules that act as multitargeted receptor tyrosine kinase inhibitors, for example imatinib, SU11248, SU6668, GW572016, EKB-569, and ZD6474. Imatinib inhibits not only the *abl* kinase but also c-*kit* and PDGFR. SU11248 targets PDGFR, VEGFR, and c-*kit*,[88] and SU6668 is a potent inhibitor of VEGFR, PDGFR and the fibroblast growth factor receptor. These are three transmembrane tyrosine kinases involved in different phases of tumour angiogenesis.[89] GW572016 and EKB-569 are small-molecule inhibitors of EGFR and erbB2 receptors.[90,91] ZD6474 is a VEGFR tyrosine kinase inhibitor, but is also able to block activation of EGFR.

An advantage of multitargeted receptor tyrosine kinase inhibitors is that several cancers can be targeted. Imatinib inhibits the *abl*-kinase, which is a main feature in CML. It also inhibits c-*kit* which is expressed in gastrointestinal cancers, AML, small-cell lung cancer, germ-cell tumours, melanoma, myeloma, and neuroblastoma.[49] Furthermore, its activity against the PDGFR tyrosine kinase may suggest an additional anti-angiogenic effect.[92] On the basis of these data, it would appear that the lack of tight molecular specificity of tyrosine kinase inhibitors might serve a good therapeutic purpose. A disadvantage of the development of multitargeted receptor tyrosine kinase inhibitors is unexpected host toxicity. As more ATP competitive inhibitors are developed, it is possible that some of them may hit other kinases whose inactivation may result in undue host toxicity. This possibility cannot be excluded and should be carefully evaluated in phase I trials.[92,93]

As well as target-molecule-specific and multitargeted small molecules, there are also humanized EGFR antibodies that can inhibit the receptor. At present it is difficult to predict which of these two anti-EGFR approaches is more effective. One advantage of small-molecule EGFR tyrosine kinase inhibitors over anti-EGFR antibodies might be the potential to inhibit the constitutive tyrosine kinase activity associated with the mutated EGFRvIII frequently detected in human glioblastomas. Another advantage is their ability to cross-react with EGFR homologous kinases like HER2, especially when it is considered that over-expression of members of the HER network confers a poor clinical outcome compared with tumours with only high levels of EFGR.[94] On the other hand, some EGFR antibodies may act by immune-effector-mediated destruction of tumour cells.[93] A possible role of antibody-dependent cellular cytotoxicity suggests a rationale for combining

EGFR antibodies with cytokines, for example with interleukin 2 (IL-2) which can stimulate immune effector cells in cancer patients. Other advantages of humanized EGFR antibodies are that they have a prolonged half-life, can induce receptor downregulation, and have no gastrointestinal toxicity.[2] A disadvantage is that antibodies need to be given parentally by injection.

The question as to whether antibodies or small-molecule inhibitors are most effective is not easy to solve. They have both their advantages. In the last 5 years, both antireceptor approaches have been investigated and enormous progress has been made. The first drugs targeted against tyrosine kinases have reached the market and numerous new tyrosine kinase targets have been identified. Currently, more than 20 tyrosine kinase targets are under evaluation worldwide.[95]

Although great successes have been achieved (imatinib), there have also been some failures. Some drugs had to be withdrawn from development (EGFR inhibitors BIBX1382BS and PKI166) owing to liver toxicity. Despite these failures, there is no doubt that with all the experience and knowledge that has been accumulated over the last few years, tyrosine kinase inhibitors will become successful in the clinic.

References

1. Fantl WJ, Johnson DE, Williams LT (1993) Signaling by receptor tyrosine kinases. *Annu Rev Biochem*, **62**, 453.
2. Ritter CA, Arteaga CL (2003) The epidermal growth factor receptor-tyrosine kinase: a promising therapeutic target in solid tumors. *Semin Oncol*, **30** (Suppl 1), 1–11.
3. Olayioye MA, Neve RM, Lane HA, *et al.* (2000) The ErbB signaling network: receptor heterodimerization in development and cancer. *EMBO J*, **19**, 3159–67.
4. Hanahan D, Weinberg RA (2000) The hallmarks of cancer. *Cell*, **100**, 57–70.
5. Baselga J (2002) Why the epidermal growth factor receptor? The rationale for cancer therapy. *Oncologist*, 7 (Suppl 4), 2–8.
6. Pinkas-Kramarski R, Soussan L, Waterman H, *et al.* (1996) Diversification of Neu differentiation factor and epidermal growth factor signaling by combinatorial receptor interactions. *EMBO J*, **15**, 2452–67.
7. Leonard WJ, O'Shea JJ (1998) Jaks and STATs: biological implications. *Annu Rev Immunol*, **16**, 293.
8. Grandis JR, Melhem MF, Gooding WE, *et al.* (1998) Levels of TGF-α and EGFR protein in head and neck squamous cell carcinoma and patient survival. *J Natl Cancer Inst*, **90**, 824–32.
9. Wells A (2000) The epidermal growth factor receptor (EGFR)-a new target in cancer therapy. *Signal*, 1, 4–11.
10. Baselga J (2000) New technologies in epidermal growth factor receptor-targeted cancer therapy. *Signal*, 1, 12–21.
11. Woodburn JR (1999) The epidermal growth factor receptor and its inhibition in cancer therapy. *Pharmacol Ther*, **82**, 241–50.
12. Brabender J, Danenberg KD, Metzger R, *et al.* (2001) Epidermal growth factor receptor and HER2-neu mRNA expression in non-small cell lung cancer is correlated with survival. *Clin Cancer Res*, 7, 1850–5.
13. Meyers MB, Shen WP, Spengler BA, *et al.* (1988) Increased epidermal growth factor receptor in multidrug-resistent human neuroblastoma cells. *J Cell Biochem*, **39**, 87–97.
14. Scheijen B, Griffin JD (2002) Tyrosine kinase oncogenes in normal hematopoiesis and hematological disease. *Oncogene*, **21**, 3314–33.
15. Baselga J, Mendelsohn J (1997) Type I receptor tyrosine kinases as targets for therapy in breast cancer. *J Mammary Gland Biol Neoplasia*, **2**, 165–74.
16. Divgi CR, Welt S, Kris M, *et al.* (1991) Phase I and imaging trial of indium 111-labeled anti-epidermal growth factor receptor monoclonal antibody 225 in patient with squamous cell lung carcinoma. *J Natl Cancer Inst*, **83**, 97–104.
17. Zwick E, Bange J, Ullrich A (2001) Receptor tyrosine kinase signaling as a target for cancer intervention strategies. *Endocr Relat Cancer*, **8**, 161–73.
18. Prenzel N, Fischer OM, Streit, *et al.* (2001) The epidermal growth factor receptor family as a central element for cellular signal transduction and diversification. *Endocr Relat Cancer*, **8**, 11–31.
19. Balcerczak E, Mirowski M, Sasor A, Wierzbicki R (2003) Expression of p65, DD3 and c-erbB2 genes in prostate cancer. *Neoplasma*, **50**, 97–101.
20. Nakamura H, Saji H, Ogata A, *et al.* (2003) Correlation between encoded protein overexpression and copy number of the HER2 gene with survival in non-small cell lung cancer. *Int J Cancer*, **103**, 61–6.
21. Fan Z, Masui H, Altas I, *et al.* (1993) Blockade of epidermal growth factor receptor function by bivalent and monovalent fragments of 225 anti-epidermal growth factor receptor monoclonal antibodies. *Cancer Res*, **53**, 4322–28.
22. Al-Obeidi FA, Lam KS (2000) Development of inhibitors for protein tyrosine kinases. *Oncogene*, **19**, 5690–701.
23. Fry DW (2000) Site-directed irreversible inhibitors of the erbB family of receptor tyrosine kinases as novel chemotherapeutic agents for cancer. *Anticancer Drug Des*, **15**, 3–16.
24. Moyer JD, Barbacci EG, Iwata KK, *et al.* (1997) Induction of apoptosis and cell cycle arrest by CP-358, 774, an inhibitor of epidermal growth factor receptor tyrosine kinase. *Cancer Res*, **57**, 4838–48.
25. Arteaga CL (2001) The epidermal growth factor receptor: from mutant oncogene in nonhuman cancers to therapeutic target in human neoplasia. *J Clin Oncol*, **19** (Suppl), 32s–40s.
26. EMEA: The European Agency for the Evaluation of Medicinal Products (2003) Glivec, Scientific Discussion, 1–61. Website http://www.emea.gov
27. Kurzrock R, Kantarjian HM, Druker BJ, Talpaz M (2003) Philadelphia chromosome-positive leukemias:

from basic mechanisms to molecular therapeutics. *Ann Intern Med*, **138**, 819–30.

28. Kantarajian H, Sawyers C, Hochhaus A, *et al.* (2000) Phase II study of ST1571, a tyrosine kinase inhibitor, in patients with resistant or refractory Philadelphia chromosome-positive chronic myeloid leukaemia. *Blood*, **96**, 470a.

29. Radford IR (2002) Imatinib Novartis. *Curr Opin Invest Drugs*, **3**, 492–9.

30. Heinrich MC, Griffith DJ, Druker BJ, Wait CL, Ott KA, Zigler AJ (2000) Inhibition of c-KIT receptor tyrosine activity by STI571, a selective tyrosine kinase inhibitor. *Blood*, **96**, 925–32.

31. Druker BJ (2002) Perspectives on the development of a molecularly targeted agent. *Cancer Cell*, **1**, 31–6.

32. Nowell PC, Hunerford DA (1960) A minute chromosome in human chronic granulocytic leukemia. *Science*, **132**, 1497–501.

33. Konopa JB, Watanabe SM, Witte ON (1984) An alteration of the human c-*abl* protein in K562 unmasks associated tyrosine kinase activity. *Cell*, **37**, 1035–42.

34. Deininger MW, Goldman JM, Melo JV (2000) The molecular biology of chronic myeloid leukemia. *Blood*, **96**, 3343–56.

35. Miettinen M, Sarlomo-Rikala M, Lasoto J (1999) Gastrointestinal stromal tumors: recent advances in understanding of their biology. *Hum Pathol*, **30**, 1213–20.

36. Fletcher CDM, Bermann JJ, Corless C, *et al.* (2002) Diagnosis of gastrointestinal tumors: a consensus approach. *Hum Pathol*, **33**, 459–65.

37. De Silva CM, Reid R (2003) Gastrointestinal stromal tumors (GIST): c-*kit* mutations, CD117 expression, differential diagnosis and targeted cancer therapy with imatinib. *Pathol Oncol Res*, **9**, 13–19.

38. Vliagoftis H, Worobec AS, Metcalfe DD (1997) The proto-oncogene c-*kit* and c-*kit* ligand in human disease. *J Allergy Clin Immunol*, **100**, 435–40.

39. Hirota S, Isozaki K, Moriyama Y, *et al.* (1998) Gain-of-function mutations of c-*kit* in human gastrointestinal stromal tumors. *Science*, **279**, 577–80.

40. Buchdunger E, Cioffi CL, Law N, *et al.* (2000) Abl protein-tyrosine kinase inhibitor STI571 inhibits *in vitro* signal transduction mediated by c- KIT and platelet-derived growth factor receptors. *J Pharmacol Exp Ther*, **295**, 139–45.

41. Ma Y, Zeng S, Metcalfe DD, *et al.* (2002) The c-KIT mutation causing human mastocytosis is resistant to STI571 and other KIT kinase inhibitors: kinases with enzymatic site mutations show different inhibitor sensitivity profiles than wild-type kinases and those with regulatory-type mutations. *Blood*, **99**, 1741–4.

42. Tuveson DA, Willis NA, Jacks T, *et al.* (2001) STI571 inactivation of the gastrointestinal stromal tumor c-KIT oncoprotein: biological and clinical implications. *Oncogene*, **20**, 5054–8.

43. Chen H, Isozaki K, Kinoshita K, *et al.* (2003) Cancer diagnosis and therapy: Imatinib inhibits various types of activating mutant kit found in gastrointestinal tumors. *Int J Cancer*, **105**, 130–5.

44. Sirvent N, Maire G, Pedeutour F (2003) Genetics of dermatofibrosarcoma protuberans family of tumors: from ring chromosomes to tyrosine kinase inhibitor treatment. *Genes Chromosom Cancer*, **37**, 1–19.

45. Okuda K, Weisberg E, Gilliland DG, Griffin JD (2001) ARG tyrosine kinase activity is inhibited by STI571. *Blood*, **97**, 2440–8.

46. Gambacorti-Passerini C, Gunby R, Piazza R, Galietta A, Rostagno R, Scapozza L (2003) Molecular mechanisms of resistance to imatinib in Philadelphia-chromosome-positive leukaemias. *Lancet Oncol*, **4**, 75–85.

47. Capdeville R, Buchdunger E, Zimmermann J, Matter A (2002) Glivec (STI571, imatinib), a rationally developed, targeted anti-cancer drug. *Nat Rev Drug Discov*, **1**, 493–502.

48. Druker BJ, Tamura S, Buchdunger E, *et al.* (1996) Effects of a selective inhibitor of the Abl tyrosine kinase on the growth of Bcr-Abl positive cells. *Nat Med*, **2**, 561–6.

49. Heinrich M, Blanke CD, Druker BJ, Corless CL (2002) Inhibition of KIT tyrosine kinase activity: a novel approach to the treatment of KIT positive malignancies. *J Clin Oncol*, **20**, 1692–1703.

50. Faderl S, Talpaz M, Estrov Z, Kantarjian HM (1999) Chronic myelogenous leukemia; biology and therapy. *Ann Intern Med*, **131**, 207–19.

51. Druker BJ, Talpaz M, Resta D, *et al.* (2001) Efficacy and safety of a specific inhibitor of the Bcr-Abl tyrosine kinase in chronic myeloid leukemia. *N Engl J Med*, **344**, 1031–7.

52. Sawyers CL, Hochhaus A, Feldman E, *et al.* (2001) Gleevec/Glivec (imatinib mesylate, ST1571) in patients with chronic myeloid leukemia (CML) in myeloid blast crisis: updated results of a phase II study. *Blood*, **98**, 845a.

53. Peng B, Hayes M, Druker B, *et al.* (2000) Clinical pharmacokinetics and pharmacodynamics of ST1571 in a phase I trial in chronic myelogenous leukemia (CML) patients. *Proc Am Assoc Cancer Res*, **41**, abstr 3468.

54. Peng B, Hayes M, Racine-Poon A, *et al.* (2001) Clinical investigation of the pharmacokinetic/pharmacodynamic relationship for Glivec (ST1571): a novel inhibitor of signal transduction. *Proc Am Soc Clin Oncol*, **20**, 280a.

55. EMEA: The European Agency for the Evaluation of Medicinal Products (2003) Glivec, Summary of product characteristics, 1–33. Website http://www.emea.gov

56. Van Oosterom AT, Judson I, Verweij J, *et al.* (2001) Safety and efficacy of imatinib (ST1574) in metastatic gastrointestinal tumours, a phase I study. *Lancet*, **358**, 1421–3.

57. Talpaz M, Silver RT, Druker B, *et al.* (2000) Phase II study of ST1571 in patients with Philadelphia chromosome-positive chronic myeloid leukemia in accelerated phase. *Blood*, **96**, 469a.

58. O'Dwyer ME, Druker BJ (2001) The role of the tyrosine kinase inhibitor ST1574 in the treatment of cancer. *Curr Cancer Drug Targets*, **1**, 49–57.

59. Mahon FX, Belloc F, Lagarde V, *et al.* (2003) MDR1 gene overexpression confers resistance to imatinib mesylate in leukemia cell line models. *Blood*, **101**, 2368–73.

60. Gorre ME, Mohammed M, Ellwood K, *et al.* (2001) Clinical resistance to STI-571 cancer therapy caused by BCR-ABL gene mutation or amplification. *Science*, **293**, 876–80.

61. Brandford S, Rudzki Z, Walsh S, *et al.* (2001) Point mutations clustered within the ATP binding region of BCR-ABL are common in patients with emerging Glivec resistance but not in Glivec non-responsive cases. *Blood*, **98**, 769a.

62. Hochhaus A, Kreil S, Muller MC, *et al.* (2001) Molecular and chromosomal mechanisms of resistance in CML patients after STI571 (Glivec) therapy. *Blood*, **98**, 435a.

63. Shah NP, Nicoll JM, Gorre ME, Paquette RL, Ford JM, Sawyers CL (2001) Resistance to Glivec: sequence analysis reveals a spectrum of Bcr/Abl kinase domain mutations in both acquired and *de novo* resistant cases of chronic myelogenous leukemia in blast crisis. *Blood*, **98**, 770a.

64. Barthe C, Cony-Makhoul P., Melo JV, Mahon JR (2001) Roots of clinical resistance to STI-571 cancer therapy. *Science*, **2163**, 293.

65. U.S. Food and Drug Administration (2003) *Iressa (gefitinib tablets)*. Washington, DC: US Government Printing Office, 1–15.

66. Herbst RS, Maddox A-M, Rothenberg ML, *et al.* (2002) Selective oral epidermal growth factor receptor tyrosine kinase inhibitor ZD 1839 is generally well-tolerated and has activity in non-small-cell lung cancer and other solid tumors: results of a phase I trial. *J Clin Oncol*, **20**, 3815–25.

67. Fukuoka M, Yano S, Giaccone G, *et al.* (2002) Final results from a phase II trial of ZD 1839 ('Iressa') for patients with advanced non-small-cell lung cancer (IDEAL 1). *Proc Am Soc Clin Oncol*, **21**, 298a.

68. Kris MG, Natale RB, Herbst RS, *et al.* (2002) A phase II trial of ZD 1839 ('Iressa') in advanced non-small cell lung cancer (NSCLC) patients who had failed platinum- and docetaxel-based regimens (IDEAL 2). *Proc Am Soc Clin Oncol*, **21**, 292a.

69. Giaconne G, Johnson DH, Manegold C, *et al.* (2002) A phase III clinical trial of ZD 1839 ('Iressa') in combination with gemcitabine and cisplatin in chemotherapy-naive patients with advanced non-small cell lung cancer (INTACT-1). *Ann Oncol*, **13** (Suppl 5), 2.

70. Johnson DH, Herbst R, Giaconne G, *et al.* (2002) ZD1839 ('Iressa') in combination with paclitaxel and carboplatin in chemotherapy-naive patients with advanced non-small cell lung cancer (NSCLC): initial results from a phase III trial (INTACT-2). *Ann Oncol*, **13** (Suppl 5), 127.

71. Ranson M (2002) ZD1839 (Iressa™): for more than just non-small cell lung cancer. *Oncologist*, 7 (Suppl 4), 16–24.

72. Arteaga CL, Johnson DH (2001) Tyrosine kinase inhibitors-ZD1839 (Iressa). *Curr Opin Oncol*, **13**, 491–8.

73. Albanell J, Rojo F, Averbuch S, *et al.* (2002) Pharmacodynamic studies of the epidermal growth factor receptor inhibitor ZD1839 in skin from cancer patients: histopathologic and molecular consequences of receptor inhibition. *J Clin Oncol*, **20**, 110–24.

74. LoRusso PM (2003) Phase I studies of ZD1839 in patients with common solid tumors. *Semin Oncol*, **30** (Suppl 1), 1–11.

75. Baselga J (2000) New therapeutic agents targeting the epidermal growth factor receptor. *J Clin Oncol*, **18** (Suppl), 54s–9s.

76. Rojo J, Tabernero E, Van Cutsem A, *et al.* (2003) Pharmacodynamic studies of tumor biopsy specimens from patients with advanced gastric carcinoma undergoing treatment with gefitinib (ZD1839). *Proc ASCO*, **22**, 191 (abstr 764).

77. Swaisland H, Laight A, Stafford L, *et al.* (2001) Pharmacokinetics and tolerability of the orally active selective epidermal growth factor receptor tyrosine kinase inhibitor ZD1839 in healthy volunteers. *Clin Pharmacokinet*, **40**, 297–306.

78. Kelly H, Ferry D, Hammond L, *et al.* (2000) ZD1839 (Iressa), an oral EGFR-TKI (epidermal growth factor receptor tyrosine kinase inhibitor): pharmacokinetic results of a phase I study in patients with advanced cancer. *Proc Am Assoc Cancer Res*, **41**, 612.

79. Kris M, Ranson M, Ferry D, *et al.* (1999) Phase I study of oral ZD1839 (Iressa), a novel inhibitor of epidermal growth factor tyrosine kinase (EGFR-TK): evidence of good tolerability and activity. *Clin Cancer Res*, 5 (Suppl), 3749s.

80. Ranson M, Hammond LA, Ferry D, *et al.* (2002) ZD1839, a selective oral epidermal growth factor receptor-tyrosine kinase inhibitor, is well tolerated and active in patients with solid, malignant tumors: results of a phase I trial. *J Clin Oncol*, **20**, 2240–50.

81. Baselga J, Rischin D, Ranson M, *et al.* (2002) Phase I safety, pharmacokinetic, and pharmacodynamic trial of ZD1839, a selective oral epidermal growth factor receptor tyrosine kinase inhibitor, in patients with five selected solid tumor types. *J Clin Oncol*, **20**, 4292–302.

82. Ciardiello F, Tortora G (2001) A novel approach in the treatment of cancer: targeting the epidermal growth factor receptor. *Clin Cancer Res*, 7, 2958–70.

83. Sauter G, Maeda T, Waldman FM, *et al.* (1996) Patterns of epidermal growth factor receptor amplification in malignant gliomas. *Am J Pathol*, **148**, 1047–53.

84. Blagosklonny MV, Darzynkiewicz Z (2003) Why Iressa failed: toward novel use of kinase inhibitors (outlook). *Cancer Biol Ther*, **2**, 137–40.

85. Bianco R, Shin I, Ritter CA, *et al.* (2003) Loss of PTEN/MMAC1/TEP in EGF receptor-expressing tumor cells counteracts the antitumor action of EGFR tyrosine kinase inhibitors. *Oncogene*, **22**, 2812–22.

86. Hidalgo M, Siu LL, Nemunaitis J, *et al.* (2001) Phase I and pharmacologic study of OSI-774, an epidermal growth factor receptor tyrosine kinase inhibitor, in patients with advanced solid malignancies. *J Clin Oncol*, **19**, 3267–79.

87. Oza AM, Townsley CA, Siu LL, *et al.* (2003) Phase II study of erlotinib (OSI-774) in patients with metastatic colorectal cancer. *Proc ASCO*, **22**, 196 (abstr 785).

88. Rosen L, Mulay M, Long J, *et al.* (2003) Phase I trial of SU11248, a novel tyrosine kinase inhibitor in advanced solid tumors. *Proc ASCO*, **22**, 191 (abstr 765).

89. Laird AD, Vajkoczy P, Shawver LK, *et al.* (2000) SU6668 is a potent antiangiogenic and antitumor agent that induces regression of established tumors. *Cancer Res*, **60**, 4152–60.

90. Spector N, Raefsky E, Hurwitz H, *et al.* (2003) Safety, clinical efficacy, and biologic assessments from EGF10004: a randomized phase IB study of GW572016 for patients with metastatic carcinomas overexpressing EGFR and erbB2. *Proc ASCO*, **22**, 193 (abstr 772).

91. Morgan JA, Bukowski RM, Xiong H, *et al.* (2003) Preliminary report of a phase I study of EKB-569, an irreversible inhibitor of the epidermal growth factor receptor (EGFR), given in combination with gemcitabine in patients with advanced pancreatic cancer. *Proc ASCO*, **22**, 197 (abstr 788).

92. Arteaga CL (2003) Molecular therapeutics: is one promiscuous drug against multiple targets better than combinations of molecule-specific drugs? *Clin Cancer Res*, **9**, 1231–2.

93. Rodeck U, Herlyn M, Herlyn D, *et al.* (1987) Tumor growth modulation by a monoclonal antibody to the epidermal growth factor receptor: immunologically mediated and effector cell-independent effects. *Cancer Res*, **47**, 3692–6.

94. Tateishi M, Ishida T, Kohdono S, *et al.* (1994) Prognostic influence of the co-expression of epidermal growth factor receptor and c-erbB-2 protein in human lung adenocarcinoma. *Surg Oncol*, **3**, 109–13.

95. Traxler P (2003) Tyrosine kinases as targets in cancer therapy—successes and failures. *Expert Opin Ther Targets*, **7**, 215–34.

15 | Anti-endocrine drugs used in cancer treatment

Per Eystein Lønning

Introduction

The discovery by Beatson a century ago that castration may cause tumour regression in premenopausal breast cancer patients marks endocrine therapy as the first successful systemic treatment strategy for malignant diseases. Although other forms of ablative surgery (orchiectomy in males suffering from prostatic carcinomas, and adrenalectomy and hypophysectomy in postmenopausal breast cancer patients) and, in the 1950s and 1960s, additive treatment with oestrogens or glucocorticoids came into

Summary

	Non-steroidal anti-oestrogens		
	Tamoxifen	Toremifene	Droloxifene
Administration	Oral	Oral	Oral
Protein binding (%)	>98	>98	Not reported
Terminal half-life	7 days	5 days	25 h

	Steroidal anti-oestrogens
	Faslodex
Administration	Intramuscular (depot)
Protein binding	Not reported
Terminal half-life	About 4 weeks[a]

	Non-steroidal aromatase inhibitors		
	Aminoglutethimide	Anastrozole	Letrozole
Administration	Oral	Oral	Oral
Protein binding (%)	25	40	60
Terminal half-life (h)	13 h or 7 h[b]	50 h	48 h

	Steroidal aromatase inhibitors	
	Formestane	Exemestane
Administration	Intramuscular	Oral
Protein binding (%)	85%	Not reported
Terminal half-life	2 h or 7 days[c]	24 h

	Luteinizing hormone-releasing hormone analogues			
	Buserelin	Goserelin	Leuprorelin	Nafarelin
Administration	Subcutaneous (depot)	Subcutaneous (depot)	Subcutaneous (depot)	Subcutaneous (depot)
Protein binding (%)	15	25–66[d]	45%	80%
Terminal half-life	75 min[e]	5 h[e]	3 h	2 h

	Progestins	
	Megestrol	Medroxyprogesterone
Administration	Oral	Oral
Protein binding	Not known	Not known
Terminal half-life (h)	14	7–60 h[f]

	Anti-androgens		
	Flutamide	Bicalutamide	Nilutamide
Administration	Oral	Oral	Oral
Protein binding (%)	95	>95	80
Terminal half-life	8 h	56 h	100 h

[a]After intramuscular dosing.
[b]Shorter half-life during multiple than during single dosing.
[c]After oral and intramuscular dosing, respectively.
[d]Different animal species.
[e]When given as single doses, not as depot formulations.
[f]See text.

clinical use,[1] the introduction of 'modern' endocrine therapy should be dated to the successful implementation of tamoxifen for treating breast cancer three decades ago. Soon after that, progestins and the first-generation aromatase inhibitor aminoglutethimide were found to be effective treatment modalities for postmenopausal and previously castrated breast cancer patients.

Over the last decade, clinical trials with these drugs have taught us two important lessons. First, tamoxifen (but also castration in premenopausal women) may improve long-term survival and therefore cure some patients when administered as adjuvant therapy in early breast cancer.[2,3] Secondly, the development of resistance towards one endocrine treatment for breast cancer does not necessarily induce resistance toward other regimens.[4] Together, these discoveries have encouraged both the development of new compounds and further research in the field of endocrine resistance.

Different drugs and their clinical uses

Anti-oestrogens

Until recently, the term 'anti-oestrogen' was synonymous with a single drug, tamoxifen. In view of the successful results reported from trials recruiting over 10 000 patients with early-stage and metastatic disease,[5,6] this triphenylethylene derivative is the contemporary gold standard for endocrine treatment of both pre- and postmenopausal breast cancer. Tamoxifen administered in the adjuvant setting for a period of 5 years has been reported to reduce relapse rate by 47% and total mortality by 26% among patients with oestrogen-receptor-positive early breast cancers.[3]

Because of the successful results obtained with tamoxifen, several other triethylene derivatives have been synthesized. An important issue with tamoxifen therapy has been possible detrimental side effects caused by its oestrogen-agonistic activity, in particular a reported elevated risk of endometrial carcinomas.[3] Thus a major aim of the search for new anti-oestrogens has been to achieve drugs with less agonistic but more potent antagonistic activities. Several new compounds, including toremifene (4-chloro-tamoxifen), droloxifene (3-hydroxy-tamoxifen), idoxifene, and raloxifene, have been synthesized and evaluated for breast cancer treatment in clinical trials (Fig. 15.1).

In addition to the triethylene anti-oestrogens, a new class of drugs, the steroidal or 'pure' anti-oestrogens, have been introduced. Chemically, these drugs are all oestradiol derivatives (Fig. 15.2) and *in vitro* data have not reveal any evidence of oestrogen agonism associated with them. The first compound in clinical trials,

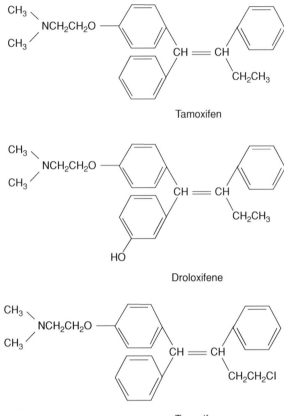

Tamoxifen

Droloxifene

Toremifene

Figure 15.1. Chemical structure of the non-steroidal anti-oestrogens tamoxifen, droloxifene, and toremifene.

faslodex (also known as 182.870), seems to be associated with clinical responses of particular long duration in patients suffering from advanced breast cancer. It is currently being evaluated in phase III trials,

Aromatase inhibitors

Aromatase inhibitors suppress postmenopausal oestrogen synthesis by inhibiting the final step in oestrogen synthesis: aromatization of androgens to oestrogens.[8] In postmenopausal women, aromatization of circulating androgens of adrenal and (to a minor extent) ovarian origin occurs in a variety of tissues such as muscle, connective tissue, skin, and liver.[9] Although peripheral aromatization also occurs in premenopausal women, its contribution is small compared with ovarian secretion. It should be noted that, while aromatase inhibitors may also influence ovarian aromatase, evidence so far suggests that this inhibition is balanced by gonadotrophin secretion,[10] and so these drugs have no place in the treatment of women with intact ovarian function. Finally, it should also be noted that aromatase inhibitors may also inhibit local oestrogen production within tumour tissue itself.[11]

The first-generation aromatase inhibitor aminoglutethimide (Fig. 15.3) was introduced for breast cancer treatment 30 years ago. While randomized studies revealed a similar clinical efficacy to tamoxifen or progestins,[4] a major reason for developing novel aromatase inhibitors is that aminoglutethimide lacks specificity (influence on other steroid-synthesizing enzymes involved in adrenal steroid synthesis) and significant side effects occur, in particular in the central nervous system.[12] Novel aromatase inhibitors developed over the last decade can be divided into steroidal and non-steroidal inhibitors; the second class consists of drugs that can be regarded as chemical derivatives of aminoglutethimide and drugs belonging to the imidazole/triazole class (Fig. 15.4).

Non-steroidal aromatase inhibitors focused on improving the 'aminoglutethimide class' have been generally unsuccessful. Thus neither roglethimide, nor the

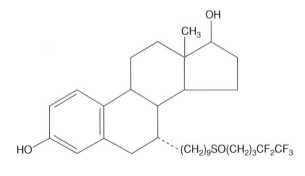

Faslodex

Figure 15.2. Chemical structure of the steroidal anti-oestrogen faslodex.

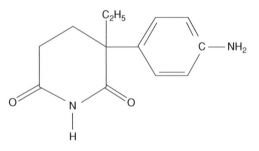

Aminoglutethimide

Figure 15.3. Chemical structure of the first-generation aromatase inhibitor aminoglutethimide.

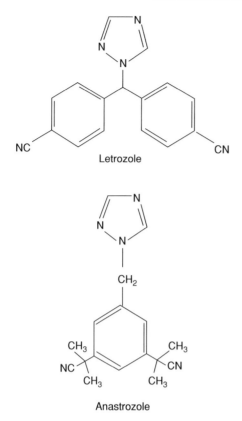

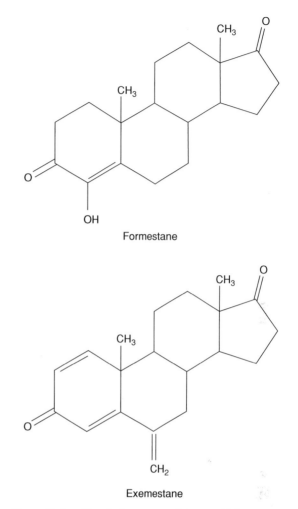

Figure 15.4. Chemical structure of non-steroidal aromatase inhibitors belonging to the triazole class currently in clinical development.

D-enantiomer of aminoglutethimide were found to be more potent than aminoglutethimide itself; in addition, both these drugs were associated with neurological side effects to a similar extent to racemic aminoglutethimide.[13,14]

Development of non-steroidal aromatase inhibitors of the imidazole/triazole class has been a far more successful approach to this form of endocrine therapy. Accordingly, new drugs like letrozole and anastrozole have both been shown to be more potent aromatase inhibitors, causing more profound plasma oestrogen suppression than aminoglutethimide.[15,16] Recent results from randomized studies show that both drugs produce a modest improvement in survival and/or increase response rate and response duration in patients with metastatic disease compared with treatment with megestrol acetate or aminoglutethimide.[17–19] In addition, treatment with these drugs is associated with only a few mild side effects.

One steroidal aromatase inhibitor (formestane, 4-hydroxyandrostenedione) is currently in clinical use, while a second drug, *exemestane*, is in clinical phase III

Figure 15.5. Chemical structure of the steroidal aromatase inhibitors formestane and exemestane.

trials (Fig. 15.5). Formestane has the disadvantage of requiring parenteral injections to be fully effective.[20,21] Interestingly, while *in vivo* tracer studies revealed that this drug caused rather less aromatase inhibition and plasma oestrogen suppression than aminoglutethimide,[14,21–24] results from different groups showed that some breast cancer patients may respond to treatment with formestane after becoming resistant to treatment with aminoglutethimide. A possible explanation of these findings could be a different influence on intra-tumour aromatase (possibly a different drug uptake). Exemestane has been shown to be a potent aromatase inhibitor with a biochemical efficacy resembling that of letrozole and anastrozole,[25] and, similarly to formestane, has also been found to be active in patients becoming resistant to therapy with a non-steroidal aromatase inhibitor.[26,27]

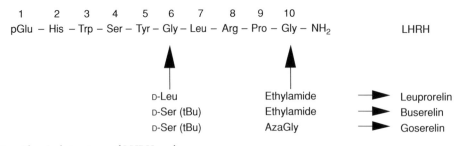

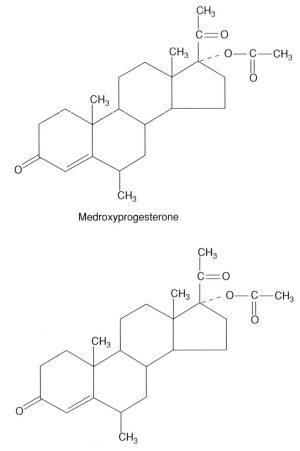

Figure 15.6.   Chemical structures of LHRH analogues.

Luteinizing hormone-releasing hormone analogues

Luteinizing hormone-releasing hormone (LHRH) triggers the secretion of gonadotrophins by acting on the pituitary gland. LHRH analogues (Fig. 15.6), such as buserelin and goserelin, also cause an initial stimulation of gonadotrophin secretion. However, these analogues have a longer half-life than LHRH itself, and this, combined with their continuous release from depot formulations, causes a sustained stimulation of the pituitary, which subsequently leads to a strong inhibition of gonadotrophin secretion in both sexes.[28,29] Goserelin and buserelin have been most extensively studied in cancer, and leuprorelin and nafarelin more extensively for treatment of benign gynaecological disorders.[30,31] However, all these drugs have now been evaluated in cancer therapy (mainly treatment of prostatic cancer). They share a mechanism of action and, with a few small differences, have similar pharmacokinetic properties.

LHRH analogues are successfully used for the treatment of advanced prostate cancer as well as breast carcinomas. A great advantage of this treatment compared with surgical or radiological castration is its reversibility, allowing return of gonadotrophin secretion upon termination of treatment. In breast cancer patients with advanced disease, a logical approach is to test for response (over a period of 3–6 months); in the case of an objective response, permanent castration (by radiotherapy or surgery) should be considered, because later sequential treatments (with drugs like aromatase inhibitors or progestins) all require elimination of ovarian function.

Progestins

Progesterone analogues are primarily used for breast cancer treatment and are administered in pharmacological doses. The common regimens are medroxyprogesterone acetate (MPA) 1000 mg daily or megestrol

Medroxyprogesterone

Megestrol

Figure 15.7. Chemical structures of the semisynthetic progestins MA and MPA.

acetate (MA) 160 mg daily. Progestins like MA and MPA (Fig. 15.7) produce clinical remission in patients suffering from advanced breast cancer; randomized studies have confirmed response rates not significantly different from those achieved with tamoxifen or aminoglutethimide.[32–34] A major limitation on their clinical use is their side effects, of which the most important are undesirable weight gain, activity-related shortness of breath (probably due to interstitial oedema in the lungs), and an increased risk of thromboembolic events.[17] Recently, the observed weight gain has led to the use of progestins for the treatment of cancer-related cachexia.

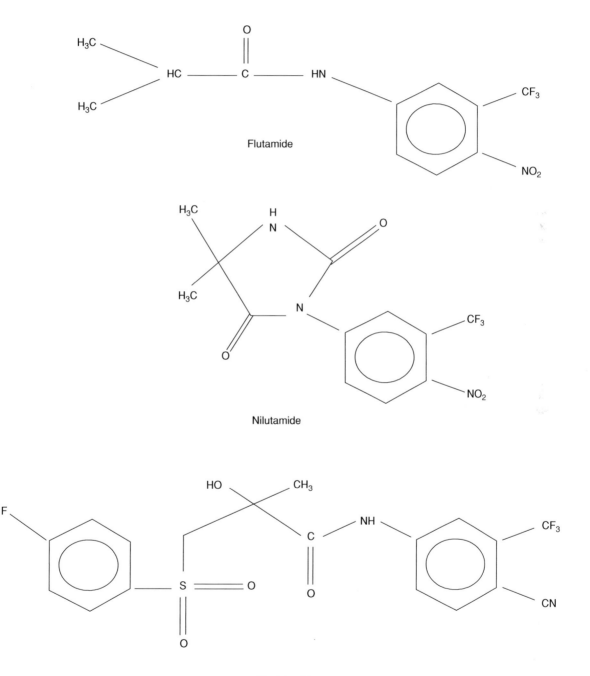

Figure 15.8. Chemical structures of non-steroidal anti-androgens used in prostate cancer therapy.

Anti-androgens

Anti-androgens can be classified as steroidal or non-steroidal.

Steroidal anti-androgens were the first anti-androgens synthesized and used clinically. The first-generation drug cyproterone acetate was introduced for clinical treatment more than 25 years ago.[35] Although this drug is effective in therapy, a major disadvantage is inhibition of gonadotrophin secretion with a subsequent drop in plasma androgen levels, leading to impotence. Thus more recent research has been focused on the development of non-steroidal anti-androgens.

Non-steroidal anti-androgens pose no intrinsic steroidal activity; thus these compounds are also known as 'pure' anti-androgens. Several drugs, such as flutamide, nilutamide, and Casodex, have been developed for clinical use (Fig. 15.8). Anti-androgens have been evaluated as monotherapy[36] as well as combined with medical or surgical castration ('total androgen blockade') in prostatic cancers.[37] While several large studies have suggested an improved overall survival for this treatment approach, a recent overview analysis did not confirm any significant influence on survival.[38]

Although non-steroidal anti-androgens like flutamide have been found to inhibit enzymes involved in androgen synthesis in the rat testis, they do not suppress plasma androgen levels in humans,[40,41] and so they are assumed to preserve sexual function better than castration. Although there is some evidence that such therapy is associated with improved sexual interest compared with castration,[42] there is limited direct support for the argument that it provides any major advantages considering sexual ability.[42,43]

A rare but serious side effect with all three non-steroidal anti-androgens in clinical use is the occurrence of hepatotoxic reactions, sometimes with a fatal outcome.[44–46] Generation of oxidative stress on the hepatocytes has been suggested as an explanation of this phenomenon.

Anti-oestrogens

Non-steroidal anti-oestrogens

Because the clinical pharmacologies of the various non-steroidal anti-oestrogens are quite similar, these drugs will be considered together. The three drugs discussed here are tamoxifen and the two other non-steroidal anti-oestrogens most extensively studied in cancer therapy to date, toremifene and droloxifene.

Pharmacology

The structures of the three compounds are shown in Figure 15.1. The anti-oestrogens act by binding to the oestrogen receptor, thereby blocking ligand stimulation by the oestradiol ligand. This topic is discussed in more detail elsewhere.[47]

All these drugs have a dual action, inasmuch as they act as partial oestrogen agonists, depending on the test system. While studies *in vitro* have revealed droloxifene to be somewhat less oestrogen agonistic compared with the other compounds,[48] *in vivo* investigations in animal models conclude that this drug also acts as an oestrogen agonist on bone metabolism.[49] Other more recent non-steroidal anti-oestrogens have been shown to have more selective actions on different tissues in this respect. Thus, while tamoxifen expresses oestrogen agonistic activities on the endometrium, the novel anti-oestrogen raloxifene was shown to express anti-oestrogen effects in tumour models and oestrogen effects on parameters like blood lipids and bone metabolism resembling those of tamoxifen, but to act as an anti-oestrogen on the endometrium.[50] The explanation could be specific binding of the drug–receptor complex generated by raloxifene to specific DNA binding sites.[51,52] The discovery of more selective actions of particular non-steroidal anti-oestrogens has resulted in the introduction of the term selective oestrogen receptor modulators (SERMs); obviously, future investigations in this field will bring in new aspects of therapy not only in breast cancer, but also in prevention of other diseases like cancers as well as osteoporosis.

Tamoxifen and the other non-steroidal anti-oestrogens have been found to interact with several other biochemical processes. Examples are induction of TGF-β secretion, suppression of plasma IGF-I, elevation of IGF-binding protein-1, downregulation of TGF-α and erbB-2, and inhibition of protein kinase C and calmodulin (reviewed by Lønning and Lien[47]). The importance of any of these effects to the antitumour effects of these drugs is currently poorly understood.

Mechanisms of drug resistance

The mechanisms of resistance to endocrine therapy are poorly understood. As endocrine therapy depends on the hormone sensitivity of the tumour, many tumours are unable to respond to any form of endocrine therapy simply because they lack expression of the oestrogen receptor. In other tumours showing primary drug resistance despite expressing the oestrogen receptor, this may be due to post-receptor events (defective responsive elements or alterations in other downstream genes). It should be noted that lack of response to tamoxifen first-line therapy in general predicts a poor response to other forms of hormone manipulation, signalling a lack of hormone sensitivity in general. A different scenario exists with respect to acquired resistance, inasmuch as these tumours often respond to second-line endocrine therapy, suggesting that a drug-specific form of resistance may have developed (reviewed by Lønning and Lien[47] and by Lønning[53]).

While different mutant oestrogen receptors have been identified in human breast cancers, so far there is little evidence supporting a major role for any of these mutants in tamoxifen resistance.[53] There is evidence suggesting that over-expression of erbB-2 as well as mutations of the TP53 gene are associated with tamoxifen resistance in human breast cancers.[54,55] Although there is no evidence pointing to alterations in total body drug pharmacokinetics as a mechanism of drug resistance, some authors have suggested that alterations in intra-tumour drug concentrations may be involved in acquired drug resistance (see below).

Clinical pharmacokinetics

Methods of drug measurement
While the concentration of tamoxifen and its metabolites in plasma are below the detection limit using standard UV detection following separation using high-performance liquid chromatography (HPLC), the molecules may be converted into highly fluorescent compounds by the UV irradiation, making detection possible. Several different HPLC methods for quantitation of tamoxifen and metabolites have been developed, and the drug has also been measured with using gas chromatography–mass spectrometry and thin-layer chromatography (GC–MS) (reviewed by Lønning et al.[56]). Similarly, HPLC methods for plasma detection of toremifene and droloxifene have been developed,[57–61] and toremifene metabolites have been detected in the urine using liqid chromatography–mass spectrometry.[62]

Absorption
Because none of these drugs have been administered to humans by the parenteral route, their exact bioavailability in humans is not known. Following administration of radioactive tamoxifen by the oral route, the bulk of radioactivity is excreted in the faeces and not the urine.[63] While this hampers an indirect estimation of the amount absorbed, the fact that the excretion occurred over 1–2 weeks suggests that the bulk of the radioactivity is absorbed and undergoes enterohepatic

recycling. It should be noted that the relative amount of radioactivity excreted in urine and faces was similar in dogs and rats following intraperitoneal and oral administration.[64]

Administration of radioactive toremifene to rats by the oral and intravenous route revealed a similar excretion pattern of radioactivity in the urine and faeces;[65] this, together with the finding of similar plasma and drug concentrations in rats and dogs following oral and intravenous drug dosing,[66] suggests good absorption and also refutes the hypothesis of any major first-pass metabolism of toremifene in these species. The drug is absorbed to a similar extent when administered as a solution or a tablet, and the AUC–drug dose relationship has been reported to be linear.[67]

Administration of radiolabelled droloxifene to different species by the oral and intravenous routes revealed that it was almost completely absorbed but with an extensive first-pass metabolism; thus the mean bioavailability of the drug following oral dosing was found to be 8% in mice, 11% in monkeys, and 18% in rats.[60] Others[68] have confirmed the bioavailability of droloxifene in rats to be about 20% following oral dosing; this effect was due to an extensive first-pass metabolism in the liver and not to poor absorption.

Metabolism and excretion
A common feature of all the three drugs mentioned above is that most of the metabolites are excreted by the faecal and not the urinary pathway.

Tamoxifen is extensively metabolized in humans. Among the different metabolites identified, several still retain biological activity. 4-Hydroxytamoxifen has a particularly high affinity for the oestrogen receptor.[69] Despite the fact that the mean plasma steady-state concentration of this metabolite is about 1–10% of the concentration of tamoxifen,[70] owing to its high receptor affinity this metabolite is thought to be the major effective form of tamoxifen *in vivo*. Most of the urine as well as the faecal metabolites appear as glucuronide conjugates in different species, including humans.[63,64,71]

Nine metabolites of toremifene have been isolated from rat faeces.[65] Some of these, like N-desmethyl-toremifene which is the main metabolite in humans, exhibit anti-oestrogen activities.[72] This metabolite, as well as 4-hydroxytoremifene, can be detected in plasma of patients treated with toremifene in common therapeutic doses,[73,74] the latter following treatment with doses in the higher range only.

The main plasma metabolites of droloxifene are N-demethyl-droloxifene and the glucuronides of this metabolite and the mother compound.[75]

Plasma and tissue pharmacokinetics

The time to C_{max} following drug ingestion has been reported to be 3–7 h, 1.5 to 6 h and 2–3 h for tamoxifen, toremifene and droloxifene, respectively.[59,60,73,76,77]

There is a major difference between tamoxifen or toremifene and droloxifene with respect to plasma pharmacokinetics. The mean terminal half-life of tamoxifen and toremifene in humans have been reported to be about 7 and 5 days respectively.[63,73,77,78] The mean half-life for droloxifene is about 25 h.[59,75] Based on AUC determinations following single drug doses,[60] a mean steady-state plasma concentration of droloxifene of about 40 ng/ml can be expected during treatment with 40 mg daily (the dose selected for ongoing clinical trials based on results from a phase II study).[79] The mean plasma concentrations of tamoxifen and its main metabolite 4-hydroxytamoxifen following 30 mg once-daily dosing are about 200 ng/ml and 6–8 ng/ml, respectively.[70] As *in vitro* investigations have revealed droloxifene to have an approximately 10-fold increased affinity for the oestrogen receptor compared with tamoxifen and an affinity resembling that of 4-hydroxytamoxifen,[48,80] this suggests that a plasma drug level of droloxifene following 40 mg once-daily dosing will achieve biological effects similar to what would be expected from use of tamoxifen. However, plasma drug concentrations may not necessarily mirror tissue concentrations for these drugs. Thus tamoxifen is found in high concentrations in different human tissues and can be detected in tissue samples obtained several months after terminating drug therapy. Tissue drug measurements have not been performed with droloxifene or toremifene. The distribution volume of droloxifene in humans is not known, but has been estimated to be 8–10 l/kg body weight after intravenous drug administration to rats, mice, and monkeys.[60] This, together with the finding of a high tissue-to-blood ratio of radioactivity in rats following administration of radioactive droloxifene,[60] suggests that high concentrations of droloxifene may be found in human tissues. Both tamoxifen and toremifene have a plasma protein binding exceeding 98%[71,81,82] and the protein binding for droloxifene has not been reported.

Drug interactions

In vitro data have suggested that tamoxifen inhibits the activity of several mixed function oxidases,[83] and the drug has been reported to inhibit its own metabolism.[78] Enhancement of the anticoagulant effect of warfarin has been reported and suggested to be caused by an impaired warfarin metabolism,[83–85] although the exact pharmacokinetic interaction has not been explored.

Considering possible interactions with other drugs used for treatment of breast cancer, drug interactions between tamoxifen and aromatase inhibitors are discussed in the section dealing with these drugs. Little is known about possible drug interactions with toremifene or droloxifene *in vivo*.

Steroidal anti-oestrogens

Pharmacology

Although several steroidal anti-oestrogens are in preclinical development,[86] only one drug, faslodex (182.780), is currently being evaluated in clinical trials.[7]

The biochemical mechanism of action of steroidal anti-oestrogens differs from that of the non-steroidal drugs. The steroidal drugs also interact with receptor shuttling and half-life to inhibit receptor folding and dimerization.[87,88] Unlike the non-steroidal anti-oestrogens, steroidal anti-oestrogens have been found to be devoid of any oestrogen agonistic effects.[89,90]

Mechanisms of drug resistance

The mechanisms of resistance to steroidal anti-oestrogens are unknown. For a consideratiom of possible mechanisms of resistance to anti-oestrogens in general as well as to oestrogen deprivation, the reader should consult the sections dealing with non-steroidal anti-oestrogens and aromatase inhibitors.

Clinical pharmacokinetics

Methods of drug measurement

Faslodex concentrations in plasma can be determined by radio-immunoassay (RIA). The sensitivity limit of this assay is 0.68 ng/ml, which allows detection of plasma levels more than 28 days after single dosing (mean concentration 3–7.5 ng/ml) and during multiple dosing (mean concentration 6–10 ng/ml).[91] Plasma levels detected with this assay were found to be in agreement with results obtained using HPLC.[91]

Absorption

Because of its poor absorption, faslodex must be administered by the parenteral route.[92] The drug is currently available as a depot formulation, allowing monthly administration.[7]

Metabolism and excretion

So far, there are no data on the metabolic pathways and excretion of faslodex in the literature.

Plasma and tissue pharmacokinetics

Plasma peak levels are seen about 8–9 days after intramuscular administration of the depot formulation.[91] Multiple dosing increased C_{max} and AUC by mean factors of 1.2 and 1.5, respectively, indicating a slight degree of drug accumulation. The plasma half-life is slow following intramuscular administration, with a mean peak plasma level of about 7.5 ng/ml following administration of a single dose of 250 mg, dropping to about 3 ng/ml after 4 weeks.[91]

So far, there are no data on plasma protein binding or tissue pharmacokinetics in the literature.

Drug interactions

So far no drug interactions with faslodex have been described.

Aromatase inhibitors

Pharmacology

Aromatase inhibitors exert their biochemical effects by inhibiting the enzymes aromatizing androgens (androstenedione and, to a lesser extent, testosterone) into their oestrogen counterparts (oestrone and oestradiol). The two classes of aromatase inhibitors, steroidal and non-steroidal drugs, bind to the substrate binding and P450 sites on the enzyme, respectively. In addition, steroidal aromatase inhibitors bind irreversibly to the enzyme complex, and thus are also known as 'suicide' inhibitors or aromatase inactivators.[8]

Mechanisms of drug resistance

Except for the mechanisms of endocrine resistance in general, the understanding of possible mechanisms of resistance to oestrogen deprivation (castration in premenopausal women and the use of aromatase inhibitors in postmenopausal women) is limited. However, a striking clinical observation is the ability of many breast cancers to respond to repeated oestrogen deprivation. Thus tumours relapsing following an initial response to medical castration may subsequently respond to an aromatase inhibitor added in concert.[92,93] Likewise, postmenopausal women expressing very low plasma oestrogen levels because of previous therapy with adreno- or hypophysectomy may subsequently respond to further oestrogen suppression from an aromatase inhibitor,[94] and patients progressing on *aminoglutethimide* administered as a 'low-dose' regimen (250 mg daily) have subsequently responded to treatment with aminoglutethimide administered in 'high doses' (1000 mg daily).[95] Finally, it has been shown that patients relapsing on *formestane* may benefit from having aminoglutethimide added in concert.[23,96] Interestingly, it has been shown that MCF-7 breast cancer cells gradually exposed to low concentrations of oestradiol *in vitro* may 'adapt' to growth stimulation by oestradiol at a concentration of 10^{-15}–10^{-14} M (the normally requirement is ~10^{-10} M).[97] This interesting finding is consistent with the hypothesis that some tumours develop resistance to oestrogen deprivation not by becoming endocrine resistant but by becoming 'hypersensitive', suggesting new therapeutic strategies such as the use of steroidal and non-steroidal aromatase inhibitors in combination to maximize oestrogen suppression.

Clinical pharmacokinetics

Methods of drug measurement

Plasma levels of *aminoglutethimide* and its major plasma metabolite N-acetylaminoglutethimide were initially measured spectrophotometrically,[98] but can now be determined using HPLC methods[99–102] or a multiple selected ion monitoring (SIM) technique.[103] An HPLC method to determine aminoglutethimide in the urine has also been reported.[104] These methods measure the (R)- and (S)-enantiomers together, but a chiral assay measuring the separate enantiomers has been developed.[105] *Formestane* can be measured in plasma by RIA or isotope dilution mass spectrometry[106,107] and in the urine by HPLC–MS,[108,109] and *exemestane* can be measured in plasma by HPLC.[109] An enzyme immunoassay and a sensitive HPLC method are available for plasma *letrozole*,[110,111] and *anastrozole* can be measured by gas–liquid chromatography (GLC).[16]

Absorption

Following oral dosing of the 'classical' non-steroidal drug aminoglutethimide labelled with ^{14}C, 80%–98% of the radioactivity was recovered from the urine.[112] Only about 1% of the dose was recovered from the faeces.[113] Based on knowledge of its plasma clearance rate, a first-pass metabolism in the order of 2%–8% has been estimated,[112] suggesting a fairly good systemic exposure following oral administration.

The steroidal aromatase inhibitor formestane was developed for both oral and parenteral use. Following oral dosing, 20%–45% of the dose can be recovered from the urine as 4-hydroxyandrostenedione glucuronide.[114] Because no study has compared drug bioavailability following parenteral and oral dosing, its exact bioavailability is not known.

Following ingestion of radioactive *exemestane*, about 40% of the radioactivity is recovered from the urine.[115] Absorption in humans is rapid, with a peak level occurring about 1 h after drug intake. The same study reported a linear dose–peak plasma drug level relationship with single doses up to 400 mg.[116]

In-house animal experiments with administration of radioactive *anastrozole* have revealed the drug to be well absorbed.[117] Bioavailability of letrozole measured by administrating the drug by the intravenous and oral routes to healthy postmenopausal women was found to be close to 100%,[118] with no influence of food administration.[119]

Metabolism and excretion

Although only the major metabolite of aminoglutethimide, N-acetyl-aminoglutethimide, has been identified in human plasma,[112,120,121] several metabolites have been identified in urine from rats and humans.[122,123] One metabolite, hydroxyaminoglutethimide, occurs in the urine only after multiple dosing, suggesting that production is induced by long-term treatment.[124] About 12%–20% of an ingested dose is excreted as unmetabolized aminoglutethimide in the urine, and 3%–7% as N-acetylaminoglutethimide.[104,121]

Formestane is extensively metabolized in humans. While there is no significant excretion of unmetabolized drug, 4-hydroxyandrostenedione glucuronide appears to be the main metabolite in human urine and rat bile.[114,124,125] Several different metabolites have been isolated and characterized from human urine,[108] but their quantitative importance is unknown.

While several metabolites of exemestane have been identified in the urine,[115] the only metabolite of exemestane reported in human plasma is 17-hydro-exemestane, which is found at about one-tenth of the concentration of the parent compound.[116]

In-house studies by the manufacturer have found anastrozole to be heavily metabolized by the liver (>85%), with only about 10% of the drug excreted unmetabolized in the urine.[117] The main metabolic pathways are N-dealkylation (cleaving the two rings of anastrozole and releasing free triazole) and hydroxylation followed by glucuronidation and excretion in the urine. The major metabolite of letrozole is its secondary alcohol; the urinary glucuronides of this when

metabolite and letrozole itself accounts for about 60–65% and 3–4% of the dose, respectively.[118]

Plasma and tissue pharmacokinetics

Following single dosing, aminoglutethimide is rapidly absorbed with the peak level appearing after 0.5–4 h. Plasma clearance (assuming a 100% bioavailability) is 1.5–6 l/h, and the half-life is 6–24 h.[98,103,112,120,126] The half-life is markedly reduced following repeated dosing owing to autoinduction of drug metabolism; however, the fact that plasma clearance rate is not increased to a similar extent as the half-life is reduced suggests there may also be a reduction in the volume of distribution.[112]

Following intramuscular administration of a formestane dose of 500 mg, peak levels of 10–30 ng/ml are seen followed by a half-life of about 7 days.[127] An interesting finding in this study was that plasma oestradiol started to rise when plasma drug levels fell below 3 ng/ml. Following ingestion of a single oral dose of 250 mg, peak levels of about 45 ng/ml were seen 1–3 h after ingestion,[127] followed by a plasma elimination half-life of about 2 h.[125] Thus, while peak levels expected to cause effective plasma oestrogen suppression are achieved following oral dosing, the short half-life of this compound makes it unsuitable for oral dosing. This was confirmed by tracer studies revealing that formestane administered as 250 mg once daily or 125 mg twice daily caused *in vivo* aromatase inhibition of only about 60%–70%.[20] However, exemestane has a terminal half-life of about 24 h, allowing once-daily dosing.[128]

The median time to peak drug level following oral dosing is about 3 h for anastrozole, although a substantial variation (2–12 h) is seen.[129] The terminal half-life of the drug is about 50 h. Consistent with that, plasma steady-state levels are reached in about 9–10 days during multiple dosing.[129] Letrozole is characterized by a rapid absorption (peak level about 1 h after oral dosing), a long half-life (about 48 h), a low plasma clearance rate (mean 2.2 l/h), and a high volume of distribution (1.87 l/kg), suggesting a rather high tissue distribution.[118,130]

Plasma protein binding, was about 25% for aminoglutethimide,[112] 85% for formestane,[106] and about 60% for letrozole.[130,131]

No information is currently available regarding tissue concentrations of any of the aromatase inhibitors except for aminoglutethimide and formestane. Tracer studies in animals and anecdotal observations from human autopsies suggest that aminoglutethimide is concentrated in the adrenal gland.[132,133] Although the drug seems to be evenly distributed in the other tissues, a volume of distribution in excess in body water suggests that some tissue binding to occur.[112,120] In contrast, a lower concentration of formestane was reported in malignant as well as benign breast tissue compared with plasma levels.[134]

Drug interactions

Aminoglutethimide is a potent inducer of mixed-function oxidases.[135] Thus, as well as enhancing the metabolism of different compounds like dexamethasone, antipyrine, theophylline and digitoxin,[136] aminoglutethimide has been found to enhance the metabolism of tamoxifen,[70] MA, and MPA.[137,138] Based on the findings that aminoglutethimide interacts with tamoxifen disposition, several investigations have been performed to evaluate possible interactions between the novel aromatase inhibitors anastrozole or letrozole and tamoxifen before implementing combined treatment with these drugs in the adjuvant setting. Although anastrozole was found to inhibit certain P450 mixed-function oxidases *in vitro*,[139] it does not influence the disposition of antipyrine,[140] and recent studies revealed that neither anastrozole nor letrozole treatment influenced plasma levels of tamoxifen.[141] However, tamoxifen was found to suppress plasma levels of letrozole by 35%–40%;[142] whether a similar phenomenon will be observed during treatment with anastrozole is under evaluation.

Luteinizing hormone-releasing hormone analogues

Pharmacology

LHRH analogues are deca- or nonapeptide analogues of the LHRH decapeptide chemically modified in the 6 and, eventually, the 10 position (Fig. 15.6). They are highly potent agonists with a high affinity for the LHRH receptor. In addition, the chemical modifications of these compounds make them less susceptible to enzyme degradation and extend their half-lives.[143,144] Continuous stimulation of the pituitary gland by these analogues leads to profound suppression of gonadotrophin secretion and 'medical castration'.[145] Notably, while the antitumour effect of these drugs has been related to oestrogen or androgen deprivation in breast and prostatic cancers respectively, high-affinity receptors for LHRH have been identified in several tissues, including breast tumours.[146]

Mechanisms of drug resistance

The mechanisms of resistance to oestrogen deprivation (castration in premenopausal women or use of aromatase inhibitors in postmenopausal women) is addressed in the section discussing resistance to aromatase inhibitors. Little is known about possible mechanisms of resistance to androgen deprivation in prostatic carcinomas.

Clinical pharmacokinetics

Drug measurement

LHRH analogues such as buserelin and goserelin can be measured in plasma and urine with RIA techniques with or without separation by HPLC.[147–152]

Absorption

Because polypeptides like LHRH analogues are poorly absorbed and undergo degradation in the gastrointestinal tract, they are administered by the parenteral route. While nasal and cutaneous administration gives unpredictable and fluctuating plasma levels, various LHRH analogues such as buserelin, goserelin, leuprorelin, and nafarelin are available as slow-release depot formulations, allowing monthly or even quarterly administration.[28,153,154]

Metabolism and excretion

LHRH analogues are metabolized in several organs including the liver, kidney, and central nervous system.[155–157] In general, these compounds are metabolized by enzymatic cleavage of the peptide bound between Tyr^5 and the amino acid in the 6 position (reviewed by Robinson and Jordan[157]).

Plasma and tissue pharmacokinetics

While the terminal half-life of LHRH in the plasma is in the range 30–60 min,[155] the half-lives of buserelin and goserelin following single-dose administration were reported to be 70–80 min[149] and 5 h,[147] respectively. The half-lives of leuprorelin and nafarelin have been reported to be about 3 h and 2 h, respectively (reviewed by Chrisp and Goa[151] and by Plosker and Brogden[158]). The plasma clearance rate for goserelin is 2–8 l/h,[147,159] and its volume of distribution is about 14 litres,[147] which is in the same range as total body content of extracellular water. Except for nafarelin, which has a protein binding of about 80%,[160] in general LHRH analogues have a low plasma protein binding.[29,144,147]

Drug interactions

So far there are no known drug interactions involving LHRH analogues.

Progestins

Pharmacology

The mechanisms of action of the synthetic progestins (MA and MPA) administered in pharmacological doses for advanced breast cancer are only partly understood (reviewed by Lønning and Lien[47]). Recently, we found that MA administered at its common therapeutic dose of 160 mg daily suppressed plasma oestrogen levels down to 18%–29% of their pretreatment levels,[160,161] which is in the same range as seen during treatment with aromatase inhibitors like aminoglutethimide. Thus one mechanism of action of these progestins could be profound suppression of plasma oestrogen levels secondary to suppression of their adrenal androgen precursors.

Mechanisms of drug resistance

As with other endocrine therapies, the mechanism(s) of drug resistance to progestins in high dose regimens is poorly understood. For possible reasons for resistance towards oestrogen suppression, the reader is referred to the section dealing with aromatase inhibitors.

Clinical pharmacokinetics

Methods of drug measurement

Several methods are available for determination of MA and MPA in plasma including RIA, GLC, enzymatic detection, and GC–MS techniques (reviewed by Lønning et al.[56]). Because several metabolites of MPA as well as MA appear in the plasma,[162] and some of

these may cross-react to the antibodies when measuring MPA or MA plasma concentrations with RIA, it is extremely important to purify samples before such analysis.[162–164]

Absorption

The exact bioavailability of the progestins following oral administration is uncertain. Comparing the bio-availability of MPA following intraperitoneal and oral administration, Camaggi et al.[165] estimated that the bioavailability of this drug after oral dosing was between 0.2% and 17.4%. Thus, not only is the bio-availability low, but there is also a substantial inter-individual variation, making plasma drug levels unpredictable. Following oral administration of radio-labelled MA, 55%–80% of the radioactivity was recovered from the urine.[166] While this does not exclude an extensive first-pass metabolism, it is noteworthy that plasma drug levels following administration of MA 160 mg daily have been found to be two to three times higher than the drug levels found after administration of MPA 1000 mg daily.[167,168]

Metabolism and excretion

The metabolism of MPA varies between species (reviewed by Lønning et al.[56]). In humans, 25%–50% of the radioactivity is excreted in the urine and 5%–10% in the stools following administration of [3H]MPA, and at least 15 different urinary metabolites are detected (reviewed by Utaaker et al.[169]). The meta-bolic reactions include hydroxylation (positions 2, 6, and 21), demethylation, reduction, and combinations of the different reactions. The bulk of urinary radioac-tivity is excreted as the enol glucuronide of MPA, with less than 3% excreted as unmetabolized MPA.[170,171]

As mentioned above the bulk of radioactivity is recovered from the urine following administration of radioactive MA by the oral route. Although three glucuronide metabolites (MA hydroxylated in the 2 position, the 6 position, or both) have been isolated from the urine in humans,[163,166] they accounted for only 3%–8% of the dose administered.

Plasma and tissue pharmacokinetics

Plasma clearance rate for MPA following intravenous administration has been determined to be between 27 and 70 l/h.[169,172] Various results for the terminal half-life of the drug, with a mean varying between 7 and 60 h, have been reported by different authors. A possible reason for this could be different sampling protocols with too short a time interval for adequate detection in some of these studies (reviewed by Lønning and Lien[173]). Thus the long estimate of 60 h is most likely to be the correct value for MPA.[174] Similarly, while the terminal half-life of MA has been reported to be about 14 h,[162] the actual half-life could be longer.

A controversial subject is whether there is any critical 'threshold' regarding plasma MPA and MA levels required to achieve an optimal therapeutic response.[56]

MPA binds slightly to albumin only.[175] As far as this author is aware, no study has determined protein binding for MA.

Both drugs have been reported to concentrate in the liver and tumour tissue in rodents.[176] Human autopsies suggest that MPA is concentrated in different tissues such as the gastrointestinal system and adipose tissue.[171]

Drug interactions

Aminoglutethimide suppresses plasma levels of both MPA and MA when administered in combination with these drugs, probably due to induction of their metabolism.[137,138,17] Progestins may further increase plasma levels of *warfarin*[178] and also metabolite X of *tamoxifen* in patients receiving the drugs in combination.[179]

Non-steroidal anti-androgens

Pharmacology

Unlike the steroidal anti-androgens, which also have progestational activity, non-steroidal anti-androgens do not suppress plasma androgen levels. In animal experiments flutamide and nilutamide (but not bicalutamide) were found to increase plasma luteinizing hormone and testosterone levels in the rat.[180] However, all these drugs elevate plasma luteinizing hormone levels in humans.[41,181,182]

Although the non-steroidal anti-androgens have been claimed to be 'pure' anti-androgens with no steroid agonist activity,[183,184] some interesting observations, like the well-documented anti-tumour responses to drug withdrawal,[185–187] still lack a biochemical explanation. Mutations in the androgen receptor[188] may influence ligand binding, and the anti-androgen flutamide has been reported to act as a growth stimulator in the LNCaP prostatic cancer cell line harbouring a mutated androgen receptor.[189] This mutation has also

been identified in human prostate cancer specimens,[190] but currently it is not known whether this may explain the withdrawal phenomenon.

Mechanisms of drug resistance

Like endocrine therapy in breast cancer, the mechanism of drug resistance to anti-androgens is poorly understood. One possibility is mutations in the androgen receptor, which make the antagonist act as an agonist, but so far we lack data from clinical investigations supporting or refuting this hypothesis.

Clinical pharmacokinetics

Methods of drug measurement

Flutamide and its active metabolite hydroxyflutamide[191] can be measured by mass spectrometry, gas chromatography, or HPLC methods.[192–194] Nilutamide and bicalutamide in plasma can be measured by HPLC,[195] and the urinary metabolites of bicalutamide by mass spectrometry.[196] Bicalutamide is a racemic drug, with the (*R*)-isomer being the active compound, and a chiral HPLC assay separating the two enantiomers has been developed.[196]

Absorption

Administration of radioactive flutamide to humans revealed that the bulk of radioactivity was excreted in the urine with only a few per cent excreted in the faeces,[192] confirming that the drug was well absorbed. Administration of radioactive nilutamide to rats by the oral and intravenous routes revealed similar plasma AUCs.[197] Similar studies conducted in rats and dogs with bicalutamide revealed almost complete absorption when the drug was administered at doses of 0.1–1 mg/kg body weight, but the absorption was gradually reduced with increasing doses to about 30% when administered at 100 mg/kg body weight.[198] In humans, there appears to be a linear increase in plasma drug levels with respect to bicalutamide doses in the range 10–50 mg/day, but there is a somewhat lower than expected increase in plasma drug levels with increasing doses in the range 50–200 mg/day.[36]

Metabolism and excretion

Flutamide, unlike the two other drugs, requires *in vivo* metabolic activation into its active compound 2-hydroxyflutamide.[199] In addition to the parent compound and its 2-hydroxylated metabolite, the hydrolysis product 3-trifluoromethyl-4-nitroaniline is detected in human plasma.[193] A total of 11 metabolites have been documented but not identified; these metabolites are excreted in the urine as glucuronides.[192]

Tracer studies of nilutamide in humans suggest that the parent compound accounts for 23%–38% of the total plasma radioactivity following oral dosing.[195] The bulk of radioactivity is excreted in the urine with only a few per cent appearing in the faeces.[195] In the urine, only about 1% of the radioactivity is excreted as unmetabolized drug; the rest is excreted as conjugated metabolites.[195] Several metabolic reactions take place, and a detailed overview of these reactions is given elsewhere.[197] The metabolites have little or no biochemical activity.[200]

Bicalutamide is eliminated mainly by the faecal route in the rat, mouse, rabbit, and human, although a substantial portion is excreted in the urine. This contrasts with the metabolic pathways in dogs, where the metabolites are excreted solely by the faecal route.[196,201] Notably, the drug is excreted to a substantial extent as unmetabolized drug, with both the unmetabolized drug and the metabolites mainly excreted as glucuronides. The metabolite profile differs somewhat between species; a detailed description of the different metabolites is given elsewhere.[196,201]

Plasma and tissue pharmacokinetics

Following oral administration of tracer flutamide, the parent compound accounts for only a few per cent of the total plasma radioactivity 1 h after dosing, with multiple polar metabolites (at least 11) accounting for the rest of the radioactivity.[192] Peak plasma concentration occurs about 2 h after drug intake, and the peak level of 2-hydroxyflutamide, the active compound, is more than 20-fold higher than the flutamide concentration.[193] The plasma curve of flutamide is bi-exponential; the mean terminal half-lives of flutamide and 2-hydroxyflutamide are about 8 h, but with a substantial inter-individual variation.[193,202] Nilutamide and bicalutamide, on the other hand, do not need metabolic activation. The half-lives of these drugs are substantially longer than that of flutamide, with a mean value of about 56 h for nilutamide[195] and about 100 h for (R)-bicalutamide (the active compound). In contrast, the mean half-life for (S)-bicalutamide is about 19 h.[196] The time to peak level was found to be about 3 h for nilutamide but as long as 6 h for bicalutamide. Owing to the different elimination rates of the bicalutamide enantiomers, the ratio of the (S)- to the (R)-enanthiomer at steady state will be low.[196] Plasma protein binding of bicalutamide, similar to flutamide, has been found to be about 95%,[198,202] while the binding of nilutamide is about 80%.[195]

Drug interactions

Nilutamide has been reported to inhibit several human as well as mouse mixed-function oxidases *in vitro*,[203] but the possible implications of this finding for the *in vivo* situation are not known.

References

1. Lønning PE, Dowsett M, Powles TJ (1989) Treatment of breast cancer with aromatase inhibitors–current status and future prospects. *Br J Cancer*, **60**, 5–8.
2. Early Breast Cancer Trialists' Collaborative Group (1996) Ovarian ablation in early breast cancer: Overview of the randomised trials. *Lancet*, **348**, 1189–96.
3. Clarke M, Collins R, Davies C, Godwin J, Gray R, Peto R (1998) Tamoxifen for early breast cancer: an overview of the randomised trials. *Lancet*, **351**, 1451–67.
4. Santen RJ, Manni A, Harvey H, Redmond C (1990) Endocrine treatment of breast cancer in women. *Endocr Rev*, **11**, 221–65.
5. Early Breast Cancer Trialists' Collaborative Group (1992) Systemic treatment of early breast cancer by hormonal, cytotoxic, or immune therapy. 133 randomised trials involving 31 000 recurrences and 24 000 deaths among 75 000 women. *Lancet*, **339**, 1–15.
6. Fossati R, Confalonieri C, Torri V, *et al.* (1998) Cytotoxic and hormonal treatment for metastatic breast cancer: A systematic review of published randomized trials involving 31,510 women. *J Clin Oncol*, **16**, 3439–60.
7. Howell A, DeFriend D, Robertson J, Blamey R, Walton P (1995) Response to a specific antioestrogen (ICI 182780) in tamoxifen-resistant breast cancer. *Lancet*, **345**, 29–30.
8. Lønning PE (1996) Pharmacology of new aromatase inhibitors. *Breast*, **5**, 202–8.
9. Lønning PE, Dowsett M, Powles TJ (1990) Postmenopausal estrogen synthesis and metabolism: Alterations caused by aromatase inhibitors used for the treatment of breast cancer. *J Steroid Biochem*, **35**, 355–66.
10. Santen RJ, Samojlik E, Wells SA (1980) Resistance of the ovary to blockade of aromatization with aminoglutethimide. *J Clin Endocrinol Metab*, **51**, 473–7.
11. Miller WR (1991) *In vitro* and *in vivo* effects of 4-hydroxyandrostenedione on steroid and tumour metabolism. *R Soc Med Int Congr Symp Ser*, **180**, 45–9.
12. Lønning PE, Kvinnsland S (1988) Mechanisms of action of aminoglutethimide as endocrine therapy of breast cancer. *Drugs*, **35**, 685–710.

13. Dowsett M, MacNeill F, Mehta A, *et al.* (1991) Endocrine, pharmacokinetic and clinical studies of the aromatase inhibitor 3-ethyl-3-(4-pyridyl)piperidine-2,6-dione ('pyridoglutethimide') in postmenopausal breast cancer patients. *Br J Cancer*, **64**, 887–94.

14. Geisler P, Lundgren S, Berntsen H, Greaves JL, Lonning PE (1998) Influence of dexaminoglutethimide, an optical isomer of aminoglutethimide, on the disposition of estrone sulfate in postmenopausal breast cancer patients. *J Clin Endocrinol Metab*, **83**, 2687–93.

15. Dowsett M, Jones A, Johnston SRD, Jacobs S, Trunet P, Smith IE (1995) *In vivo* measurement of aromatase inhibition be letrozole (CGS 20267) in post menopausal patients with breast cancer. *Clin Cancer Res*, **1**, 1511–15.

16. Geisler J, King N, Dowsett M, *et al.* (1996) Influence of anastrozole (Arimidex®), a selective, non-steroidal aromatase inhibitor, on *in vivo* aromatisation and plasma oestrogen levels in postmenopausal women with breast cancer. *Br J Cancer*, **74**, 1286–91.

17. Buzdar AU, Jonat W, Howell A, *et al.* (1998) Anastrozole versus megestrol acetate in the treatment of postmenopausal women with advanced breast carcinoma: results of a survival update based on a combined analysis of data from two mature phase III trials. *Cancer*, **83**, 1142–52.

18. Dombernowsky P, Smith I, Falkson G, *et al.* (1998) Letrozole, a new oral aromatase inhibitor for advanced breast cancer: double-blind randomized trial showing a dose effect and improved efficacy and tolerability compared with megestrol acetate. *J Clin Oncol*, **16**, 453–61.

19. Gershanovich M, Chaudri HA, Campos D, *et al.* (1998) Letrozole, a new oral aromatase inhibitor: randomised trial comparing 2.5 mg daily, 0.5 mg daily and aminoglutethimide in postmenopausal women with advanced breast cancer. *Ann Oncol*, **9**, 639–45.

20. MacNeill FA, Jacobs S, Dowsett M, Lønning PE, Powles TJ (1995) The effects of oral 4-hydroxyandrostenedione on peripheral aromatisation in postmenopausal breast cancer patients. *Cancer Chemother Pharmacol*, **36**, 249–54.

21. Jones AL, MacNeill F, Jacobs S, Lønning PE, Dowsett M, Powles TJ (1992) The influence of intramuscular 4-hydroxyandrostenedione on peripheral aromatisation in breast cancer patients. *Eur J Cancer*, **28A**, 1712–16.

22. MacNeill FA, Jones AL, Jacobs S, Lønning PE, Powles TJ, Dowsett M (1992) The influence of aminoglutethimide and its analogue rogletimide on peripheral aromatisation in breast cancer. *Br J Cancer*, **66**, 692–7.

23. Geisler J, Johannessen DC, Anker G, Lønning PE (1996) Treatment with formestane alone and in combination with aminoglutethimide in heavily pretreated cancer patients: clinical and endocrine effects. *Eur J Cancer*, **32A**, 789–92.

24. Geisler J, Lien EA, Ekse D, Lønning PE (1997) Influence of aminoglutethimide on plasma levels of estrone sulphate and dehydroepiandrosterone sulphate in postmenopausal breast cancer patients. *J Steroid Biochem Mol Biol*, **63**, 53–8.

25. Geisler J, King N, Anker G, *et al.* (1998) *In vivo* inhibition of aromatization by exemestane, a novel irreversible aromatase inhibitor, in postmenopausal breast cancer patients. *Clin Cancer Res*, **4**, 2089–93.

26. Thurlimann B, Paridaens R, Serin D, *et al.* (1997) Third-line hormonal treatment with exemestane in postmenopausal patients with advanced breast cancer progressing on aminoglutethimide: a phase II multicentre multinational study. *Eur J Cancer*, **33**, 1767–73.

27. Lonning PE, Bajetta E, Murray R, Tubiana-Hulin M, *et al.* (2000) Activity of exemestane in metastatic breast cancer after failure of nonsteroidal aromatase inhibitors: a phase II trial. *J Clin Oncol*, **18**, 2234–44.

28. Brogden RN, Buckley MM-T, Ward A (1990) Buserelin: a review of its pharmacodynamic and pharmacokinetic properties, and clinical profile. *Drugs*, **39**, 399–437.

29. Chrisp P, Goa KL (1991) Goserelin: a review of its pharmacodynamic and pharmacokinetic properties, and clinical use in sex hormone-related conditions. *Drugs*, **41**, 254–88.

30. Zhau SZ, Arguelles LM, Wong JM, Davis MB, Gersh GE, Struthers BJ (1998) Cost comparison between nafarelin and leuprorelide in the treatment of endometriosis. *Clin Ther*, **20**, 592–602.

31. Emons G, Ortmann O, Becker M, *et al.* (1993) High affinity binding and direct antiproliferative effects of LHRH analogues in human ovarian cancer cell lines. *Cancer Res*, **53**, 5439–46.

32. Lundgren S, Gundersen S, Klepp R, Lønning PE, Lund E, Kvinnsland S (1989) Megestrol acetate versus aminoglutethimide for metastatic breast cancer. *Breast Cancer Res Treat*, **14**, 201–6.

33. Canney PA, Priestman TJ, Griffiths T, Latief TN, Mould JJ, Spooner D (1988) Randomized trial comparing aminoglutethimide with high-dose medroxyprogesterone acetate in therapy for advanced breast carcinoma. *J Natl Cancer Inst*, **80**, 1147–51.

34. Sørensen JB, Boas J, Brünner N, *et al.* (1991) Randomized trial of aminoglutethimide plus hydrocortisone versus megestrol acetate versus all three drugs in postmenopausal patients with advanced breast cancer. *Eur J Cancer*, **27**, S67.

35. Fotherby K, James F (1972) Metabolism of synthetic steroids. *Adv Steroid Biochem Pharmacol*, **3**, 67–165.

36. Tyrrell CJ, Denis L, Newling D, Soloway M, Channer K, Cockshott ID (1998) Casodex™ 10–200 mg daily, used as monotherapy for the treatment of patients with advanced prostate cancer. *Eur Urol*, **33**, 39–53.

37. Janknegt R.A. (1993) Total androgen blockade with the use of orchiectomy and nilutamide (Anandron) or placebo as treatment of metastatic prostate cancer. Androgen International Study Group. *Cancer*, **72**, 3874–7.

38. Group, P.C.T.C. (1995) Maximum androgen blockade in advanced prostate cancer: an overview of 22 randomised trials with 3283 deaths in 5710 patients. *Lancet*, **346**, 265–9.

39. Ayub M, Levell MJ (1987) Inhibition of rat testicular 17α-hydroxylase and 17,20-lyase activities by anti-androgens (flutamide, hydroxyflutamide, RU23908, cyproterone acetate) *in vitro*. *J Steroid Biochem*, **28**, 43–7.

40. Eri LM, Haug E, Tveter KJ (1995) Effects on the endocrine system of long-term treatment with the non-

steroidal anti-androgen Casodex in patients with benign prostatic hyperplasia. *Br J Urology*, 75, 335–40.

41. Verhelst J, Denis L, VanVliet P, *et al.* (1994) Endocrine profiles during administration of the new non-steroidal anti-androgen Casodex in prostate cancer. *Clinical Endocrinol*, 41, 525–30.

42. Iversen P, Tyrrell CJ, Kaisary AV, *et al.* (1998) Casocex (bicalutamide) 150-mg monotherapy compared with castration in patients with previously untreated non-metastatic prostate cancer: results from two multicenter randomized trials at a median follow-up of 4 years. *Urology*, 51, 389–96.

43. Iversen P, Tveter K, Varenhorst E (1996) Randomised study of Casodex 50 mg monotherapy vs orchidectomy in the treatment of metastatic prostate cancer. *Scand J Urol Nephrol*, 30, 93–8.

44. Fau D, Berson A, Eugene D, Fromenty B, Fisch C, Pessayre D (1992) Mechanism for the hepatotoxicity of the antiandrogen, nilutamide. Evidence suggesting that redox cycling of this nitroaromatic drug leads to oxidative stress in isolated hepatocytes. *J Pharmacol Exp Ther*, 263, 69–77.

45. Wysowski DK, Freiman JP, Tourtelot JB, Horton ML (1993) Fatal and nonfatal hepatotoxicity associated with flutamide. *Ann Intern Med*, 118, 860–4.

46. Dawson LA, Chow E, Morton G (1997) Fulminant hepatic failure associated with bicalutamide. *Urology*, 49, 283–4.

47. Lønning PE, Lien E (1995) Mechanisms of action of endocrine treatment in breast cancer. *Crit Rev Oncol Hematol*, 21, 158–93.

48. Löser R, Seibel K, Roos W, Eppenberger U (1985) *In vivo* and *in vitro* antiestrogenic action of 3-hydroxy-tamoxifen, tamoxifen and 4-hydroxytamoxifen. *Eur J Cancer Clin Oncol*, 21, 985–90.

49. Ke HZ, Simmons HA, Pirie CM, Crawford DT, Thompson DD (1995) Droloxifene, a new estrogen antagonist/agonist, prevents bone loss in ovariectomized rats. *Endocrinology*, 136, 2435–41.

50. Delmas PD, Bjarnason NH, Mitlak BH, *et al.* (1997) Effects of raloxifene on bone mineral density, serum cholesterol concentrations, and uterine endometrium in postmenopausal women. *N Engl J Med*, 337, 1641–7.

51. Yang NN, Venugopalan M, Hardikar S, Glasebrook A (1996) Identification of an estrogen response element activated by metabolites of 17 beta-estradiol and raloxifene. *Science*, 273, 1222–5.

52. Yang NN, Venugopalan M, Hardikar S, Glasebrook A (1997) Correction: raloxifene response needs more than an element. *Science*, 275, 1249.R

53. Lønning PE (1997) Resistance to endocrine therapy in breast cancer. In *Drug Resistance in Oncology*. New York: Marcel Dekker.

54. Newby JC, Johnston SRD, Smith IE, Dowsett M (1997) Expression of epidermal growth factor receptor and c-erbB2 during the development of tamoxifen resistance in human breast cancer. *Clin Cancer Res*, 3, 1643–51.

55. Berns EMJJ, Klijn JGM, vanPutten WLJ, *et al.* (1998) p53 protein accumulation predicts poor response to tamoxifen therapy of patients with recurrent breast cancer. *J Clin Oncol*, 16, 121–7.

56. Lønning PE, Lien EA, Lundgren S, Kvinnsland S (1992) Clinical pharmacokinetics of endocrine agents used in advanced breast cancer. *Clin Pharmacokinet*, 22, 327–58.

57. Holleran WM, Gharbo SA, DeGregorio MW (1987) Quantitation of toremifene and its major metabolites in human plasma by high-performance liquid chromatography following fluorescent activation. *Anal Lett*, 20, 871–9.

58. Webster LK, Crinis NA, Stokes K, Bishop JF (1991) High-performance liquid chromatographic method for the determination of toremifene and its major human metabolites. *J Chromatogr*, 565, 482–7.

59. Grill HJ, Pollow K (1991) Pharmacokinetics of droloxifene and its metabolites in breast cancer patients. *Am J Clin Oncol*, 14, S21–9.

60. Tanaka Y, Sekiguchi M, Sawamoto T, *et al.* (1994) Pharmacokinetics of droloxifene in mice, rats, monkeys, premenopausal and postmenopausal patients. *Eur J Drug Metab Pharmacokinet*, 19, 47–58.

61. Lien EA, Anker G, Lønning PE, Ueland PM (1995) Determination of droloxifene and two metabolites in serum by high-pressure liquid chromatography. *Ther Drug Monit*, 17, 259–65.

62. Watanabe N, Irie T, Koyama M. (1989) Liquid chromatographic atmospheric pressure ionization mass spectrometric analysis of toremifene metabolites in human urine. *J Chromatogr*, 497, 169–80.

63. Fromson JM, Pearson S, Bramah S (1973) The metabolism of tamoxifen (I.C.I. 46.474) part II: in female patients. *Xenobiotica*, 3, 711–14.

64. Fromson JM, Pearson S, Bramah S (1973) The metabolism of tamoxifen (I.C.I. 46.474) part I: in laboratory animals. *Xenobiotica*, 3, 693–709.

65. Sipila H, Kangas L, Vuorilehto L, *et al.* (1990) Metabolism of toremifene in the rat. *J Steroid Biochem*, 36, 211–15.

66. Kangas L (1990) Review of the pharmacological properties of toremifene. *J Steroid Biochem*, 36, 191–5.

67. Anttila M, Valavaara R, Kivinen S, Maenpaa J (1990) Pharmacokinetics of toremifene. *J Steroid Biochem*, 36, 249–52.

68. Nickerson DF, Tess DA, Toler SM (1997) First-pass metabolism and biliary recirculation of droloxifene in the female Sprague–Dawley rat. *Xenobiotica*, 27, 257–64.

69. Jordan VC, Collins MM, Rowsby L, Prestwick G (1977) A monohydroxylated metabolite of tamoxifen with potent antiestrogenic activity. *J Endocrinol*, 75, 305–16.

70. Lien EA, Anker G, Lønning PE, Solheim E, Ueland PM (1990) Decreased serum concentrations of tamoxifen and its metabolites induced by aminoglutethimide. *Cancer Res*, 50, 5851–7.

71. Lien EA, Solheim E, Lea OA, Lundgren S, Kvinnsland S, Ueland PM (1989) Distribution of 4-hydroxy-N-desmethyltamoxifen and other tamoxifen metabolites in human biological fluids during tamoxifen treatment. *Cancer Res*, 49, 2175–83.

72. Kangas L (1990) Biochemical and pharmacological effects of toremifene metabolites. *Cancer Chemother Pharmacol*, 27, 8–12.

73. Kohler PC, Hamm JT, Wiebe VJ, DeGregorio MW, Shemano I, Tormey DC (1990) Phase I study of the tolerance and pharmacokinetics of toremifene in patients with cancer. *Breast Cancer Res Treat*, **16** (Suppl), s19–26.

74. Wiebe VJ, Benz CC, Shemano I, Cadman TB, DeGregorio MW (1990) Pharmacokinetics of toremifene and its metabolites in patients with advanced breast cancer. *Cancer Chemother Pharmacol*, **25**, 247–51.

75. Stamm H, Roth R, Huber H-J, *et al.* (1986) Preliminary data on a phase-I trial of the new antiestrogen droloxifene: tolerance, pharmacokinetics and metabolism. *Contrib Oncol*, **23**, 73–8.

76. Fabian C, Sternson L, Barnett M (1980) Clinical pharmacology of tamoxifen in patients with breast cancer: comparison of traditional and loading dose schedules. *Cancer Treat Rep*, **64**, 765–73.

77. Tominaga T, Abe O, Izuo M, Nomura Y (1990) A phase I study of toremifene. *Breast Cancer Res Treat*, **16** (Suppl), s27–29.

78. Adam HK, Patterson JS, Kemp JV (1980) Studies on the metabolism and pharmacokinetics of tamoxifen in normal volunteers. *Cancer Treat Rep*, **64**, 761–4.

79. Bruning PF (1992) Droloxifene, a new anti-oestrogen in postmenopausal advanced breast cancer: preliminary results of a double-blind dose-finding phase II trial. *Eur J Cancer*, **28A**, 1404–7.

80. Roos W, Oeze L, Löser R, Eppenberger U (1983) Antiestrogenic action of 3-hydroxytamoxifen in the human breast cancer cell line MCF-7. *J Natl Cancer Inst*, **71**, 55–9.

81. Lien EA, Solheim E, Ueland PM (1991) Distribution of tamoxifen and its metabolites in rat and human tissues during steady-state treatment. *Cancer Res*, **51**, 4837–44.

82. Sipilä H, Namo V, Kangas L, Anttila M, Halme T (1988) Binding of toremifene to human serum proteins. *Pharmacol Toxicol*, **63**, 62–4.

83. Meltzer NM, Stang P, Sternson L (1984) Influence of tamoxifen and its N-desmethyl and 4-hydroxy metabolites on rat liver microsomal enzymes. *Biochem Pharmacol*, **33**, 115–23.

84. Lodwick R, McConkey B, Brown AM, Beeley L (1987) Life threatening interaction between tamoxifen and warfarin. *Br Med J*, **295**, 1141.

85. Ritchie LD, Grant SMT (1989) Tamoxifen–warfarin interaction: the Aberdeen hospital drug file. *Br Med J*, **298**, 1253.

86. Martel C, Labrie C, Belanger A, *et al.* (1998) Comparison of the effects of the new orally active antiestrogen EM-800 with ICI 182 780 and toremifene on estrogen-sensitive parameters in the ovariectomized mouse. *Endocrinology*, **139**, 2486–92.

87. Dauvois S, Danielian PS, White R, Parker MG (1992) Antioestrogen ICI 164384 reduced cellular estrogen receptor content by increasing its turnover. *Proc Natl Acad Sci USA*, **89**, 4037–41.

88. Fawell SE, White R, Hoare S, Sydenham M, Page M, Parker MG (1990) Inhibition of oestrogen receptor DNA-binding by the 'pure' antioestrogen ICI 164, 384 appears to be mediated by impaired receptor dimerization. *Proc Natl Acad Sci USA*, **87**, 6883–7.

89. Dukes M, Waterton JC, Wakeling AE (1993) Anti-uterotrophic effects of the pure antioestrogen ICI 182,780 in adult female monkeys (*Macaca nemestrina*): quantitative magnetic resonance imaging. *J Endocrinol*, **138**, 203–9.

90. Gallagher A, Chambers TJ, Tobias JH (1993) The estrogen antagonist ICI 182,780 reduces cancellous bone volume in female rats. *Endocrinology*, **133**, 2787–91.

91. Howell A, Defriend DJ, Robertson JFR, *et al.* (1996) Pharmacokinetics, pharmacological and anti-tumour effects of the specific anti-oestrogen ICI 182780 in women with advanced breast cancer. *Br J Cancer*, **74**, 300–8.

92. DeFriend DJ, Howell A, Nicholson RI, *et al.* (1994) Investigation of a new pure antiestrogen (ICI 182780) in women with primary breast cancer. *Cancer Res*, **54**, 408–14.

93. Dowsett M, Stein RC, Coombes RC (1992) Aromatization inhibition alone or in combination with GmRH agonists for the treatment of premenopausal breast cancer patients. *J Steroid Biochem Mol Biol*, **43**, 155–9.

94. Samojlik E, Santen RJ, Worgul TJ (1984) Suppression of residual oestrogen production with aminoglutethimide in women following surgical hypophysectomy or adrenalectomy. *Clin Endocrinol*, **20**, 43–51.

95. Murray R, Pitt P (1985) Low-dose aminoglutethimide without steroid replacement in the treatment of postmenopausal women with advanced breast cancer. *Eur J Cancer Clin Oncol*, **21**, 19–22.

96. Lønning PE, Dowsett M, Jones A, *et al.* (1992) Influence of aminoglutethimide on plasma oestrogen levels in breast cancer patients on 4-hydroxyandrostenedione treatment. *Br Cancer Res Treat*, **23**, 57–62.

97. Masamura S, Santner SJ, Heitjan DF, Santen RJ (1995) Estrogen deprivation causes estradiol hypersensitivity in human breast cancer cells. *J Clin Endocrinol Metab*, **80**, 2918–25.

98. Murray FT, Santner S, Samojlik E, Santen RJ (1979) Serum aminoglutethimide levels; studies of serum half-life, clearance and patient compliance. *J Clin Pharmacol*, **19**, 704–11.

99. Adam AM, Bradbrook ID, Rogers HJ (1985) High-performance liquid chromatographic assay for simultaneous estimation of aminoglutethimide and acethylamidoglutethimide in biological fluids. *Cancer Chemother Pharmacol*, **15**, 176–8.

100. Menge G, Dubois JP (1984) Determination of aminoglutethimide and N-acetylaminoglutethimide in human plasma by high-performance liquid chromatography. *J Chromatogr*, **310**, 431–7.

101. Robinson BA, Cornell FN (1983) Liquid-chromatographic determination of aminoglutethimide in plasma. *Clin Chem*, **29**, 1104–8.

102. Schanche J-S, Lønning PE, Ueland PM, Kvinnsland S (1984) Determination of aminoglutethimide and N-acetylaminoglutethimide in human plasma by reversed-phase liquid chromatography. *Ther Drug Monit*, **6**, 221–6.

103. Sirtori CR, DeFabiani E, Caruso D, Malavasi B, Galli G, Galli-Kienle M (1988) Single dose pharmacokinetics of aminoglutethimide by a rapid SIM methodology. *Int J Clin Pharmacol Ther Toxicol*, 26, 380–4.

104. Coombes RC, Foster AB, Harland SJ, Jarman M, Nice EC (1982) Polymorphically acetylated aminoglutethimide in humans. *Br J Cancer*, 46, 340–5.

105. Aboul-Enein HY, Islam MR (1988) Direct liquid chromatographic resolution of racemic aminoglutethimide and its acetylated metabolite using a chiral alpha1-acid glycoprotein column. *J Chromatogr Sci*, 26, 616–19.

106. Khubieh J, Aherne GW, Chakraborty J (1990) Radioimmunoassay of the anticancer agent 4-hydroxyandrostenedione in body fluids. *J Steroid Biochem*, 35, 377–82.

107. Guarna A, Moneti G, Prucher D, Salerno R, Serio M (1989) Quantitative determination of 4-hydroxyandrostene-3,17-dione (4-OHA), a potent aromatase inhibitor, in human plasma, using isotope dilution mass spectrometry. *J Steroid Biochem*, 32, 699–702.

108. Poon GK, Jarman M, Rowlands MG, Dowsett M, Firth J (1991) Determination of 4-hydroxyandrost-4-ene-3,17-dione metabolism in breast cancer patients using high-performance liquid chromatography-mass spectrometry. *J Chromatogr*, 565, 75–88.

109. Breda M, Pianezzola E, Benedetti MS (1993) Determination of exemestane, a new aromatase inhibitor, in plasma by high-performance liquid chromatography with ultraviolet detection. *J Chromatogr*, 620, 225–31.

110. Pfister CU, Duval M, Godbillon J, et al. (1994) Development, application and comparison of an enzyme immunoassay and a high-performance liquid chromatography method for the determination of the aromatase inhibitor cgs 20 267 in biological fluids. *J Pharm Sci*, 83, 520–4.

111. Marfil F, Pineau V, Sioufi A, Godbillon J (1996) High-performance liquid chromatography of the aromatase inhibitor, letrozole, and its metabolite in biological fluids with automated liquid-solid extraction and fluorescence detection. *J Chromatogr*, 683, 251–8.

112. Lønning PE, Schanche JS, Kvinnsland S, Ueland PM (1985) Single-dose and steady-state pharmacokinetics of aminoglutethimide. *Clin Pharmacokinet*, 10, 353–64.

113. Nicholls PJ (1982) Pharmacokinetic and balance studies of aminoglutethimide in animals and man. *R Soc Med Int Congr Symp Ser*, 53, 23–4.

114. Goss PE, Jarman M, Wilkinson JR, Coombes RC (1986) Metabolism of the aromatase inhibitor 4-hydroxyandrostenedione *in vivo*: identification of the glucuronide as a major urinary metabolite in patients and biliary metabolite in the rat. *J Steroid Biochem*, 24, 619–22.

115. Cocchiara G, Allievi C, Berardi A, Zugnoni P, Benedetti MS, Dostert P (1994) Urinary metabolism of exemestane, a new aromatase inhibitor, in rat, dog, monkey and human volunteers. *J Endocrinol Invest*, 17 (Suppl 1), 78.

116. Evans TRJ, Salle ED, Ornati G, et al. (1992) Phase I and endocrine study of exemestane (FCE 24304), a new aromatase inhibitor, in postmenopausal women. *Cancer Res*, 52, 5933–9.

117. Plourde PV, Dyroff M, Dukes M (1994) Arimidex: a potent and selective fourth-generation aromatase inhibitor. *Breast Cancer Res Treat*, 30, 103–11.

118. Sioufi A, Gauducheau N, Pineau V, et al. (1997) Absolute bioavailability of letrozole in healthy postmenopausal women. *Biopharm Drug Dispos*, 18, 779–89.

119. Sioufi A, Sandrenan N, Godbillon J, et al. (1997) Comparative bioavailability of letrozole under fed and fasting conditions in 12 healthy subjects after a 2.5 mg single oral administration. *Biopharm Drug Dispos*, 18, 489–97.

120. Adam AM, Rogers HJ, Amiel SA, Rubens RD (1984) The effect of acetylator phenotype on the disposition of aminoglutethimide. *Br J Clin Pharmacol*, 28, 495–505.

121. Coombes RC, Jarman M, Harland S, et al. (1980) Aminoglutethimide: metabolism and effects on steroid synthesis *in vivo*. *J Endocrinol*, 87, 31–2.

122. Egger H, Bartlett F, Itterly W, Rodebaugh R, Shimanskas C (1982) Metabolism of aminoglutethimide in the rat. *Drug Metab Dispos*, 10, 405–12.

123. Foster AB, Griggs LJ, Howe I, et al. (1984) Metabolism of aminoglutethimide in humans. *Drug Metab Dispos*, 12, 511–16.

124. Jarman M, Foster AB, Goss PE, Griggs LJ, Howe I (1983) Metabolism of aminoglutethimide in humans: identification of hydroxylaminoglutethimide as a induced metabolite. *Biomed Mass Spectrom*, 10, 620–5.

125. Dowsett M, Lloyd P (1990) Comparison of the pharmacokinetics and pharmacodynamics of unformulated and formulated 4-hydroxyandrostenedione taken orally by healthy men. *Cancer Chemother Pharmacol*, 27, 67–71.

126. Thompson TA, Vermeulen JD, Wagner WE, LeSher AR (1981) Aminoglutethimide bioavailability, pharmacokinetics, and binding to blood constituents. *J Pharm Sci*, 70, 1040–3.

127. Dowsett M, Goss PE, Powles TJ, et al. (1987) Use of the aromatase inhibitor 4-hydroxyandrostenedione in postmenopausal breast cancer: optimization of therapeutic dose and route. *Cancer Res*, 47, 1957–61.

128. Lønning PE, Paridaens R, Thürlimann B, Piscitelli G, Salle Ed (1997) Exemestane experience in breast cancer treatment. *J Steroid Biochem Mol Biol*, 61, 151–5.

129. Yates RA, Dowsett M, Fisher GV, Selen A, Wyld PJ (1996) Arimidex (ZD 1033): a selective, potent inhibitor of aromatase in postmenopausal female volunteers. *Br J Cancer*, 73, 543–8.

130. Pfister C, Dowsett M, Iveson T, Mueller P, Sioufi A, Trunet PF (1993) Pharmacokinetics of new aromatase inhibitor CGS 20267. *Eur J Drug Metab Pharmacokinet*, 18 (Suppl), 117.

131. Colussi DM, Parisot CY, Lefevre GY (1998) Plasma protein binding of letrozole, a new nonsteroidal aromatase enzyme inhibitor. *J Clin Pharmacol*, 38, 727–35.

132. Appelgren L-E, Brittebo E, Carlstrøm K, Theve NO, Wilking N (1985) Distribution and metabolism of 14C-labelled aminoglutethimide in mice. *Abstr 2nd Scandinavian Breast Cancer Symposium, Bergen, Norway, May 23–24, 1985*.

133. Cash R, Brough AJ, Cohen MNP, Satoh PS (1967) Aminoglutethimide (Elipten-Ciba) is an inhibitor of

adrenal steroidogenesis: mechanism of action and therapeutic trial. *J Clin Endocrinol Metab*, **27**, 1239–48.

134. Reed MJ, Aherne GW, Ghilchik MW, Patel S, Chakraborty J (1991) Concentrations of oestrone and 4-hydroxyandrostenedione in malignant and normal breast tissue. *Int J Cancer*, **49**, 562–5.

135. Murray M, Cantrill E, Farrell GC (1993) Induction of cytochrome P450 2B1 in rat liver by the aromatase inhibitor aminoglutethimide. *J Pharmacol Exp Ther*, **265**, 477–81.

136. Lønning PE (1990) Aminoglutethimide enzyme induction: pharmacological and endocrinological implications. *Cancer Chemother Pharmacol*, **26**, 241–4.

137. van Deijk WA, Blijham GH, Mellink WAM, Meulenberg PMM (1985) Influence of aminoglutethimide on plasma levels of medroxyprogesterone acetate: its correlation with serum cortisol. *Cancer Treat Rep*, **69**, 85–90.

138. Lundgren S, Lønning PE, Aakvaag A, Kvinnsland S (1990) Influence of aminoglutethimide on the metabolism of medroxyprogesterone acetate and megestrol acetate in post-menopausal patients with advanced breast cancer. *Cancer Chemother Pharmacol*, **27**, 101–5.

139. Grimm SW, Dyroff MC (1997) Inhibition of human drug metabolizing cytochromes P450 by anastrozole, a potent and selective inhibitor of aromatase. *Drug Metab Dispos*, **25**, 598–602.

140. St Peter J, Pharm D, Thyrum P, Yeh C, Dyroff M, Selen A (1997) Lack of effect of anastrozole, an aromatase inhibitor, on antipyrine pharmacokinetics in postmenopausal women. *Clin Pharmacol Ther*, **61**, 172.

141. Dowsett M, Yates R, Wong YWJ (1998) Arimidex (anastrozole): lack of interactions with tamoxifen, antipyrine, cimetidine and warfarin. *Eur J Cancer*, **34** (Suppl 1), s39–40.

142. Dowsett M, Pfister CU, Johnston SRD, *et al.* (1997) Pharmacokinetic interaction between letrozole and tamoxifen in postmenopausal patients with advanced breast cancer. *Breast*, **6**, 245.

143. Nestor JJ Jr (1984) Development of agonistic LHRH analogs. In Vickery BH *et al.* (eds) *LHRH and its Analogs: A New Class of Contraceptive and Therapeutic Agents*. Lancaster.

144. Sandow J (1987) Pharmacology of LHRH agonists. *Pharmacology and Clinical Uses of Inhibitors of Hormone Secretion and Action*. London: Bailliére Tindall.

145. Nillius SJ (1981) The therapeutic uses of gonadotrophin-releasing hormone and its analogues. *Clinical Endocrinology I*. London: Butterworths.

146. Eidne KA, Flanagan CA, Millar RP (1985) Gonadotropin-releasing hormone binding sites in human breast carcinoma. *Science*, **229**, 989–92.

147. Clayton RN, Bailey LC, Cottam J, Arkell D, Perren TJ (1985) A radioimmunoassay for GnRH agonist analogue in serum of patients with prostate cancer treated with D-Ser (tBu)6 AZA Gly10 GnRH. *Clin Endocrinol*, **22**, 453–62.

148. Holland FJ, Fishman L, Costigan DC, Luna L, Leeder S (1986) Pharmacokinetic characteristics of the gonadotropin-releasing hormone analog D-Ser (TBU)-

6EA-10 luteinizing hormone-releasing hormone (buserelin) after subcutaneous and intranasal administration in children with central precocious puberty. *J Clin Endocrinol Metab*, **63**, 1065–70.

149. Kiesel L, Sandow J, Bertges K, Jerabek Sandow G, Trabant H, Runnebaum B (1989) Serum concentration and urinary excretion of the luteinizing hormone-releasing hormone agonist buserelin in patients with endometriosis. *J Clin Endocrinol Metab*, **68**, 1167–73.

150. Perren TJ, Clayton RN, Blackledge G, Bailey LC, Holder G (1986) Pharmacokinetic and endocrinological parameters of a slow-release depot preparation of the GnRH analogue ICI 118630 (Zoladex) compared with a subcutaneous bolus and continuous subcutaneous infusion of the same drug in patients with prostatic cancer. *Cancer Chemother Pharmacol*, **18**, 39–43.

151. Chrisp P, Goa KL (1990) Nafarelin: a review of its pharmacodynamic and pharmacokitetic properties, and clinical potential in sex hormone-related conditions. *Drugs*, **39**, 523–51.

152. Ueno H, Matsuo S (1991) High-performance liquid chromatography followed by radioimmunoassay for the determination of a luteinizing formone-releasing analogue, euprorelin, and its metabolite. *J Chromatogr*, **566**, 57–66.

153. del Moral PF, Dijkman GA, Debruyne FMJ, Witjes WPJ, Kolvenbag GJCM (1996) Three-month depot of goeserelin acetate: clinical efficacy and endocrine profile. *Urology*, **48**, 894–900.

154. Wechsel HW, Zerbib M, Pagano F, Coptcoat MJ (1886) Randomized open labelled comparative study of the efficacy, safety and tolerability of leuprorelin acetate IM and 3M depot in patients with advanced prostatic cancer. *Eur Urol*, **30** (Suppl 1), 7–14.

155. Bennet HPJ, McMartin C (1979) Peptide hormones and their analogues: distribution, clearance from the circulation, and inactivation *in vivo*. *Pharmacol Rev*, **30**, 247–92.

156. Parker CR, Foreman MM, Porter JC (1979) Subcellular localization of luteinizing hormone-releasing hormone degrading activity in the hypothalamus. *Brain Res*, **174**, 221–8.

157. Robinson SP, Jordan VC (1988) Metabolism of steroid-modifying anticancer agents. *Pharmacol Ther*, **36**, 41–103.

158. Plosker GL, Brogden RN (1994) Leuprorelin. A review of its pharmacology and therapeutic use in prostatic cancer, endometriosis and other sex hormone-related disorders. *Drugs*, **48**, 930–67.

159. Adam HK, Barker Y, Hutchinson FG, Milsted RAV, Moore RH (1988) Zoladex: a one-month duration LH-RH agonist. *Pharm Weekbl Sci Ed*, **10**, 57 (abstr 8964).

160. Chan RL, Chaplin MD (1985) Plasma binding of LHRH and nafarelin acetate, a highly potent LHRH agonist. *Biochem Biophys Res Com*, **127**, 673–9.

161. Lundgren S, Helle SI, Lønning PE (1996) Profound suppression of plasma estrogens by megestrol acetate in postmenopausal breast cancer patients. *Clin Cancer Res*, **2**, 1515–21.

162. Adlercreutz H, Eriksen PB, Christensen MS (1983) Plasma concentration of mgestrol acetate and medroxy-

progesterone acetate after single oral administration to healthy subjects. *J Pharm Biomed Anal*, **1**, 153–62.

163. Martin F, Adlercreutz H (1977) Aspects of megestrol acetate and medroxyprogesterone acetate metabolism. In *Pharmacology of Steroid Contraceptive Drugs*. New York: Raven Press.

164. Milano G, Carle G, Renee N, Boublil JL, Namer M (1982) Determination of medroxyprogesterone acetate in plasma by high-performance liquid chromatohraphy. *J Chromatogr*, **232**, 413–17.

165. Camaggi CM, Strocchi E, Costanti B, Beghelli P, Ferrari P, Pannuti F (1985) Medroxyprogesterone acetate bioavailability after high-dose intraperitoneal administration in advanced cancer. *Cancer Chemother Pharmacol*, **14**, 232–4.

166. Cooper JM, Kellie AE (1968) The metabolism of megestrol acetate (17-a-acetoxy-6-methylpregna-4,6-diene-3,20-dione) in women. *Steroids*, **11**, 133–49.

167. Lundgren S, Lønning PE (1990) Influence of progestins on serum hormone levels in postmenopausal women with advanced breast cancer II: a differential effect of megestrol acetate on serum estrone sulfate and sex hormone binding globulin. *J Steroid Biochem*, **36**, 105–9.

168. Lundgren S, Lønning PE, Utaaker E, Aakvaag A, Kvinnsland S (1990) Influence of progestins on serum hormone levels in postmenopausal women with advanced breast cancer-I. General findings. *J Steroid Biochem*, **36**, 99–104.

169. Utaaker E, Lundgren S, Kvinnsland S, Aakvaag A (1988) Pharmacokinetics and metabolism of medrxytprogesterone acetate in patients with advanced breast cancer. *J Steroid Biochem*, **31**, 437–41.

170. Slaunwhite WR, Sandberg AA (1961) Disposition of radioactive 17a-hydroxyprogesterone, 6a-methyl-prednisolone in human subjects. *J Clin Endocrinol Metab*, **21**, 753–64.

171. Pannuti F, Camaggi CM, Strocchi E, et al. (1984) Medroxyprogesterone acetate pharmacokinetics. In *Role of Medroxyprogesterone in Endocrine-Related Tumors*. New York: Raven Press.

172. Gupta C, Osterman J, Santen R, Bardin CW (1979) *In vivo* metabolism of progestins. V. Effect of protocol design on the estimated metabolic clearance rate and volume of distribution of medroxyprogesterone acetate in women. *J Clin Endocrinol Metab*, **48**, 816–20.

173. Lønning PE, Lien EA (1993) Pharmacokinetics of anti-endocrine agents. *Cancer Surv*, **17**, 343–70.

174. Pannuti F, Camaggi CM, Strocchi E, Giovannini M, Do Marco AR, and Costanti B (1982) Medroxyprogesterone acetate (MAP) relative bioavailability after single high-dose administration in cancer patients. *Cancer Treat Rep*, **66**, 2043–9.

175. Mathrubutham M, Fotherby K (1981) Medroxyprogesterone acetate in human serum. *J Steroid Biochem*, **14**, 783–6.

176. Kinci FA, Angee I, Chang CL, Rudel HW (1970) Plasma levels and accumulation into various tissue of 6-methyl-17a-acetoxy-4,6-pregnandiene-3,20-dione after oral administration or absorption from poly-dimethyl-siloxane implants. *Acta Endocrinol*, **64**, 508–18.

177. Halpenny O, Bye A, Cranny A, Feely J, Daly PA (1990) Influence of aminoglutethimide on plasma levels of medroxyprogesterone acetate. *Med Oncol Tumor Pharmacother*, **7**, 241–7.

178. Lundgren S, Kvinnsland S, Utaaker E, Bakke O, Ueland PM (1986) Effect of high dose progestins on the disposition of antipyrune, sigitoxin and warfarin in patients with advanced breast cancer. *Cancer Chemother Pharmacol*, **18**, 270–5.

179. Camaggi CM, Strocchi E, Canova N, Costani BPF (1985) Medroxyprogesterone acetate (MAP) and tamoxifen (TMX) plasma levels after simultaneous treatment with 'low' TMX and 'gifg' MAP doses. *Cancer Chemother Pharmacol*, **14**, 229–31.

180. Furr BJA, Valcaccia B, Curry B, Woodburn JR, Chesterson G, Tucker H (1987) ICI 176,334: a novel non-steroidal, peripherally selective antiandrogen. *J Endocrinol*, **113**, R7–9.

181. Hellman L, Bradlow HL, Freed S, et al. (1977) The effect of flutamide on testosterone metabolism and plasma levels of androgens and gonadotropin. *J Clin Endocrinol Metab*, **45**, 1224–9.

182. Moguilewsky M, Bertagna C, Hucher M (1987) Pharmacological and clinical studies of the anti-androgen Anandron. *J Steroid Biochem*, **27**, 871–5.

183. Harris MG, Coleman SG, Faulds D, Chrisp P (1993) Nilutamide: a review of its pharmacodynamic and pharmacokinetic properties, and therapeutic efficacy in prostate cancer. *Drugs Aging*, **3**, 9–25.

184. Kolvenbag GJCM, Blackledge GRP, Gotting-Smith K (1998) Bicalutamide (Casodex) in the treatment of prostate cancer: history of clinical development. *Prostate*, **34**, 61–72.

185. Scher HI, Kelly WK (1993) Flutamide withdrawal syndrome: its impact on clinical trials in hormone-refractory prostate cancer. *J Clin Oncol*, **11**, 1566–72.

186. Huan SD, Gerridzen RG, Yau JC, Stewart DJ (1997) Antiandrogen withdrawal syndrome with nilutamide. *Urology*, **49**, 632–4.

187. Nieh PT (1995) Withdrawal phenomenon with the antiandrogen Casodex. *J Urol*, **153**, 1070–3.

188. Taplin M-E, Bubley GJ, Shuster TD, et al. (1995) Mutation of the androgen-receptor gene in metastatic androgen-independent prostate cancer. *N Engl J Med*, **332**, 1393–8.

189. Young CY-F, Montgomery BT, Andrews PE, Qiu S, Bilhartz DL, Tindall DJ (1991) Hormonal regulation of prostate-specific antigen messenger RNA in human prostatic adenocarcinoma cell line LNCaP. *Cancer Res*, **51**, 3748–52.

190. Gaddipati JP, McLeod DG, Heidenberg HB, et al. (1994) Frequent detection of codon 877 mutation in the androgen receptor gene in advanced prostate cancers. *Cancer Res*, **54**, 2861–4.

191. Gaillard Moguilewsky M (1991) Pharmacology of anti-androgens and value of combining androgen suppression with antiandrogen therapy. *Urology*, **37** (Suppl), 5–12.

192. Katchen B, Buxbaum S (1975) Disposition of a new, nonsteroid, antiandrogen, a,a,a,trifluoro-2-methyl-4'-nitro-m-propionotoluidide (flutamide), in men fol-

lowing a single oral 200 mg dose. *J Clin Endocrinol Metab*, **41**, 373–9.

193. Schulz M, Schmoldt A, Donn F, Becker H (1988) The pharmacokinetics of flutamide and its major metabolites after a single oral dose and during chronic treatment. *Eur J Clin Pharmacol*, **34**, 633–6.

194. Belanger A, Labrie F, Dupont A, Brochu M, Cusan L (1988) Endocrine effects of combined treatment with an LHRH agonist in association with flutamide in metastatic prostatic carcinoma. *Clin Invest Med*, **11**, 321–6.

195. Pendyala L, Creaven PJ, Huben R, Tremblay D, Bertagna C (1988) Pharmacokinetics of Anandron in patients with advanced carcinoma of the prostate. *Cancer Chemother Pharmacol*, **22**, 69–76.

196. McKillop D, Boyle GW, Cockshott ID, Jones DC, Phillips PJ, Yates RA (1993) Metabolism and enantioselective pharmacokinetics of Casodex in man. *Xenobiotica*, **23**, 1241–53.

197. Creaven PJ, Pendyala L, Tremblay D (1991) Pharmacokinetics and metabolism of nilutamide. *Urology*, **37** (Suppl), 13–19.

198. Cockshott ID, Plummer GF, Cooper KJ, Warwick MJ (1991) The pharmacokinetics of Casodex in laboratory animals. *Xenobiotica*, **21**, 1347–55.

199. Neri R, Peets E, Watnick A (1979) Anti-androgenicity of flutamide and its metabolite Sch 16423. *Biochem Soc Trans*, **7**, 565–9.

200. Tournemine C, Coussediere D, Cousty C, Tremblay D, Pottier J (1987) Pharmacological activity of four metabolites of Anandron. *Eur J Cancer Clin Oncol*, **23**, 1250.

201. Boyle GW, McKillop D, Phillips PJ, Harding JR, Pickford R, McCormick AD (1993) Metabolism of Casodex in laboratory animals. *Xenobiotica*, **23**, 781–98.

202. Radwanski ER, Perentesis G, Symchowicz S, Zampaglione N (1989) Single and multiple dose pharmacokinetic evaluation of flutamide in normal geriatric volunteers. *J Clin Pharmacol*, **29**, 554–9.

203. Babany G, Tinel M, Letterson P, *et al.* (1989) Inhibitory effects of nilutamide, a new androgen receptor antagonist, on mouse and human liver cytochrome p-450. *Biochem Pharmacol*, **38**, 941–7.

16 | *The clinical application of tumour biology*

D. Paul Harkin and Patrick G. Johnston

Introduction

Cellular growth and division is a carefully regulated process that depends on the precise interaction of multiple regulatory factors. Cancer represents a deregulation of this process, in which some of the normal constraints on cell growth and division have been lost. How this deregulation occurs has been the focus of intense interest over the last three decades. However, it is now generally accepted that tumours arise through the accumulation of several genetic changes affecting the control of cellular growth. Recent advances in molecular biology have made it possible to define some of the molecular changes that regulate the mechanisms by which certain tumours arise.

Three major classes of genes have now been implicated in the development of cancer. The first class, termed *oncogenes*, are mutated or over-expressed forms of normal cellular genes called proto-oncogenes and tend to function as positive regulators of cell growth. Oncogenes were first discovered in transducing RNA tumour viruses, which acquired cellular genes by transduction. When these cellular genes are incorporated into the viral genome they become activated oncogenes. Oncogene activation has also been shown to occur by retroviral insertion near a proto-oncogene chromosomal translocation, resulting in abnormal expression of the gene, activating point mutations and gene amplification. Examples of this include n-*myc* in neuroblastoma, k-*ras* in pancreatic cancer, and c-*erb*-B2 in breast cancer.

The second class of genes, termed tumour suppressor genes (TSGs), act as negative regulators of cell growth. Loss or inactivation of a TSG results in loss of growth inhibition and results in a selective growth advantage for the cell. The observed recessive nature of TSGs means that both copies of a TSG must be lost or inactivated in order for the malignant phenotype to be expressed.[1] In the case of hereditary forms of cancer such as retinoblastoma one of these mutations may be inherited through the germline. A number of mechanisms by which TSGs are lost or inactivated have been identified. These include deletions, resulting in complete loss, translocations which interrupt the coding sequence, point mutations, which inhibit gene function or result in protein truncation, and imprinting which may result in abnormal gene expression.

A third class of genes, termed DNA repair genes have more recently been implicated in the genesis of cancer. The initial observation that an association may exist between DNA repair deficiencies and cancer came approximately 20 years ago with the report of an elevated risk of skin cancer in the human disease xeroderma pigmentosum. However, the major breakthrough in this field was the cloning of a human mismatch repair gene hMSH2, identified on the basis of its homology to the *Saccharomyces cerevisiae* MSH2 gene. It was subsequently shown that this gene was mutated in families with hereditary non-polyposis colorectal cancer (HNPCC), resulting in what has been described as a mutator phenotype.[2] Conceptually, inactivation of DNA repair genes can be considered as initiation events in tumour development, but they are not rate limiting. Mutations within DNA repair genes tend to result in an intrinsic genetic instability, which subsequently leads to additional mutational events such as inactivation of TSGs.

The majority of tumours arise through a combination of genetic events, which involve both activation of oncogenes and inactivation of DNA repair or TSGs. In the last decade remarkable progress has been made in understanding the underlying genetic defects giving rise to a variety of tumour types. This new information has paved the way for the development of new early detection techniques, in addition to radical new strategies for the treatment of cancer. In this chapter we review our current knowledge regarding the molecular basis of cancer and how this is being used in developing ideas that are emerging for cancer diagnosis, treatment, and cure.

Molecular basis of cancer

Oncogenes

The signalling pathways which control whether a cell divides or remains quiescent involve a complex array of growth factors, growth factor receptors, intracellular transducers, and transcription factors (Fig. 16.1). Tumorigenesis reflects a malfunction in one or more of these pathways, caused in part by the action of oncogenes. To gain an overall insight as to how oncogenes disrupt normal cellular growth controls, it is necessary to examine oncogene function in the context of these signalling pathways.

Growth factors

Historically, the first growth factor to be described was nerve growth factor, which was identified in mouse

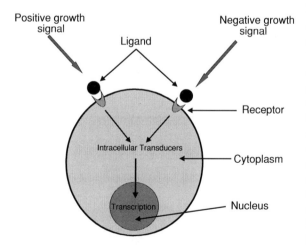

Figure 16.1. Cellular proliferation is regulated by both positive and negative growth signals. These signals are relayed to the nucleus via receptor ligand interactions which activate intracellular transduction pathways. These intracellular transducers transmit this signal to the nucleus where the appropriate transcription factor and hence genes are activated.

sarcoma cells and shown to stimulate the growth of chick embryo nerve cells. Since then a large variety of growth factors have been identified, including platelet-derived growth factor (PDGF), insulin like growth factors (IGFs), and epidermal growth factor (EGF) and its structural and functional homologue transforming growth factor-α (TGF-α), to name but a few. Growth factors mediate their mitogenic effect by binding to specific receptors on the cell surface. This results in the upregulation of a cascade of genes, termed immediate early genes, such as *fos*, *myc*, and *jun*. Some of these genes are themselves pleiotropic regulators of growth. A characteristic of tumour cells is their ability to grow in an autonomous fashion, lacking dependence on one or more growth factors whose presence is required for growth of their normal counterparts.[3,4] The potential of growth factor genes to contribute to the process of transformation became apparent with the observation that PDGF-β, which is the cellular homologue of the v-*sis* oncogene, functions as a PDGF-β receptor agonist and stimulates a cascade of immediate early genes that result in cellular transformation. Proof of growth factor autonomy by this direct autocrine pathway was provided when it was demonstrated that the *sis* oncogene is unable to transform cells that lack the PDGF receptor.[5]

Growth factor receptors

One of the best studied growth factor receptors, the EGF receptor, was initially characterized as a ligand-stimulated protein tyrosine kinase. The receptor was subsequently shown to consist of an extracellular EGF binding domain, a cytoplasmic domain with tyrosine specific protein kinase activity, and a transmembrane region of 23 amino acids, and to be a member of the *erb*-B receptor family. Functional studies of an EGF receptor mutant demonstrated that the diverse biochemical effects exhibited by this receptor, such as the alteration of intracellular calcium levels and activation of transcription and receptor downregulation, were dependent on the protein's intrinsic tyrosine kinase activity.[6] Mutations within the protein tyrosine kinase domain of c-*erb*-B2 were shown to abrogate its transforming potential, indicating that receptor tyrosine kinase (RTK) activity was necessary for neoplastic transformation.[7]

The discovery that the v-*erb*-B oncogene was the viral homologue of the EGF receptor added increasing weight to the argument that deregulation of a normal growth-controlling pathway results in neoplastic transformation. The importance of protein tyrosine kinases (PTKs) in normal signalling pathways is highlighted by a number of other studies. For example, the oncogenic effect of c-*erb*-B2, the second member of the *erb*-B2 family, is mediated by increased PTK activity caused by a point mutation in the transmembrane region.[6] The c-*erb*-B2 oncogene is amplified in approximately 30% of breast cancers. Over-expression of this oncogene correlates with lymph node involvement and poor survival, suggesting that it plays an important role in the development and progression of breast cancer in these patients.

Intracellular transducers

The discovery of cyclic adenosine-3′,5-monophosphate (cAMP) more than 30 years ago gave rise to the idea that hormones can regulate cells by activating the production of intracellular second messengers. Since then a number of other intracellular molecules, including calcium and the products of phosphoinositide metabolism, have been discovered. In most cases second-messenger production is stimulated via a family of small heterotrimeric G proteins [called G proteins because they bind guanosine 5′-triphosphate (GTP)]. The speci-

ficity with which a receptor can bind a particular G proteins defines the range of responses a cell is capable of making to a particular stimulus. G proteins are comprised of three subunits: an α subunit that binds and hydrolyses GTP and a combined βγ subunit that exists as a dimer.[8] The *ras* family of proto-oncogenes encodes a group of closely related 21 kDa proteins that control regulatory pathways critical for normal proliferation and differentiation. *ras* gene products bind guanine nucleotides, have GTPase activity, and have amino terminal sequence homology with GTP-binding proteins.

The discovery that *ras* proteins could bind GTP and guanosine 5′-triphosphate (GDP) and were localized to the inner surface of the plasma membrane led to the suggestion that *ras* proteins and G proteins may have functional similarities.[9] Direct evidence to support this hypothesis was obtained when it was shown that normal Ha-*ras* possessed intrinsic GTPase activity, which was dramatically enhanced by the binding of a protein called GTPase-activating protein (GAP). This GTPase activity was subsequently shown to be reduced 500-fold in oncogenic mutants compared with normal *ras* proteins, resulting in an accumulation of the active GTP bound *ras*. These observations led to a model of *ras* action whereby the oncogenic effect of a *ras* protein

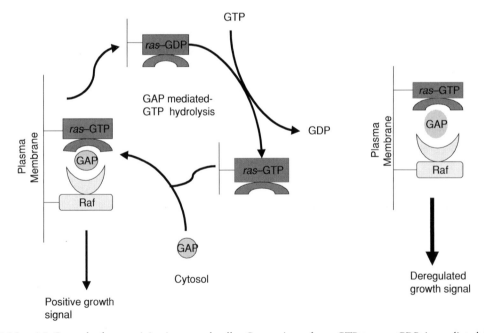

Figure 16.2. (a) Control of *ras* activity in normal cells. Conversion of *ras*–GTP to *ras*–GDP is mediated by binding of GAP. *ras*–GTP is in the active state and regulates the next component in the pathway, represented here as Raf. (b) Activity of mutant *ras*. Oncogenic *ras* is maintained in the active GTP bound state and thereby sends a continuous unregulated signal to the cell.

strongly correlates with its reduced GTPase activity[10] (Fig. 16.2).

ras family genes are mutated in approximately 30% of all cancers. This has lead to intense study aimed at defining the mechanism through which oncogenic *ras* functions. These studies suggest that the *ras* proteins act as conduits between growth factor receptor activation and gene regulation via mitogen-activated protein kinase (MAPK) cascades. These MAPK cascades result in phosphorylation and activation of specific transcription factors.[11] Activation of growth factor receptors results in the recruitment of the nucleotide exchange factor Sos to the plasma membrane, where it catalyses the transient formation of *ras*-GTP. The active *ras*-GTP form then recruits the serine–threonine kinase Raf to the plasma membrane where it becomes activated and in turn activates the MAPK pathway. Mutations, which activate the *ras* proteins, result in chronic over-stimulation of this pathway, which in turn leads to malignant transformation.

Nuclear oncogenes (transcription factors)

A number of proto-oncogene products are located in the nucleus where it has been suggested that they provide the final stage in the signalling pathway governing cellular proliferation. The first example of an oncogenic transcription factor was v-*jun*, the transforming gene of the chicken sarcoma virus ASV17.[12] It was subsequently demonstrated that the cellular homologue c-*jun*, could dimerize with a second proto-oncogene called c-*fos* and that the *fos*–*jun* heterodimer represented the components of the AP-1 transcription factor.[13] Several lines of evidence suggest that the AP-1 transcription factor is an important component of mitogenic signal transduction. First, upon stimulation with serum growth factors, many cells display an increase in both *jun* and *fos* mRNA levels that is associated with an increase in AP-1 activity. In addition, pre-existing AP-1 complexes are further activated through post-translational modifications, including phosphorylation and dephosphorylation.[14] Further evidence linking *jun* and *fos* proteins with cellular proliferation comes from the demonstration that these proteins can transform cells in culture, either directly or in co-operation with other oncogenes. However, it should be noted that the target of these oncogenic transcription factors is still a matter of debate.

Another nuclear transcription factor that has been shown to play an important role in cellular transformation is the c-*myc* oncogene. This oncogene was first identified as the homologue of the transforming sequence of the avian myelocytomatosis virus MC29,[15] and has subsequently been shown to be amplified in a variety of cancer types including colon carcinoma, small-cell lung carcinoma, and breast cancer.

A number of related genes have been discovered based on their homology to c-*myc*. The two best described family members are n-*myc* and l-*myc*, both of which are amplified in certain types of tumours. c-*myc* is a nuclear phosphoprotein that is localized to chromosome 8q24 and spans about 5 kb of genomic DNA. In Burkitt's lymphoma, c-*myc* is involved in a translocation to one of the three chromosomes that carry the immunoglobulin light- or heavy-chain genes. Translocations involving c-*myc* and the heavy-chain locus on chromosome 14 are the most common, occurring in approximately 90% of these tumours. This juxtaposition of the c-*myc* gene with the immunoglobulin gene loci is thought to result in the aberrant expression of c-*myc* and ultimately to give rise to neoplastic transformation. The expression of the c-*myc* gene is regulated by both positive and negative growth signals, while in transformed cells c-*myc* expression is consistently elevated and not responsive to external growth factors. The biological activity of the c-Myc protein is dependent on two conserved domains. The first is an amino terminal transactivation domain, and the second is a carboxy terminal helix–loop–helix–leucine zipper motif that functions as an interface for protein–protein interactions. The activity of c-Myc is regulated by its ability to bind its partner protein called Max. The Myc–Max heterodimer binds DNA in a sequence-specific manner and activates transcription from promoters containing the sequence CACGTG. Although c-Myc can homodimerize, its oncogenic potential has been shown to be dependent on its ability to bind Max.[16] Max can homodimerize and also heterodimerize with another protein called Mad. The Mad–Mad homodimer and the Mad–Max heterodimer are thought to act as transcriptional repressors that modulate the transcriptional activity of c-Myc.[17] c-Myc expression is highly regulated throughout the cell cycle and has a very short half-life of approximately 45 min. In comparison, Max is constitutively expressed and has a very long half-life in excess of 18 h. Induction of c-Myc by upstream events induces a shift from Max–Max or Max–Mad complexes to Myc–Max complexes, which results in a switch from transcriptional repression to transcriptional activation (Fig. 16.3). In tumours in which c-Myc is over-expressed it is likely that the Myc–Max heterodimer would represent the

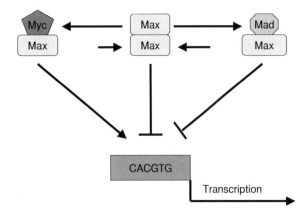

Figure 16.3. The ability of Myc to activate transcription is dependent on its ability to bind its partner Max. When Myc is induced the predominant complex will be Myc–Max and therefore will result in upregulation of specific target genes. When Myc is downregulated a shift to Max–Max or Max–Mad complexes occurs, leading to transcriptional repression.

predominant species and would therefore result in constitutive upregulation of specific target genes. This may form the basis of the oncogenic effect of c-Myc over-expression in tumours.

Tumour suppressor genes

Over the last three decades it has become apparent that a frequent and often necessary genetic alteration occurring during tumour development is the inactivation or loss of function of one or more TSGs. Three independent lines of evidence have converged to support this idea and to help in the identification of the initial members of this class of genes: (i) somatic and microcell genetic studies; (ii) analysis of families with an apparent underlying genetic predisposition to cancer; (iii) loss of heterozygosity studies.

Somatic and microcell genetic studies

The first suggestion that cancer may occur as a recessive event came from the fusion of malignant and non-malignant mouse cells. The resultant hybrid clones exhibited a reduction in tumorigenicity, indicating that malignancy acts as a recessive trait.[18] Subsequent studies in which human carcinoma cells (HeLa cells) were fused to normal human diploid fibroblasts confirmed these observations, with hybrid clones showing total suppression of tumour-forming ability. Follow-up studies revealed a statistical correlation between loss of a single normal chromosome 11 from these hybrids and re-

expression of the malignant phenotype.[19] Direct evidence for the presence of a TSG on chromosome 11 came with the reintroduction of a normal copy of chromosome 11 into HeLa cells by microcell-mediated transfer. The resultant microcell hybrids were found to be non-tumorigenic.[20] These studies indicated that specific chromosomes contained genes capable of suppressing tumour growth and that at least one event in the development of cancer was loss or inactivation of these genes. Microcell-mediated chromosome transfer has implicated a number of chromosomes in a variety of cancer types, and in some cases these genes have now been identified.

Familial cancers as indicators of TSGs

Knudson and others have stressed the importance of genetic inheritance in the search for cancer related genes.[1] The first step towards isolation of a disease gene is its localization to a specific chromosomal region. The observation of specific chromosomal abnormalities associated at high frequency with particular hereditary conditions has proved invaluable in this search. The paradigm of this approach is the retinoblastoma gene (RB), which was initially localized to chromosome 13q14 when cytogenetic analysis of a proportion of hereditary tumours exhibited a deletion of this region. Similarly, the first locus to be implicated in the WAGR syndrome of Wilm's tumour, aniridia, genitourinary anomalies, and mental retardation was chromosome 11p13, based on the observation that most WAGR patients carry a cytogenetically detectable constitutional deletion of this region. In the absence of detectable cytogenetic abnormalities, localization of a particular disease gene will usually rely on linkage analysis which allows the ordering of inherited markers relative to each other. This process has been revolutionized by the ability to detect variation between individuals at the DNA sequence level, in the form of restriction fragment length polymorphisms (RFLPs).[21] More recently, polymorphisms in the length of tandemly repeated simple sequences such as microsatellites have provided a source of easily detectable highly polymorphic markers for genetic analysis. For example, the gene predisposing to early-onset breast and ovarian cancer (BRCA1) was localized to chromosome 17q21 by a combination of these two methods.[22]

Loss of heterozygosity studies

The location of putative TSGs may also be discovered by the use of RFLP or microsatellite analysis to search for chromosome losses that lead to allelic homozygosity or hemizygosity.[23] Consistent allelic loss of a specific chromosomal region in a particular cancer type is taken as evidence for the location of a putative TSG in that region. In looking for loss of heterozygosity (LOH) at a particular locus, it is sufficient to compare DNAs from normal and tumour-derived cells of the same patient. By using this method it was demonstrated that the region on chromosome 17p that was commonly deleted in colorectal cancer was the site of the p53 TSG. LOH at a variety of chromosomal sites has now been described in many different types of tumour, and for some tumour types more than one area of LOH has been identified indicating that more than one gene is involved.

The RB paradigm

Retinoblastoma, which has an incidence of approximately one in 20 000, occurs in cells of the embryonal neural retina in young children up to age 5 and exhibits both sporadic and familial forms. Between the ages of 5 and 7 the retinoblasts terminally differentiate, cell division stops, and consequently no more tumours develop. The observation that as many as one-third of retinoblastomas appear to arise from a genetic predisposition with a dominant mode of inheritance led Knudson to postulate the now classical 'two-hit' theory.[1] He suggested that retinoblastoma is caused by two mutational events. In the dominantly inherited form one mutation is inherited through the germ line and the second mutation is somatic. In the sporadic form of the disease both mutations are somatic. It was subsequently shown that in retinoblastoma the target of these mutational events was the RB tumour suppressor gene.[24] The RB gene is comprised of 27 exons spanning 200 kb of genomic DNA and encodes a nuclear phosphoprotein, suggesting that it plays a role in the regulation of transcription. It has been demonstrated that the phosphorylation state of RB is cell-cycle dependent, with the unphosphorylated form predominating in G_0 and G_1, and progressively more phosphorylated forms appearing as the cells enter the S phase. It has now been clearly demonstrated that RB exerts its tumour suppressor effect by binding to and inactivating the E2F/DP transcription factor family when in the unphosphorylated state. The E2F/DP transcription factors are responsible for the upregulation of a number of genes such as dihydrofolate reductase (DHFR), thymidylate synthase (TS), and DNA polymerase-α (POL), which are essential for S-phase entry. Therefore loss of RB in tumours removes this negative block on entry into the S phase of the cell cycle and results in a selective growth advantage for the tumour cell. The phosphorylation state of the RB protein is tightly regulated by the activity of cyclin D and the cyclin-dependent kinases 4 and 6 (cdk4/6), which in turn are regulated by CDK inhibitors such as p16 and p21. Therefore the RB pathway serves as a major checkpoint on S-phase entry, and the majority of

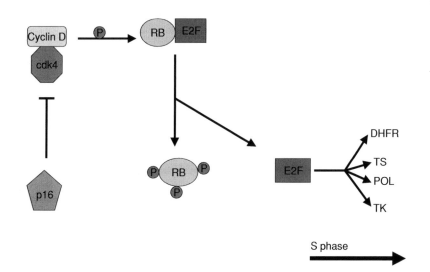

Figure 16.4. The RB protein binds to and inhibits the activity of the E2F transcription factor. RB is phosphorylated by the action of the cyclin D–cdk4 complex with the result that E2F is released and activates transcription of essential S-phase genes. Cdk4 is inhibited by the peptide p16, which acts to regulate the pathway negatively.

tumour types will have a mutation in at least one component of this pathway (Fig. 16.4).

The p53 tumour suppressor gene

The p53 gene was initially identified by the ability of its encoded protein to complex with the SV40 large T antigen in SV40-transformed cells. It was later localized to chromosome 17p13.1 and shown to span approximately 20 kb of genomic DNA. The p53 cDNA encodes a 393 amino acid, 53 kda phosphoprotein, which is predominantly localized to the nucleus.

The protein can be divided into four regions: (i) a highly charged acidic amino terminal region which functions as a transactivation domain; (ii) a DNA binding domain encompassing residues 102–292, which is required for sequence-specific DNA binding; (iii) an oligomerization domain between residues 324 and 355 which facilitates formation of an active p53 tetramer in solution; (iv) a carboxy terminal domain that is thought to modulate its ability to bind DNA. It is now estimated that approximately 50% of all tumours carry a p53 gene mutation, making p53 the most frequently mutated gene in human cancers. Moreover, 90% of these mutations fall within the DNA binding domain. In most tumours where p53 is mutated, one allele contains a missense mutation and the second allele is lost by deletion, thereby fulfilling the essential criteria for its classification as a TSG originally proposed by Knudson.[25] The number of viruses which have evolved a mechanism capable of inactivating p53 highlights the importance of this gene; these include the herpes simplex virus (HPV) and the human adenovirus. The HPV E6 protein binds to and promotes the proteolytic degradation of p53, while the adenovirus E1B 55Kd protein binds to and inactivates p53, preventing p53-mediated apoptosis. The biochemical properties of the p53 protein have been the focus of a large number of studies in recent years. Two consistent observations have prevailed: first, p53 is a transcription factor; secondly, it acts as a regulator of the cell cycle in response to DNA damage. The majority of p53 transcriptional targets identified to date have been implicated in either cell-cycle arrest or apoptotic pathways.

p53-mediated cell-cycle regulation

In response to various types of DNA damage the p53 protein is activated and induces expression of a number of target genes, two of which have been implicated in cell-cycle control. These are p21 (waf1/cip1) which,

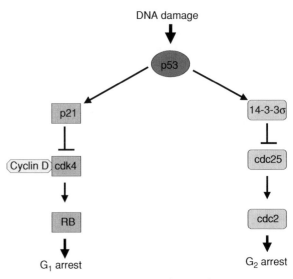

Figure 16.5. In response to DNA damage the p53 protein is stabilized and induces expression of p21 and 14-3-3σ. p21 inhibits the activity of cdk4, thus preventing phosphorylation of RB with the result that it remains complexed with E2F and thereby inhibits S-phase progression. p53-mediated transactivation of 14-3-3σ results in inhibition of cdc25 which is an essential activator of CDK1, the predominant G2 cyclin-dependent kinase, with the result that the cells arrest at the G_2–M checkpoint. 14-3-3σ inhibits cdc25 by binding to it and sequestering it in the cytoplasm.

when upregulated by p53, induces a G_1–S cell-cycle arrest and 14-3-3σ, which can induce a G_2–M cell-cycle arrest. p21 binds to and inhibits the function of a number of cyclin–cdk complexes including cyclin D–cdk4, cyclin A–cdk2 and cyclin E–cdk2.[26] The net effect of p21 upregulation is cell-cycle arrest mediated through inhibition of the RB pathway (Fig. 16.5). Induction of 14-3-3σ induces a G_2–M arrest by binding to cdc25 and sequestering it in the cytoplasm.[26] Cdc25 is a phosphatase, which activates the cyclin-B-dependent kinase CDK1 (cdc2), the activity of which is essential for mitosis to proceed (Fig. 16.5).

p53-mediated apoptosis

Several experimental lines of study have clearly demonstrated that p53 plays a role in initiating apoptosis under various physiologically stressful conditions such as gamma irradiation, oxygen deficiency, and altered ribonucleotide pools. Some of these experiments have been carried out in thymocytes from p53–/– mice and the corresponding normal counterparts. In this system it has been shown that while the normal thymocytes undergo apoptosis in response to DNA damage, those from p53-null animals fail to initiate apoptosis under the same stimulus. In addition, p53 has been shown to regulate the expression of genes implicated in apoptosis, including BAK and Fas/APO1; however, neither gene has been shown to be required for p53-dependent apoptosis. Recently, a model for p53-mediated apoptosis has been proposed which suggests that p53 induces apoptosis through a three-step process: (i) the transcriptional induction of redox genes; (ii) the formation of reactive oxygen species; (iii) The oxidative degradation of mitochondrial components, culminating in death. The p53-induced redox genes were identified by SAGE analysis and were shown in general to encode proteins that could generate or respond to oxidative stress. These p53-induced genes then collectively increase the cellular content of reactive oxygen species, which in turn leads to mitochondrial damage. Leakage of cytochrome c from damaged mitochondria then activates the cysteine aspartate proteases (caspases), which are the early effectors of apoptosis.[27,28]

The breast cancer susceptibility genes BRCA1 and BRCA2

Few gene-cloning strategies have generated as much interest in the last few years as that generated by the identification of first BRCA1 and subsequently BRCA2.[29,30] Mutations within these two genes account for practically all cases of hereditary breast cancer. BRCA1 is also mutated in early-onset breast and ovarian families and in some cases of sporadic ovarian cancer, while BRCA2 mutations have been found in male breast cancer and to a lesser extent in prostate and pancreatic cancer.

While the exact function of these two genes remains elusive, recent data suggests a role in transcriptional regulation and maintenance of genome integrity. The products of both genes are localized to the nucleus and contain transactivation domains, suggesting a role in the regulation of transcription. In addition, BRCA1 has been shown to be a component of the RNA polymerase-11 holoenzyme complex via its interaction with RNA helicase A. This interaction is mediated through the C-terminal BRCT motif, a previously undescribed motif which is conserved in genes involved in DNA repair and cell-cycle regulation.[31] Co-localization and immunoprecipitation studies have shown that BRCA1 and BRCA2 bind to Rad 51, a gene required for the repair of double-stranded DNA breaks. Furthermore, knockout studies in mice have demonstrated that BRCA1- and BRCA2-null cells exhibit hypersensitivity to gamma irradiation and other agents which cause double-stranded DNA breaks.[32,33] BRCA1 and BRCA2

have become the focus of intense research, both to elucidate fully their function and how it relates to tumour progression and to evaluate the potential for gene therapeutic strategies in tumours in which they are inactivated through mutation. In addition, their identification has heightened the public awareness of the availability of genetic screening as a predictive measure for cancer risk (see later in this chapter).

DNA repair genes

Mammalian cells have evolved highly regulated mechanisms for dealing with DNA damage incurred through spontaneous mutation, nucleotide mismatch during DNA synthesis, exposure to ultraviolet or gamma radiation, or exposure to reactive metabolites that cause oxidation and alkylation of DNA. A complete review of the various DNA repair strategies employed by eukaryotic cells to combat this continual assault on DNA integrity is beyond the scope of this chapter. However, two repair mechanisms, namely nucleotide excision repair and mismatch repair, will be discussed as these have clearly been implicated in the development of cancer. Both repair mechanisms maintain genomic integrity in mammalian cells and work in concert with various cell-cycle regularity proteins to induce cell-cycle arrest in response to DNA damaging agents. This cell-cycle arrest is necessary in order for the cell to repair any DNA damage incurred, thereby preventing propagation of mutations.

Nucleotide excision repair

Nucleotide excision repair (NER) is the process whereby DNA damage is removed and replaced with new DNA using the intact wild-type strand as a template. It is one of the most extensively studied and complicated of the excision repair processes, involving up to 30 gene products. The NER machinery has broad specificity and is able to recognize a wide variety of chemical alterations to DNA which result in distortion of the DNA structure. A typical lesion repaired by this mechanism is the pyrimidine dimer, which is induced by the photochemical fusion of two adjacent pyrimidines in response to ultraviolet radiation. It is estimated that skin cells would acquire thousands of pyrimidine dimers each day in response to sunlight exposure if they were not removed by excision repair. There are several pathways of excision repair in which a damaged base or backbone segment of DNA is removed. All lead to the same intermediate product:

either a single-strand break or a gap in the DNA at the site of damage which provides a 3′-hydroxyl end from which DNA polymerase can initiate synthesis to replace the damaged segment. A large number of the genes implicated in NER have been shown to be involved in transcription regulation, and mutations affecting different domains of these multifunctional proteins can lead to widely differing clinical phenotypes.[34] The best described cancer syndrome caused by mutation of genes involved in excision repair is the human skin disease xeroderma pigmentosum (XP), which is characterized by hypersensitivity to sunlight (ultraviolet radiation) and predisposition to skin cancer. Some of the genes implicated in the development of XP have now been identified as subunits of the TF11H transcription complex, which serves as a further demonstration of the link between transcription and DNA repair.[33]

Mismatch repair

It has been known for some time that mismatch repair (MMR) plays an essential role in the correction of replicative mismatches that escape proofreading polymerases and in the processing of recombination intermediates. Therefore MMR acts as an important failsafe mechanism to ensure the fidelity of DNA replication. More recently it has been suggested that MMR may play a role in some types of nucleotide excision repair pathways, as part of a cell-cycle checkpoint control system, by recognizing certain types of DNA damage and triggering cell-cycle arrest. Studies in *Escherichia coli* have provided much of the fundamental information on how the MMR system works. In *E.coli*, three gene products, MutS, MutL, and MutH, are involved in the initial stages of DNA repair. These three genes act in concert to recognize DNA mismatches and orchestrate the repair process. In eukaryotes the situation is more complex. Three homologues of the MutS gene [hMSH2, hMSH3 and GTBP (hMSH6)] and three homologues of the MutL gene (hMLH1, hPMS1 and hPMS2) have been identified.[35] To date, no homologue of the *E.coli* MutH gene has been discovered.

Interest in this field received a considerable boost with the observation that the underlying genetic defect in hereditary nonpolyposis colorectal cancer (HNPCC) could be attributed to mutations within various members of the MMR genes, particularly hMSH2 and hMLH1.[36] Phenotypically, patients with mutations of MMR genes exhibit a mutator phenotype which manifests itself as instability within simple repeat sequences.

The majority of tumours with MMR mutations contain frequent deletions and insertions within CA repeat sequences, and have been characterized as replication error positive (RER+). These microsatellite repeat sequences are found in non-coding and coding regions of the genome, and have been described in a number of genes including HPRT, APRT, APC, type 11 TGF-β and BAX.[34] In MMR-deficient cells there is an increased rate of mutation at these loci, which is presumably due to the inability of these cells to carry out efficient MMR. In addition to HNPCC, mutations within MMR genes have also been observed in numerous forms of sporadic cancer, including endometrial, pancreatic, gastric, ovarian, and breast cancer to name but a few.

Mutations within MMR genes appear to follow the classical Knudson 'two-hit' hypothesis. This has led to the suggestion that DNA repair genes should also be classified as TSGs, a subject of current debate.

Recently it has been suggested that DNA repair genes should be regarded as 'caretakers' of the genome and TSGs should be regarded as 'gatekeepers'.[37] The difference between caretakers and gatekeepers is that mutations in caretaker genes do not represent a rate-limiting step in tumour formation, while mutations in gatekeeper genes do.

Genes which fall into the caretaker class include the NER genes implicated in XP, the MMR genes involved in HNPCC, and probably the ATM, *BRCA1*, and BRCA2 genes. Gatekeeper genes generally function as negative regulators of cell growth, and include the Rb, p53, APC, and WT1 genes. The impact of the loss of a given gatekeeper gene exhibits a certain degree of tissue specificity, and inactivation of both copies of a gatekeeper gene represents the rate-limiting step for a given tumour type. As only two mutational events are required to initiate tumour formation, individuals predisposed to a particular cancer type inherit one mutant copy of a gatekeeper gene from a carrier parent, and somatically acquire a second mutation within the same gene in the tumour. Conversely, inactivation of DNA repair genes (caretaker genes) does not promote tumour progression directly, but rather results in a 'mutator' phenotype, characterized by genetic instability, which ultimately leads to an increased overall mutation rate affecting all genes including gatekeeper genes. In this latter scenario an individual would need to acquire four separate mutations in order to facilitate tumour progression. The first two mutational events would represent inactivation of both copies of a caretaker gene, which would result in general genetic instability, eventually leading to inactivation of both copies of a particular gatekeeper gene—the rate-limiting step.

Clinical implications and the way forward

The important questions that now need to be addressed are what recent insights into the molecular basis of cancer mean in terms of better treatment for cancer patients, and how we can translate these findings into everyday clinical practice. This information is already being used to design and test a variety of novel and exciting new strategies for cancer treatment. These strategies are based on an understanding of tumour initiation and progression at the molecular, and therefore most basic, level. The approach taken to developing a treatment for a particular tumour type is dependent on an understanding of the underlying genetic defects giving rise to that tumour. Unfortunately, cancer is a multistep process, with most tumours having undergone a series of mutational events during transition to malignancy, and therefore the challenge is to identify the rate-limiting step for each tumour and use that information to design the appropriate countermeasures. Most tumours will have acquired mutations in one or all of the classes of genes described above, making the task of devising an appropriate therapy extremely difficult. However, in a number of cases it has been possible to identify the critical changes responsible and to develop radical new therapies based on that information. The strategy employed for various tumour types is dependent on the nature of the gene implicated in the development of the specific tumour. Other strategies are focusing on the identification of novel chemotherapeutic targets and further defining interactions between known chemotherapeutic drugs and their intracellular targets in order to improve therapeutic efficacy.

Genetic risk analysis

The cloning of the BRCA1 and BRCA2 genes has resulted in an increased awareness among the general public about the availability of genetic screening to assess the risk of developing breast cancer. This heightened interest has created a situation in which a curious public is demanding more information about the genetic cause of disease from a medical system which is not equipped to handle the genetic information available nor the impact that that information might have on the patient. Genetic screening has been carried out for some time for other inherited cancer syndromes, such as multiple endocrine neoplasia type 2 (MEN-2), retinoblastoma, and familial adenomateous polyposis. The genes underlying the defects in these three cancer types have been well described, but more importantly protocols exist to provide a specific treatment based on the genetic information provided.

Multiple endocrine neoplasia

A good example of genetic risk analysis is the predictive testing for patients at risk of developing MEN-2A, MEN-2B, or familial medullary thyroid carcinoma (FMTC). All three diseases are caused by mutations within the RET oncogene, which encodes a transmembrane receptor tyrosine kinase. The three diseases are clinically distinct but share a common characteristic, the development of medullary thyroid carcinoma.[37] All mutations associated with MEN-2A or FMTC affect cysteine residues in the extracellular domain of the receptor, while MEN-2B is associated with mutation of the intracellular tyrosine kinase domain.[38] The localization of predisposing mutations to a specific region of the gene has facilitated the use of genetic testing to identify patients at risk of developing MEN-2. The risk to MEN-2A patients of developing medullary thyroid carcinoma (MTC), in cases where a predisposing mutation has been identified by genetic screening, is 100%.[37] It is now standard procedure to provide prophylactic thyroidectomy to patients based on the results of this genetic screen to prevent the development of MTC. A medium-term follow-up of the first 18 patients having prophylactic thyroidectomy for MEN-2A based on direct DNA testing has concluded that this is a safe and effective way of managing MTC in patients with MEN-2A.[39]

Hereditary colorectal cancer

A similar strategy is being proposed for the treatment of familial adenomateous polyposis (FAP) and for hereditary non-polyposis colorectal carcinoma (HNPCC). Currently, patients at risk of developing colon cancer are identified based on family history, physical examination, testing for occult blood, or colonoscopy. Despite these measures, patients typically present with late-stage disease and the overall 5-year survival rate is only 37%.[40] The possibility of genetically screening patients at risk of developing familial forms of colon cancer became a reality with the cloning of the adenomateous polyposis coli gene (APC) and the demonstration that mutations within this gene predispose to FAP.[41] FAP accounts for approximately 1% of all colorectal tumours; it is characterized by the development of hundreds of colorectal adenomas and leads to the development of colorectal cancer usually by age 50. The majority of mutations within the APC gene result in a prematurely truncated protein, and thus it is particularly suited to screening by the *in vitro* synthesized protein assay (IVSP).[42]

These discoveries have made presymptomatic molecular diagnosis possible for patients from high-risk families and, in approximately 80% of cases, allow the unambiguous identification of those family members who carry the mutant allele. In situations where the predisposing mutation within a family has already been identified, at-risk relatives can be tested with an almost 100% positive or negative predictive value.[43] This information can have a profound effect on the patient; a negative result in the case where the predisposing mutation has already been identified assures the patient that his or her overall risk is now that of the general population and negates the need for regular physical examinations. In addition, it allows the patient to plan for a family without the risk of passing the mutation on to any offspring. Conversely, a positive test result carries with it the certainty of developing colon cancer at a relatively young age and the associated lifestyle changes that go along with this knowledge. The positive aspect of knowing that a patient carries a mutation is the ability to carry out the appropriate preventative measures such as regular screening for polyps and pre-emptive surgery.

The situation for HNPCC is not as clear cut, which is unfortunate since this disease accounts for approximately 6% of all colorectal cancers.[42] Unlike FAP, which is characterized by hundreds of polyps, HNPCC is usually characterized by the occurrence of a single tumour and may be associated with a variety of other cancers, especially cancer of the endometrium. HNPCC is caused by mutations in any one of five MMR genes (see above), although hMSH2 and hMLH1 are most frequently involved.[33,34] Patients with MMR gene mutations also exhibit a replication error phenotype (RER+) which is characterized by microsatellite instability. Therefore these patients can be screened genotypically or phenotypically, depending on the preferred technique. The situation for HNPCC is further complicated by the observation that gene penetrance is only 70%–80%, unlike FAP where it is virtually 100%.[42]

This effectively means that 30% of patients having a mutation in one of the MMR genes will never develop colorectal cancer. Despite these problems, genetic testing for HNPCC can provide valuable information for both the patient and the clinician. It allows informed decision-making in terms of which patients need regular screening and what preventative measures should be taken.

Hereditary breast and ovarian cancer

Public awareness of the power of genetic testing received a huge boost with the cloning of the BRCA1 TSG, which predisposes to early-onset breast and ovarian cancer.[28] The subsequent cloning of the second breast cancer gene BRCA2[29] added fuel to the perception that a major breakthrough had been made in the fight against breast cancer. While the cloning of these two genes represents a major advance in our ability to begin to understand the development of breast cancer at a molecular level, it has also raised public expectations of what this means in terms of breast cancer treatment to an unrealistic level.

The first problem is that hereditary breast cancer only accounts for approximately 5%–10% of all breast cancers and, unlike the situation for other TSGs such as RB or p53 which are also implicated in sporadic cancers, the link between BRCA1 or BRCA2 and sporadic breast cancer is unclear. Secondly, while mutational analysis of these two genes in families predisposed to breast cancer will allow the identification of patients who are specifically at risk, the clinical application of this information remains unclear. Although prophylactic surgery, such as mastectomy or oophorectomy, is an option for patients who have tested positive for a BRCA1 or BRCA2 mutation, there is no evidence to suggest that this surgical intervention improves outcome.[44]

Thus the isolation of these two genes has served to highlight the benefits and problems that are associated with predictive genetic testing in general. When we look at the cases of MEN-2 and APC genetic testing, where the mutations identified are practically 100% penetrant and a defined clinical response is in place to act upon the information provided by the test, the benefits are obvious. However, the benefits of BRCA1 and BRCA2 genetic testing are not so clear cut. The lifetime risk of developing breast cancer is approximately 80% for those patients who have inherited a mutant BRCA1 allele in a family in which that mutation clearly segregates with the disease.[45] However, these families are not a good reflection of a typical breast cancer family, but rather reflect a minority of families in which the particular mutation involved is highly penetrant. It has been suggested that the real risk will be somewhat lower when one takes into account the large number of different mutations that have been identified to date in BRCA1 families. In addition, it is reasonable to assume that penetrance may vary depending on the nature of the mutation and the genetic background of the individual.[44]

The complex nature of cancer genetics has also served to highlight the problems regarding the use of genetic counselling for patients and families undergoing genetic tests, and in the misinterpretation of genetic test results.[46] These are important issues which need to be resolved through better education as to what genetic testing can and cannot do. Despite these problems, the future of genetic testing as an integral part in the assessment of patient risk is secure. More research is required for a full understanding of the implications of mutational heterogeneity in the genetically more complex diseases, and how these relate to predictive risk assessment for individual patients. In addition, guidelines should be introduced so that patients and clinicians clearly understand the implications of acquiring this new genetic information, particularly for those cancers in which a clear clinical response to the information is not in place.

Novel therapeutics from understanding tumour biology

Oncogene-based strategies

'Know your enemy' is an oft repeated phrase among military strategists, and is a phrase which can also be applied to the fight against cancer. Information obtained from years of basic research is finally being used to engineer new and conceptually simple approaches to cancer treatment. Although still in their infancy, oncogene-based therapies which attack cancer at its most basic level hold out the promise of revolutionizing cancer treatment in the future. In devising a new means of cancer treatment, it is imperative to understand the molecular phenotype of a given cancer. The type of defect underlying a particular tumour type defines the strategy that can be employed to counteract its harmful effect. Activation of oncogenes represents a critical event in the genesis of many types of tumours and, as has been described previously, these activated oncogenes tend to drive a cell towards cell growth. Ident-

ification of the critical regulatory function and locus of action of a particular oncogene has permitted the development of novel therapeutic strategies. Oncogenes belonging to two groups, cell surface receptors and intracellular transducers, have been the primary focus of this type of research to date.

Cell surface receptors as targets for novel therapies

The first line of attack for investigators has been directed towards oncogenes which encode cell surface receptors. These receptors normally interact with specific ligands such as growth factors to transmit a signal from the extracellular environment to the intracellular transduction machinery. In some cancers these receptors are over-expressed or are mutated, resulting in an excessive growth signal being transmitted to the cell. As long as 15 years ago scientists began exploring the possibility of targeting these receptors using specific antibodies as antagonists.

The c-*erb*-B2 oncogene is amplified in approximately 30% of breast cancers, and represents one such receptor which has been the target of this type of approach.

Antibodies against the c-*erb*-B2 receptor have been generated in an effort to block its function in tumour cells in which it was over-expressed. These antibodies were shown to inhibit the growth of *breast cancer* cells which over-express c-*erb*-B2, and a series of clinical trials aimed at evaluating their activity in patients were performed. Investigations in larger-scale trials have demonstrated improved survival in women with advanced breast cancer treated with c-*erb*-B2 antibodies and chemotherapy.[47]

The production of antibodies is costly and time consuming, and has led some scientists to begin searching for other alternatives that may have the same end result. This has precipitated the search for small synthetic molecules that may have the same effect. Rather than target the outer extracellular domain, these strategies have focused on the development of molecules against the inner cytoplasmic effector domain. The majority of these cell surface receptors encode a tyrosine kinase which comprises the intracellular domain. As previously described, the function of this motif is to bind to and phosphorylate specific intracellular components of the signalling pathway. Therefore the rationale behind this approach is to design specific synthetic compounds which will bind to and inhibit the phosphorylation of the specific target signal transduction molecule.

The predicted problem with tyrosine kinase inhibitors is the specificity of the synthetic molecule for a specific receptor. The tyrosine kinase domains of many of these receptors are conserved and this may lead to non-specific blocking of non-target receptors. However, in practice this has not been the case, as some molecules exhibit high specificity for the intended kinase. A number of these tyrosine kinase inhibitors function by blocking the site of interaction between the kinase and ATP, which supplies the phosphate group for activation of the target molecule. Several of these compounds are now in clinical trials. The first of these inhibitors, SU-101 which is a PDGF antagonist, has been evaluated on 150 patients and has shown responses in patients with glioblastoma.[46]

Intracellular transducers as targets for novel therapeutics

Of the genes that we ascribe to this class of signalling molecule, the most frequently mutated in cancer is the *ras* gene family (Ha-*ras*, K-*ras*, and N-*ras*) (see above), reflecting the central role that this family of genes plays in a variety of signalling pathways. Because of their central role in signal transduction pathways and the high frequency of their mutation in cancer, the *ras* genes have been the focus of intense research aimed at

devising a means of blocking their transforming action. Clues as to how this might be achieved were obtained with the observation that the *ras* protein is synthesized as an immature precursor which must undergo a series of post-translational modifications in order to be converted to its mature active form.[48] The post-translational modifications allow the *ras* protein to be anchored to the inner face of the plasma membrane where it is activated and in turn activates its target molecules (Fig. 16.6). The first and most critical step in post-translational modification of *ras* is the addition of a 15-carbon farensyl moiety to its C-terminal CAAX motif (C, cysteine; A, an aliphatic residue; X, any other amino acid). This reaction is catalysed by an enzyme called farnesyltransferase and is essential for *ras* function. The subsequent steps are not necessary for *ras* membrane association or its ability to transform cells.[48]

One strategy for inhibiting the action of the *ras* proteins is to generate inhibitors of farnesyltransferase and thus prevent post-translational modification of *ras*, and a number of farnesyltransferase inhibitors have now been generated. One such inhibitor has been designed to function as a CAAX analogue which can effectively compete with *ras* for binding to farnesyltransferase.

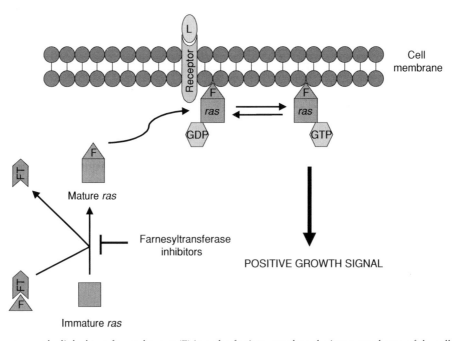

Figure 16.6. *ras* must be linked to a farnesyl group (F) in order for it to attach to the inner membrane of the cell. This attachment is necessary for *ras* to be activated by a tyrosine kinase receptor. Once *ras* has been activated to the GTP bound state it activates the next molecule in the signalling pathway. The transfer of a farnesyl group to the immature *ras* protein is catalysed by the enzyme farnelystransferase (FT). Farnesyltransferase inhibitors prevent this reaction and thereby inhibit the essential post-translational modification of *ras*.

This compound, called L-731,735, has been shown to be a potent and selective inhibitor of farnesyltransferase *in vitro*.[49] This and related compounds have been shown to inhibit the tumorigenic phenotype of *ras*-transformed cells, human tumour cell lines, and in animal models. Fortunately, farnesyltransferase inhibitors appear to be quite specific and do not affect normal cells or cells transformed by other oncogenes.

Indeed, the specificity of these inhibitors suggests that side effects may be minimal, and initial experiments indicate that even when given at high doses (enough to eliminate tumours in mouse models) there appears to be no toxicity towards normal tissue.[50]

In summary, these farnesyltransferase inhibitors represent the first of a new wave of synthetic chemotherapeutic agents which may revolutionize our approach to cancer treatment. Although there are many pitfalls that can be expected with such a fundamental change in our concept of how we should treat cancer, these approaches have their roots in decades of high-quality basic research and therefore represent a solid foundation on which to build.

Strategies based on tumour suppressor genes

Unlike the blocking of inappropriately expressed oncogenes, the inactivation of TSGs represents a more complex hurdle to overcome in the development of new cancer therapies. TSGs act as negative regulators of cell growth and their loss or inactivation results in the release of a particular cell from this type of growth restraint. Conceptually, the aim here is to replace the defective or missing gene with a normal copy, a process termed gene therapy. Although on the surface this sounds like a straightforward idea, in reality it has proved to be a more formidable challenge. The principal problems to be overcome are threefold: (i) delivery of the gene of interest; (ii) targeting of the gene to all tumour cells; (iii) appropriate long-term expression of the transferred gene. Although an in-depth study of the strategies being developed to overcome these problems is beyond the scope of this chapter, we will briefly describe some of the potential benefits and pitfalls with this type of approach.

Delivery methods

A variety of approaches have been devised to facilitate the transfer of a specific gene of interest from the test tube to the patient. Essentially, research has focused on the use of either viral or non-viral vectors. Viral vectors tend to be modified forms of either DNA viruses, such

as adenovirus, or RNA viruses, such as retroviruses, into which the gene of interest has been inserted. In addition, various structural genes have been removed to make the viruses replication defective in the target cell, or such that they can only replicate in a specific tumour cell and not in the surrounding normal tissue. The advantage of using viral vectors is that they have evolved specifically for this purpose and are extremely efficient at transducing human cells, particularly those cells which are actively dividing, such as tumour cells. Some of the drawbacks include immunogenicity of vectors, low viral titres< particularly for retrovirus-based vectors, and cellular toxicity from background expression of viral genes leading to cell death, which results in limited expression of the transgene.[51]

The non-viral vectors that have been most extensively studied are liposomes, which are a mixture of lipid and DNA, forming lipid–DNA complexes capable of delivering the complexed DNA to many cell types. Liposomes are positively charged and readily fuse with the negatively charged cell membrane resulting in transfer of the DNA into the cells. Liposome vectors are extremely flexible and there is no limit to the size of the DNA fragment to be transferred. In addition, they are capable of delivery to many different cell types and are not dependent on the mitotic index of the target cell. The principal drawback to liposomes is the lack of specificity for a particular cell type and the low transduction efficiency compared with viral vectors.[50] The final method of delivery is by directly introducing the gene of interest to a specific tumour by mechanical means, such as injection, or by high-velocity bombardment of tissue with DNA attached to gold particles.[52] Although this strategy has been successfully employed in a number of cases, the main problem is that the therapeutic benefit is restricted to the site of injection only and in some cases requires surgical procedure in order to gain access to the target organ.

Tumour targeting

One of the areas of vector design, which is crucial to the success of gene therapy as a viable therapeutic approach, is that of targeting the vector exclusively to a specific tumour cell. Some viruses exhibit, to varying degrees, a tissue-specific tropism. For example, adenovirus preferentially infects lung epithelium and can also mediate high-level transduction of the liver parenchyma, while retroviruses exhibit no such tissue-specific tropism. A number of strategies are currently under development to address this issue. One approach has been to attach synthetic ligands to the viral coat which will recognize a particular cell surface receptor expressed only on the target cell.[53] Similar approaches are being employed to target non-viral vector systems through, for example, the generation of protein–DNA complexes. In one such study an EGF–DNA complex was generated to target lung cancer cells which over-express the EGF receptor.[54] Another method of achieving specificity is by using tissue-specific promoters to drive expression of the gene of interest. A number of reports have been published using this principle, which represents an exciting avenue for further study.[50]

Appropriate gene expression

The effectiveness of any gene therapy strategy is determined by the ability not only of targeting the therapeutic gene to the correct cell type, but also by the appropriate long-term expression of the transferred gene. Retrovirus-based vectors in particular can integrate into the host genome, providing the potential for long-term expression, but they may also have the associated problem of gene toxicity. This potential problem has focused attention on the need for regulated expression of the transferred gene rather than the constitutive expression systems currently available. One example of the application of regulated gene expression is the discovery that ionizing radiation can induce transcription from the promoter regions of various genes including *jun–fos*, NF-KB, and the early growth response gene family (EGR-1), and this information has been used to design a gene therapy strategy for a radioresistant human squamous cell carcinoma xenograph model. A radiosensitizing cytokine, TNF-α, was transfected into the HL525 cell line under the control of the Egr-1 promoter, and the resultant clones were then injected into nude mice and the effect of radiation on tumour growth assayed. It was shown that in this model the combination of gene therapy and radiation therapy produced an increase in tumour cures without an increase in toxicity.[55] Another potential strategy involves the use of tetracycline-regulated promoters to regulate gene expression in an *in vivo* setting. The utility of this approach has recently been demonstrated in a rat system in which expression of enhanced green fluorescent protein (EGFP) in the rat central nervous system could be switched on or off by the addition or removal of the tetracycline analogue doxycycline from the animal's drinking water.[56]

p53 as a target for gene therapy

As previously discussed the p53 TSG is found to be mutated in approximately 50% of all human cancers

and therefore represents an obvious target for gene therapy. Indeed, a number of groups are in the process of devising methods of replacing p53 in tumours in which this gene is defective, and some of these strategies are now in clinical trials. One approach, which aims to selectively kill tumour cells with a mutant p53, is based on the understanding of the relationship between adenoviral infection and p53 function. Adenovirus forces its host cell into the cell cycle in order that it may harness the cell's replication machinery to replicate its own genome. In order to achieve this, adenovirus has evolved a number of genes which specifically allow the virus to drive this forced replication. The product of one of these genes, E1A, binds to and inactivates the RB TSG product, thereby releasing its inhibitory effect on the E2F transcription factor, expression of which drives the cells into the S phase of the cell cycle. The cell responds by inducing p53-mediated apoptosis in response to E1A expression. However, the virus has also evolved a means to counteract this response by expression of a second gene called E1B-55KD, the product of which binds to and inhibits the function of p53. An understanding of this relationship has formed the basis of a gene therapy strategy which makes use of an adenovirus mutant for E1B-55KD.

The mutant form of adenovirus cannot inhibit the function of p53 and therefore cannot replicate in cells with a wild-type p53 gene. However, the mutant virus can replicate efficiently and kill cells with mutant p53 (Fig. 16.7). The benefit of this type of approach is immediately obvious when one remembers that approximately 50% of cancers have mutant p53.[56]

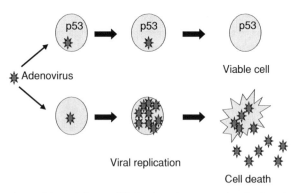

Figure 16.7. The modified adenovirus can infect both p53 wild type and p53 mutant cells but can only replicate in the mutant cells. Therefore, in theory, once the virus has gained access to a p53 mutant cell, it should replicate killing the tumour cell and release additional viral particles which can subsequently infect and kill neighbouring tumour cells.

Results in culture and in tumour-bearing mice have indicated that the mutant adenovirus replicates 100 times less efficiently in cells expressing wild-type p53. One of the major problems with this strategy, as is the case with many other gene therapy protocols, is efficient delivery of the adenovirus to the tumour. Despite these problems, a gene therapy protocol based on this approach has entered phase I clinical trials in patients with p53 mutant squamous cell carcinoma of the head and neck. The problem of delivery in this instance has been overcome by the direct injection of the virus into the tumour mass.[57]

Strategies based on DNA repair genes

DNA repair genes represent the third category of genes that provide an attractive target for gene therapeutic approaches. The main function of these genes is to maintain DNA integrity and ensure the fidelity of DNA replication. This is still a relatively new field in terms of gene therapy, but similar applications to those being explored for TSGs are being proposed. Some of the TSGs previously described, such as p53 and BRCA1, have also been implicated in DNA damage response pathways. These genes function as DNA damage sensors which in turn signal to the cell-cycle machinery. This is certainly true for p53, and evidence is accumulating to suggest a similar role for BRCA1. However, it is not clear whether these genes are themselves actively involved in the repair of DNA or whether their primary role is the activation of specific DNA repair genes.

Although the genes involved in HNPCC represent obvious targets for gene therapeutic approaches, little has been published to date on this topic. One might anticipate that an approach similar to that devised for various TSGs would prove to be effective. However, some progress has been made in designing therapeutic strategies for XP, which is characterized by hypersensitivity to ultraviolet radiation caused by a defect in one of seven genes involved in NER (see above). These seven genes, designated XPA to XPG, have become the focus for gene therapeutic strategies aimed at correcting NER defects. In one such study a recombinant retroviral vector, LXSN, was used to transfer cDNAs encoding the XPA, XPB, and XPC genes into primary and immortalized fibroblasts from XP patients. Analysis of these clones revealed that the recombinant retroviruses are extremely efficient at transducing the XP primary fibroblasts, while functional analysis of the transduced clones indicated that the defect in the XP cells had been corrected.[58] These experiments have

paved the way for future protocols aimed at bringing this technology into the clinical arena.

Chemotherapeutic targets

While current approaches to the development of new therapies for patients with cancer have primarily focused on the development of innovative therapeutic targets, another important strategy has been to determine the impact on chemotherapeutic targets during treatment. The development of new biological or pharmacological agents based on sound preclinical principles will ultimately lead to more effective therapies for patients with cancer. One example of using biomarker analysis to optimize therapy is the pyrimidine antagonist 5-fluorouracil. As described in Chapter 6, 5-fluorouracil is activated by multiple enzymes to inhibit thymidylate synthase or incorporate into RNA or DNA. Alternatively, the drug is degraded to inactive metabolites by dihydropyrimidine dehydrogenase.

Thymidylate synthase

Thymidylate synthase (TS) is a folate-dependent enzyme that catalyses the methylation of 2′-deoxyuridine 5′-monophosphate (dUMP) using 5,10- methylene tetrahydrofolate as a one-carbon donor for the reductive methylation to deoxythymidine monophosphate (dTMP), which is required for *de novo* thymidylate synthesis, and DNA replication and repair.[58] TS is also a critical target for fluoropyrimidine drugs as well as novel antifolate drugs used in the treatment of breast, gastrointestinal, and head and neck cancers. Fluorouracil (5-FU) is converted intracellularly to fluorodeoxyuridine monophosphate (FdUMP), and in the presence of 5,10-methylene tetrahydrofolate forms a stable covalent TS ternary complex (TS–FdUMP-5,10-methylene tetrahydrofolate) resulting in TS inhibition.[59,60] In addition to 5-FU, several novel antifolate inhibitors of thymidylate synthase have recently been synthesized and found to have potent antitumour activity *in vitro* and *in vivo*.[61,62] Thus the central role of TS in the *de novo* synthesis of dTMP, and hence DNA synthesis, has made it a major target for antitumour drug development.

Thymidylate synthase as a determinant of chemotherapeutic resistance

The major limitation to use of TS-directed chemotherapy has been the development of clinical resistance. Clinically achievable concentrations of 5-FU have been shown to result in an approximately four- to fivefold increase in the level of TS protein over a 24 h period in a H630 human colon carcinoma cell line.[63] The use of interferon-γ was associated with repression of the acute induction of TS protein and potentiated the cytotoxic effect of 5-FU by approximately 20-fold. This increase in cytotoxicity ordinarily occurs with exposure to fluoropyrimidine.

Increased TS expression would also appear to play a significant role in the development of resistance to folate-based TS inhibitors. Several investigators have shown in human tumour cell lines that increased TS expression is one of the major determinants of resistance to these novel antifolates.[64,65]

Recently, Chu *et al.*[66] demonstrated that cells efficiently adjust their level of TS through an autoregulatory feedback mechanism whereby TS enzyme binds to its own messenger RNA, resulting in a diminished translational efficiency. Furthermore, the ability of TS protein to bind to its mRNA depends on the occupancy of the enzyme. When TS is occupied by either its physiological substrates deoxyuridylate and 5,10-methylene hydrofolate or by FdUMP, the enzyme is incapable of binding its own RNA. Therefore TS mRNA is translated with an enhanced efficiency yielding increased levels of cellular TS protein.[66] Additional investigations have revealed at least two sites on TS mRNA capable of binding TS protein.[67] One occurs at the translational start site, which is predicted to have a stem–loop structure by a computer-assisted RNA folding algorithm, while the second is located within the protein-coding region. Taken together, these observations support the critical role of TS in defining sensitivity to antifolate- and fluoropyrimidine-based drugs, and suggest that the determination of TS levels in tumour tissues would help to clarify the relationship between pretreatment TS levels, prognosis, and a response to TS-directed therapies.

Given the importance of TS as a chemotherapeutic target, it has been important to develop sensitive methods for measuring it in patient tumour samples. To this end Johnston *et al.*[68] developed human murine monoclonal antibodies against recombinant human TS protein. These were found to be highly specific and have been used to develop a number of sensitive immunoassays capable of measuring the level of TS protein in cell lines and tumour tissues. Investigation using a variety of immunoquantitative techniques have shown that these antibodies are capable of accurately quantitating TS levels down to approximately 30 amol of protein.[69] A major advantage of this technology compared with traditional assays is that these antibodies

facilitate the measurement of TS on the basis of individual cells and formalin-fixed and paraffin-embedded tissues, and therefore are applicable to retrospective analysis of archival material. Moreover, a reverse transcriptase polymerase chain reaction assay (RT–PCR) capable of measuring tissue levels of TS mRNA has also recently been developed by investigators at the University of Southern California who have shown, using this assay, that TS mRNA levels are associated with responsiveness to fluoropyrimide-based therapy in patients with colorectal and gastric carcinoma.[70] Patients with relatively low levels of TS mRNA responded to fluoropyrimidine-based therapy, as might be predicted from preclinical data. These sensitive monoclonal antibody and RT–PCR based assays have now proved useful in assessing the long-term prognosis for patients with gastrointestinal malignancies as well as breast cancer and head and neck cancer.

Clinical relevance of TS expression

Recent studies examining the level of TS expression in clinical tumour samples suggest that TS expression predicts for overall clinical outcome and response to fluoropyrimidine-based therapy. Using the TS monoclonal antibodies Johnston *et al.*[71] have shown that TS protein levels predict for disease-free survival and survival in patients with rectal cancer independent of Dukes' stage. These investigators have also found that lower TS expression in patients with node-positive primary breast cancer correlates with improved event-free and overall survival, independent of other established prognostic factors in this disease.[72] In both these lstudies adjuvant chemotherapy had the greatest impact on survival and disease-free survival in tumours expressing higher TS levels. Other studies have also shown that the level of TS staining in primary tumour sections may not necessarily correlate with the chemosensitivity of subsequent metastases, suggesting that changes in TS expression may occur with tumour spread and evolution.[73]

More recently, Lenz *et al.*[74] have reported that increased pretreatment TS expression together with expression of mutant p53 identified a subgroup of primary stage II colon carcinoma patients with an overall poor prognosis. In the setting of advanced metastatic disease both high TS mRNA, quantified by RT–PCR, and high TS protein expression, quantitated by cytochemical techniques, have been shown to predict poor response to fluoropyrimidine-based therapy in colorectal, gastric, head and neck, and breast cancer.[75-77] Considerable overlap between responders and non-responders was often present in the low-TS categories, but patients with TS levels above the median do not tend to respond to fluoropyrimidine- or antifolate-based therapy. In the adjuvant and advanced disease setting, TS levels predicted outcome of therapy not only for TS inhibitors such as 5-FU but also when other agents, which are cytotoxic to cancer cells through other mechanisms, were used in combination. That such correlations should emerge is interesting and suggest that TS might be a marker for overall tumour sensitivity for a number of therapeutic approaches.

Thus these clinical studies evaluating the expression of TS in human tumours suggest that an ability to predict response and outcome based upon TS expression may provide the opportunity in the future to select patients most likely to benefit from TS-directed therapy.

Dihydropyrimidine dehydrogenases

Dihydropyrimidine dehydrogenase (DPD, EC1.5.1.3) is an important rate-limiting enzyme involved in the catabolic degradation of 5-FU to fluoro-β-alanaline.[77] DPD accounts for the elimination of at least 80% of an administered dose of 5-FU and has received considerable attention as a potential target for pharmacological manipulation. DPD is present in the liver, but is also found in bowel, pancreas, lung, kidney, lymphocytes, and other tissues. DPD activity in normal tissues exhibits diurnal variation with an inverse relationship with plasma 5-FU concentrations which vary up to fivefold over 24 h; DPD activity is highest at night with peak activity around 1 a.m. Cellular division in normal proliferating tissues also exhibits cyclical variations in activity with peak rates during the daytime.[78]

Similar studies in tumour cells harvested from patients have shown that tumours also possess circadian fluctuations in proliferative activity. These observations have given rise to the concept that a cell-cycle-specific drug such as 5-FU would affect normal tissues less if given at night, when DNA synthesis and proliferation are lower and catabolic pathways for the drug are more active. Thus chronomodulation of infusional 5-FU has been designed to exploit these diurnal variations in 5-FU catabolism as described above. There have been recent attempts to develop novel approaches to fluoropyrimidine therapy through the use of DPD-resistant prodrugs or the design of DPD inhibitors which can be administered with oral 5-FU.[79] A number of orally stable active 5-FU prodrugs such as tegafur are now in various stages of clinical evaluation. These

have been combined with uracil in molar ratios of 1:4, which result in saturation of DPD and a greatly enhanced oral bioavailability.[80,81] DPD inhibitors have made oral 5-FU dosing an attractive alternative for future trials, some of which are underway, which compare established regimens of intravenous infusional 5-FU with oral formulations.

There have also been several studies looking at DPD activity in patients in both normal blood mononuclear cells and tumour material. DPD activity in monocytes has been shown to correlate with that found in normal functioning liver, and this information is now being applied to population studies.[82] Such studies have suggested that levels of DPD can vary considerably among individuals and between sexes.

Recently, Etienne *et al.*,[83] in a study of 185 consecutive cancer patients, reported an eightfold difference in DPD activity and a 15% lower mean level of enzyme activity in females, but no variation with age. Moreover, peripheral blood mononuclear DPD activity correlated poorly with 5-FU clearance and the incidence of toxicity in this group. Consequently, peripheral blood mononuclear DPD activity could not be used for the 5-FU dose adaptation. However, the ability to measure DPD in peripheral blood mononuclear cells has facilitated the monitoring of the biochemical efficacy of the more potent recent inhibitors of DPD in clinical trials.[83] Etienne *et al.*[84] have also studied the prognostic importance of DPD in head and neck cancer and shown that patients with lower tumour to normal tissue DPD ratios were more likely to respond to 5-FU-based regimens. This observation has raised the possibility that the selective inhibition of tumour DPD may make tumour cells more susceptible to 5-FU.

Future directions

The inhibition of TS and DPD has been a major focus for the development of novel therapeutic strategies. Moreover, the biomodulation of 5-FU by leucovorin, inhibition of 5-FU degradation by DPD inhibitors, and the clinical introduction of rationally designed TS inhibitors have begun to show great clinical promise. The introduction of novel assays for the quantitation of TS has, for the first time, allowed the target to be analysed prior to and during treatment. The ability to measure chemotherapeutic targets such as TS and DPD in clinical material will allow the importance of these targets in clinical drug resistance to be assessed, which should ultimately lead to improved therapeutic strategies for patients with cancer.

Conclusions

This review has highlighted some of the advances that have been made over the last 20 years in understanding the nature of cancer and how this information can be used to develop new strategies for cancer treatment. There has been a rapid expansion in our knowledge of how cell growth and death pathways are regulated, and the mechanisms by which cancer cells subvert these normal regulatory processes to achieve inappropriate clonal expansion. One of the main observations to emerge from this accumulation of data is the realization that in the majority of cancers the route to immortality is complex and involves both positive and negative regulatory pathways. Nevertheless, for some cancer types it has been possible to identify the major rate-limiting step, which appears critical for tumour growth. This information is now being used in a variety of ways to attack cancer cells at the molecular level, through both earlier detection methods and the design of novel gene therapeutic strategies. In tandem with these new developments have come various associated problems, especially problems involving predictive genetic testing and the design of some gene therapy protocols.

The initial optimism and high expectation which followed in the wake of these new developments has been replaced by an acceptance that an easy solution is unlikely. This is clearly seen in the case of predictive genetic testing, where our ability to detect mutations far exceeds our ability to define a clear clinical response to the information obtained. The hype which surrounded the cloning of the breast cancer genes BRCA1 and BRCA2 is partly responsible for raising public expectations regarding the power of genetic testing to an unrealistic level. However, the fact remains that genetic testing is a powerful tool in the fight against cancer, allowing at least an improved chance of earlier detection with the result that conventional therapies have a greater chance of success. More importantly, in situations where absolute predictive tests are possible, genetic testing can remove a lifetime of worry and offer the chance of a normal life to those who do not carry predisposing genes. It is the responsibility of scientists and clinicians to provide proper guidelines for the use of genetic testing, which should include appropriate counselling regarding the possible interpretation of any result, whether positive or negative.

The initial wave of euphoria which accompanied the first gene therapy protocols has also given way to a more protracted struggle. A criticism levelled at some of the initial gene therapy protocols is that they were rushed through to clinical trials without first having undergone exhaustive preclinical trials in appropriate model systems. The same is not true of recent trial designs, which tend to be based on solid preclinical research. However, the single major obstacle to effective gene therapy protocols is design of a reliable delivery system, and this remains an area of intensive research.

Dramatic progress will not occur overnight; rather, as has been the case for conventional cancer treatment, we can expect slow steady progress. Moreover, it is likely that some of these new approaches will be most effective when given in combination with more traditional therapies rather than acting alone. What is clear, however, is that gene therapy is here to stay and has the potential over time to revolutionize our approach to cancer treatment. Exploring the scientific rationale of novel treatments in patients has also begun to prove beneficial in the development of therapeutic strategies for target patient groups. The quantification of chemotherapeutic targets such as TS has already begun to identify specific patient populations most likely to benefit from currently available chemotherapeutic regimens.

The past decade has clearly witnessed important advances in the development of novel therapeutic strategies for treating cancer patients. Innovative therapies using biological reagents may prove to be very important. The continued development of these strategies must be based on sound preclinical principles that ultimately result in less toxic and more effective methods for diagnosis and treatment of cancer patients.

References

1. Knudson AG Jr (1971). Mutation and cancer: statistical study of retinoblastoma. *Proc Natl Acad Sci USA*, **68**, 820–3.
2. Cleaver JE (1994) It was a very good year for DNA repair. *Cell*, **76**, 1–4.
3. Holley RW (1975) Control of growth of mammalian cells in cell culture. *Nature*, **258**, 487–90.
4. Heldin CH, Westermark B (1984) Growth factors: mechanisms of action and relation to oncogenes. *Cell*, **37**, 9–20.
5. Leal F, Williams LT, Robbins KC, Aaronson SA (1985) Evidence that the v-*sis* gene product transforms by interaction with the receptor for platelet-derived growth factor. *Science*, **230**, 327–30.
6. Chen WS, Lazar CS, Poenie M, Tsien RY, Gill GN, Rosenfield MG (1987) Requirement for intrinsic protein tyrosine kinase in the immediate and late action of the EGF receptor. *Nature*, **328**, 820–3.

7. Bargmann CJ, Hung MC, Weinberg RA (1986) Multiple independent activations of the *neu* oncogene by a point mutation altering the transmembrane domain. *Cell*, **45**, 649–57.

8. Neer EJ (1995) Heterotrimeric G proteins: organizers of transmembrane signals. *Cell*, **80**, 249–57.

9. Scolnick EM, Papageorge AG, Shih TY (1979) Guanine nucleotide-binding activity as an assay for src protein of rat-derived murine sarcoma virus. *Proc Natl Acad Sci USA*, **76**, 5355–9.

10. Trahey M, McCormick F (1987) A cytoplasmic protein stimulates normal N-*ras* P21 GTPase, but does not affect oncogenic mutants. *Science*, **238**, 542–5.

11. Marshall CJ (1995) Specificity of receptor tyrosine kinase signalling: transient versus sustained extracellular signal-regulated kinase activation. *Cell*, **80**, 179–85.

12. . Maki Y, Bos TJ, Davis C, Starbuck M, Vogt PK (1987) Avian sarcoma virus carries the *jun* oncogene. *Proc Natl Acad Sci USA*, **84**, 2848–52.

13. Smeal T, Angel P, Meek J, Karin M (1989) Different requirements for formation of *jun:jun* and *jun:fos* complexes. *Genes Dev*, **3**, 2091–100.

14. Smeal T, Binetruy B, Mercola DA, Birrer M, Karin M (1991) Oncogenic and Transcriptional cooperation with Ha-*ras* requires phosphorylation of c-*jun* on serines 63 and 73. *Nature*, **354**, 494–6.

15. Donner P, Greiser-Wilke I, Moelling K (1982) Nuclear localization and DNA Binding of the transforming gene product of the avian myelocytomatosis virus. *Nature*, **296**, 262–5.

16. Amati B, Brooks MW, Naomi L, Littlewood TD, Evan G, Land H. (1993) Oncogenic activity of the c-Myc protein requires dimerization with Max. *Cell*, **72**, 233–45.

17. Ayer DE, Kretzner L, Eisenman RN (1993) Mad: a heterodimeric partner for Max that antagonizes Myc transcriptional activity. *Cell*, **72**, 211–22.

18. Harris H, Miller OJ, Klein G, Worst P, Tachibana T (1969) Suppression of malignancy by cell fusion. *Nature*, **223**, 363–8.

19. Stanbridge EJ, Flandemeyer R, Daniels D, Nelson-Rees R (1981) Specific chromosome loss associated with the expression of tumorigenicity in human cell hybrids. *Somat Cell Genet*, **7**, 699–712.

20. Saxon PJ, Srivatsan ES, Stanbridge EJ (1986) Introduction of human chromosome 11 via microcell transfer controls tumorigenic expression of HeLa cells. *EMBO J*, **5**, 3461–6.

21. Yunis JJ (1983) The chromosomal basis of human neoplasia. *Science*, **221**, 227–36.

22. Hall JM, Lee MK, Newman B, Morrow JE, Anderson LA, Huey B, King MC (1990) Linkage of early-onset familial breast cancer to chromosome 17q21. *Science*, **250**, 1684–9.

23. Hansen MF, Cavenee WK (1987) Genetics of cancer predisposition. *Cancer Res*, **47**, 5518–27.

24. Cavenee WK, Hansen MF, Nordenskjold M, Kock E, Maumenee I (1985) Genetic origin of mutations predisposing to retinoblastoma. *Science*, **228**, 501–3.

25. Levine AJ, Momand J, Finlay CA (1991) The p53 tumour suppressor gene. *Nature*, **351**, 453–6.

26. El-Deiry WS, Tokino T, Velculescu VE, *et al.* (1993) WAF1, a potential mediator of p53 tumour suppression. *Cell 75*, 817–25.

27. Hermeking H, Longauer C, Polyak K, *et al.* (1997) 14-3-3σ is a p53-regulated inhibitor of G2/M progression. *Mol Cell*, **1**, 3–11.

28. Polyak K, Xia Y, Zweier JL, Kinzler KW, Vogelstein B (1997) A model for p53-induced apoptosis. *Nature*, **389**, 300–5.

29. Miki Y, Swensen J, Shattuck-Eidens D, *et al.* (1993) A strong candidate for the breast and ovarian cancer susceptibility gene BRCA1. *Science*, **266**, 66–71.

30. Wooster R, Bignell G, Swift S, *et al.* (1995) Identification of the breast cancer susceptibility gene BRCA2. *Nature*, **378**, 789–92.

31. Anderson SF, Schlegel BP, Nakajima T, Wolpin ES, Parvin JD (1998) BRCA1 protein is linked to the RNA polymerase 11 holoenzyme complex via RNA helicase A. *Nat Genet*, **19**, 254–6.

32. Gowen LC, Avrutskaya AV, Latour AM, Koller BH, Leadon SA (1998) BRCA1 required for transcription-coupled repair of oxidative DNA damage. *Science*, **281**, 1009–12.

33. Sharan SK, Morimatsu M, Albrecht U, *et al.* (1997) Embryonic lethality and radiation hypersensitivity mediated by Rad51 in mice lacking BRCA2. *Nature*, **386**, 804–10.

34. Lehmann AR (1998) Dual functions of DNA repair genes: molecular, cellular, and clinical implications. *Bioessays*, **20**, 146–55.

35. Fink D, Aebi S, Howell SB (1998) The role of DNA mismatch repair in drug resistance. *Clin Cancer Res*, **4**, 1–6.

36. Fishel R, Lescoe MK, Rao MRS, *et al.* (1993) The human mutator gene homologue MSH2 and its association with hereditary nonpolyposis colon cancer. *Cell*, **75**, 1027–38.

37. Kinzler KW, Vogelstein B (1997) Gatekeepers and caretakers. *Nature*, **386**, 761–3.

38. Lips CJM, Landsvater RM, Hoppener JWM, *et al.* (1994) Clinical screening as compared with DNA analysis in families with multiple endocrine neoplasia type 2A. *N Engl J Med*, **31**, 828–35.

39. Wells SA, Skinner MA (1998) Prophylactic thyroidectomy, based on direct Genetic testing, in patients at risk for multiple endocrine neoplasia type 2 syndromes. *Exp Clin Endocrinol Diabetes*, **106**, 29–34.

40. Cunningham C, Dunlop MG (1996) Molecular genetic basis of colorectal cancer susceptibility. *Br J Cancer*, **83**, 321–9.

41. Groden J, Thliveris A, Samowitz W, *et al.* (1991) Identification and characterization of the familial adenomatous polyposis coli gene. *Cell*, **66**, 589–600.

42. Powell SM, Petersen GM, Krush AJ, *et al.* (1993) Molecular diagnosis of familial adenomatous polyposis. *N Engl J Med*, **329**, 1982–7.

43. Giardiello FM (1997) Genetic testing in hereditary colorectal cancer. *JAMA*, **278**, 1278–81.

44. Burke W, Daly M, Garber J, *et al.* (1997) Recomendations for follow-up care of individuals with an inherited predisposition to cancer. 11. BRCA1 and BRCA2. Cancer Genetics Studies Consortium. *JAMA*, **277**, 997–1003.

45. Kahn P (1996) Coming to grips with genes and risk. *Science*, **274**, 496–8.

46. Giardiello FM, Brensinger JD, Petersen GM, *et al.* (1997) The use and interpretation of commercial APC gene testing for familial adenomatous polyposis. *N Engl J Med*, 336 823–7.

47. Barinaga M (1997) From benchtop to bedside. *Science*, 278, 1036–9.

48. Hancock JF, Magee AI, Childs JE, Marshall CJ (1989) All *ras* proteins are polyisoprenylated but only some are palmitoylated. *Cell*, 57, 1167–77.

49. Kohl NE, Mosser SD, deSolms SJ, *et al.* (1993) Selective inhibition of *ras*-dependent transformation by a farnesyl-transferase inhibitor. *Science*, 260, 1934–7.

50. Gibbs JB, Oliff A (1997) The potential of farnesyltrans-ferase inhibitors as cancer chemotherapeutics. *Annu Rev Pharmacol Toxicol*, 37, 143–66.

51. Roth JA, Cristiano RJ (1997) Gene therapy for cancer. What have we done and where are we going? *J Natl Cancer Inst*, 89, 21–39.

52. Cheng L, Ziegelhoffer PR, Yang NS (1993) *In vivo* pro-moter activity and transgene expression in mammalian somatic tissues evaluated by using particle bombardment. *Proc Natl Acad Sci USA*, 90, 4455–9.

53. Kasahara N, Dozy AM, Kan YW (1994) Tissue-specific targeting of retroviral vectors through ligand-receptor interactions. *Science*, 266, 1373–6.

54. Cristiano R, Roth J (1996) Epidermal growth factor mediated DNA delivery into lung cancer cells via the epi-dermal growth factor receptor. *Cancer Gene Ther*, 3, 4–10.

55. Weichselbaum RR, Hallahan DE, Beckett MA, *et al.* (1994) Gene therapy targeted by radiation preferentially radiosensitizes tumour cells. *Cancer Res*, 54, 4266–9.

56. Harding TC, Geddes BJ, Murphy D, Knight D, Uney JB (1998) Switching transgene expression in the brain using an adenoviral tetracycline regulatable system. *Nat Bio-technol*, 16, 553–5.

57. Bischoff JR, Kirn DH, Williams A, *et al.* (1996) An aden-ovirus mutant that replicates selectively in p53 deficient human tumour cells. *Science*, 274, 373–6.

58. Zeng L, Quilliet X, Chevallier-Lagente O, Eveno E, Sarasin A, Mezzina M (1997) Retrovirus-mediated gene transfer corrects DNA repair defect of xeroderma pig-mentosum cells of complementation groups A, B and C. *Gene Ther*, 4, 1077–84.

59. Danenberg PV (1977) Thymidylate synthase—a target enzyme in cancer chemotherapy. *Biochem Biophys Acta*, 473, 73–92.

60. Grem, JL (1990) Fluorinated pyrimidines. In: Chabner BA, Collins, JM (eds) *Cancer Chemotherapy: Principles and Practice*. Philadelphia, PA: JB. Lippincott, 180–224.

61. Jackman AL, Taylor GA, Gibson W, *et al.* (1991) ICI D1694, A quinazoline antifolate thymidylate synthase inhibitor that is a potent inhibitor of L1210 tumour growth *in vitro* and *in vivo*. A new agent for clinical study. *Cancer Res*, 51, 5579–86.

62. Zalcberg JR, Cunningham D, Van Cutsern E, *et al.* (1996) ZD 1694: a novel thymidylate synthase inhibition with substantial activity in the treatment of patients with advanced colorectal cancer. *J Clin Oncol*, 14, 716–21.

63. Chu E, Koeller D, Johnston PG, Zinn S, Allegra CJ (1993) The regulation of thymidylate synthase in human

colon cancer cells treated with 5-fluorouracil and inter-feron gamma. *Mol Pharmacol*, 433, 527–33.

64. Jackman AL, Kelland LR, Kimbell R, *et al.* (1995) Mechanisms of acquired resistance to the quinazoline thymidylate synthase inhibitor ZD1694 (Tomudex) in one mouse and three human cell lines. *Br J Cancer*, 71, 914–24.

65. Drake JC, Allegra CJ, Moran RG, Johnston PG (1996) Resistance to tomudex (ZD1694) multifactorial in human breast and colon carcinoma cell lines. *Biochem Pharmacol*, 51, 1349–55.

66. Chu E, Voeller D, Koeller DM (1993) Identification of an RNA binding site for human thymidylate synthase. *Proc Natl Acad Sci USA*, 90, 517–21.

67. Chu E, Koeller DM, Casey JL (1991) Autoregulation of human thymidylate synthase mRNA translation by thymidylate synthase. *Proc Natl Acad Sci USA*, 88, 8977–8981.

68. Johnston PG, Liang CM, Henry S, Chaber BA, Allegra CJ (1991) The production and characterisation of mono-clonal antibodies that localise human thymidylate syn-thase in the cytoplasm of human cells and tissues. *Cancer Res*, 51, 6668–76.

69. Johnston PG, Drake JC, Trepel J, Allegra CJ (1992) Immunological quantitation of thymidylate synthase using the monoclonal antibody TS 106 in 5-fluorouracil-sensitive and resistant human cancer cell lines. *Cancer Res*, 52, 4306–12.

70. Horikoshi T, Danenberg KD, Stadlbauer THW, *et al.* (1992) Quantitation of thymidylate synthase. dihydro-folate reductase and DT-diaphorase gene expression human tumours using the polymerase chain reaction. *Cancer Res*, 52, 108–16.

71. Johnston PG, Fisher ER, Rockett HE, *et al.* (1994) The role of thymidylate synthase expression prognosis and outcome of adjuvant chemotherapy in patients with rectal cancer. *J Clin Oncol*, 12, 2640–7.

72. Pestalozzi BC, Peterson HF, Gelber RD, *et al.* (1997) Prognostic importance of thymidylate synthase expres-sion in early breast cancer. *J Clin Oncol*, 15, 1923–31.

73. Findlay MPN, Cunningham D, Morgan G, Clinton S, Hardcastle A, Aherne GW. (1997) Lack of correlation between thymidylate synthase levels in primary colorectal tumours and subsequent response to chemotherapy. *Br J Cancer*, 75, 903–9.

74. Lenz H, Danenberg KD, Leichman CG, *et al.* (1997) p53 and Thymidylate Synthase (TS) Expression in untreated state II colon cancer: association with recurrence, sur-vival and tumour site. *Proc Am Assoc Cancer Res*, 38, 614.

75. Johnston PG, Lenz HJ, Leichman CG, *et al.* (1995) Thymidylate synthase gene and protein expression cor-relate and are associated with response to 5-fluorouracil in human colorectal and gastric tumors. *Cancer Res*, 55, 1407–12.

76. Leichman CG, Lenz H, Leichman L, *et al.* (1997) Quantitation of intratumoral thymidylate synthase expression predicts for disseminated colorectal cancer response and resistance to protracted-infused fluorouracil and weekly leucovorin. *J Clin Oncol*, 15, 3223–9.

77. Johnston PG, Mick R, Recant W, *et al.* (1997) Thymidylate synthase expression predicts for response to

neoadjuvant induction chemotherapy in advanced head and neck cancers. *J Natl Cancer Inst*, **89**, 308–13.

78. Daher G, Harris BE, Diasio RB, Powis G (eds) (1994) *Anticancer Drugs: Antimetabolite Metabolism and Natural Anticancer Agents*. Vol. 2: *Metabolism of Pyrimidine Analogues and their Nucleotides*. Oxford: Pergamon, 55–94.

79. Harris BE, Soong R, Soong S, Diasio RB (1996) Relationship between dihydropyrimidine dehydrogenase activity and plasma 5-fluorouracil levels with evidence for circadian variaton of enzyme activity and plasma drug levels in cancer patients receiving 5-fluorouracil by protracted continuous infusion. *Cancer Res*, **50**, 197–201.

80. Chazal M, Etienne MC, Renee N, Bourgeon A, Richelme H, Milano G (1996) Link between dihydropyrimidine dehydrogenase activity and peripheral blood mononuclear cells and liver. *Clin Cancer Res*, **2**, 507–10.

81. Pazdur R, Lassere Y, Rhodes V, *et al.* (1994) Phase II trial of uracil and tegafur plus oral leucovorin: an effective oral regimen in the treatment of metastatic colorectal carcinoma. *J Clin Oncol*, **12**, 2296–300.

82. Etienne MC, Cheradame S, Fischel JL, Formento P, Dassonville O, Renee N (1995) Response to fluorouracil therapy in cancer patients: the role of tumoral dihydropyrimidine dehydrogenase activity. *J Clin Oncol*, **13**, 1663–70.

83. Etienne MC, Milano G, Lagrange JL, Bajard F, Francois E, Thyss A (1993) Marked Fluctuations in drug plasma concentrations caused by use of portable pumps for fluorouracil continuous infusion. *J Natl Cancer Inst*, **85**, 1005–7.

84. Etienne MC, Cheradame S, Fischel JL, *et al.* (1995) Response to fluorouracil therapy in cancer patients: the role of tumoral dihydropyrimidine dehydrogenase activity. *J Clin Oncol*, **13**, 1663–70.

Index